NEW TECHNIQUES IN THORACIC IMAGING

NEW TECHNIQUES IN THORACIC IMAGING

edited by

PHILLIP M. BOISELLE
Harvard Medical School and Beth Israel Deaconess Medical Center
Boston, Massachusetts

CHARLES S. WHITE
University of Maryland School of Medicine
Baltimore, Maryland

MARCEL

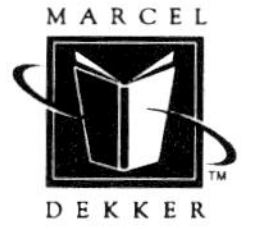

DEKKER

MARCEL DEKKER, INC.   NEW YORK • BASEL

ISBN: 0-8247-0640-4

This book is printed on acid-free paper.

Headquarters
Marcel Dekker, Inc.
270 Madison Avenue, New York, NY 10016
tel: 212-696-9000; fax: 212-685-4540

Eastern Hemisphere Distribution
Marcel Dekker AG
Hutgasse 4, Postfach 812, CH-4001 Basel, Switzerland
tel: 41-61-261-8482; fax: 41-61-261-8896

World Wide Web
http://www.dekker.com

The publisher offers discounts on this book when ordered in bulk quantities. For more information, write to Special Sales/Professional Marketing at the headquarters address above.

Current printing (last digit):
10 9 8 7 6 5 4 3 2 1

PRINTED IN THE UNITED STATES OF AMERICA

To my wife, Ellen, and my parents, Phil and Dee

—PMB

To my wife, Ellen, and my three children,
Billy, Rachel, and Danny

—CSW

Preface

This book is the first of a series of volumes designed to provide a focused update on new and emerging techniques in radiology. *New Techniques in Thoracic Imaging* is primarily intended for practicing radiologists, but will also prove useful to pulmonologists, thoracic surgeons, and physicians training in these specialties.

The primary goals of this book are three-fold. The first is to provide a pragmatic compendium of the state of the art in the imaging of thoracic disorders commonly encountered in daily practice. Toward this end, several chapters focus on the subjects of imaging the solitary pulmonary nodule, thoracic lymph nodes, pulmonary embolism, emphysema, and aortic abnormalities.

Second, it is our goal to familiarize the reader with new technologies that are playing an increasingly important role in thoracic imaging. With this objective in mind, we have included several technology-based chapters devoted to CT fluoroscopy, multidetector helical CT, and digital radiography. Although high-resolution CT is a firmly established imaging method, we have also included a chapter on this subject in order to provide the reader with an update on this important technique. A separate chapter devoted to positron emission tomography was not included because this technique is reviewed in the chapters on imaging the solitary pulmonary nodule and thoracic lymph nodes.

Our final goal is to introduce the reader to emerging techniques that are not yet standard practice but will likely play an important role in thoracic imaging in the near future. Chapters on the subjects of lung cancer screening, magnetic resonance ventilation imaging, magnetic resonance assessment of pulmonary embolism, and virtual bronchoscopy are designed to familiarize the reader with the potential contributions and challenges of these emerging technologies.

This book is a collaborative project that has benefited from the help of many. We are especially grateful to the expert contributing authors of this book, including: Drs. Suzanne Aquino, Michael Blake, Timothy Carroll, Qun Chen, J. Richard Choi, Cesario Ciccotosto, Jannette Collins, Eric Crotty, Lane Donnelly, Jeremy Erasmus, Matthew Freedman, Lawrence Goodman, Curtis Green, Hiroto Hatabu, Ella Kazerooni, Jeffrey Klein, Vu Ming Mai, James MacFall, Holman Page McAdams, and Lacey Washington. We would also like to thank Geoffrey Greenwood, Ph.D., Consulting Managing Director at Marcel Dekker, Inc., for providing us the opportunity to edit the first edition of this series; Herbert Kressel, M.D., and Philip Templeton, M.D., our departmental chairmen, for encouragement and support; Richard Johnson, for outstanding editorial assistance; and Nancy Williams, for administrative assistance.

We hope that the information provided in this book proves useful to its readers in the practice of thoracic radiology now and in the future.

Phillip M. Boiselle
Charles S. White

Contents

Contributors

Suzanne L. Aquino, M.D. Assistant Professor of Radiology, Harvard Medical School, and Associate Radiologist, Massachusetts General Hospital, Boston, Massachusetts

Michael A. Blake, F.F.R. (R.C.S.I.), F.R.C.R. Instructor of Radiology, Harvard Medical School, and Assistant Radiologist, Massachusetts General Hospital, Boston, Massachusetts

Phillip M. Boiselle, M.D. Assistant Professor of Radiology, Harvard Medical School, and Director of Thoracic Imaging, Department of Radiology, Beth Israel Deaconess Medical Center, Boston, Massachusetts

Timothy John Carroll, M.D., Ph.D. Resident in Radiology, Fletcher Allen Health Care, University of Vermont College of Medicine, Burlington, Vermont

Qun Chen, Ph.D. Assistant Professor of Radiology, Northwestern University Medical School, and Director of Magnetic Resonance Physics Laboratory, Evanston Northwestern Healthcare, Evanston, Illinois

J. Richard Choi, Sc.D., M.D. Major, United States Army Medical Corps, and Chief, Computed Tomography, Department of Radiology, Walter Reed Army Medical Center, Washington, DC

Cesario Ciccotosto, M.D. Assistant Professor of Radiology, and Director of Thoracic Imaging, Instituto di Scienze Radiologiche, Università "G. D'Annunzio," Chieti, Italy

Jannette Collins, M.D., M.Ed. Associate Professor of Radiology, Affiliate Associate Professor of Medicine, and Assistant Dean for Graduate Medical Education, University of Wisconsin Medical School, Madison, Wisconsin

Eric Crotty, M.D. Fellow, Pediatric Radiology, Children's Hospital Medical Center, Cincinnati, Ohio

Lane F. Donnelly, M.D. Associate Professor of Radiology and Pediatrics, College of Medicine, University of Cincinnati, and Associate Director, Department of Radiology, Program Director, Pediatric Radiology Fellowship Program, Children's Hospital Medical Center, Cincinnati, Ohio

Jeremy J. Erasmus, M.D. Associate Professor of Radiology, MD Anderson Cancer Center, University of Texas, Houston, Texas

Matthew Freedman, M.D., M.B.A. Associate Professor of Radiology, and Clinical Director, Division of Imaging Science and Information Systems, Department of Radiology, Georgetown University, Washington, DC

Lawrence R. Goodman, M.D., F.A.C.R. Professor of Diagnostic Radiology and Pulmonary Medicine, and Director of Thoracic Imaging, Medical College of Wisconsin and Froedtert Memorial Lutheran Hospital, Milwaukee, Wisconsin

Curtis E. Green, M.D. Professor of Radiology, Fletcher Allen Health Care, University of Vermont College of Medicine, Burlington, Vermont

Hiroto Hatabu, M.D., Ph.D. Associate Professor of Radiology and Director, Pulmonary Functional Imaging Research, Hospital of the University of Pennsylvania, Philadelphia, Pennsylvania

Ella A. Kazerooni, M.D., M.S. Associate Professor of Radiology and Director, Division of Thoracic Radiology, University of Michigan Health System, Ann Arbor, Michigan

Jeffrey S. Klein, M.D. Professor of Radiology and Chief of Thoracic Radiology, Fletcher Allen Health Care, University of Vermont College of Medicine, Burlington, Vermont

Vu Ming Mai, Ph.D. Research Assistant Professor of Radiology, Northwestern University Medical School, and Evanston Northwestern Healthcare, Evanston, Illinois

James R. MacFall, Ph.D. Associate Professor of Radiology, Duke University Medical Center, Durham, North Carolina

Holman Page McAdams, M.D. Associate Professor of Radiology, Duke University Medical Center, Durham, North Carolina

Lacey Washington, M.D. Assistant Professor of Radiology, Medical College of Wisconsin and Froedtert Memorial Lutheran Hospital, Milwaukee, Wisconsin

Charles S. White, M.D. Professor of Radiology, Director, Thoracic Imaging, and Acting Chair, Department of Diagnostic Radiology, University of Maryland School of Medicine, Baltimore, Maryland

1

Lung Cancer Screening: Past, Present, and Future

Charles S. White
University of Maryland School of Medicine
Baltimore, Maryland

Phillip M. Boiselle
Harvard Medical School and
Beth Israel Deaconess Medical Center
Boston, Massachusetts

I. INTRODUCTION

Lung cancer remains the leading cause of mortality from cancer. In 1999, there were approximately 170,000 new cases of lung cancer [1]. The 5-year survival rate from the disease is 14% and has increased only slightly since the early 1970s despite an extensive and costly research effort to find effective therapy. The disparity in survival between early- and late-stage lung cancer is substantial, with a 5-year survival rate of approximately 70% in stage 1A disease compared to less than 5% in stage IV disease according to the recently revised Lung Cancer Staging criteria [2]. Unfortunately, as many as 60% of patients present with advanced-stage lung cancer.

The disproportionately high prevalence and mortality of advanced lung cancer has encouraged attempts to detect early lung cancer with screening programs aimed at smokers. Smokers have an incidence rate of lung cancer that is 10 times that of nonsmokers and account for greater than 80% of lung cancer cases in the United States [3]. Until recently, two main approaches have been used to screen for lung cancer: chest radiography and sputum cytology. The first section of this chapter describes the evolution and results of screening studies using these techniques and the controversies that developed surrounding the results of these studies. The following section describes several emerging technologies for early lung cancer detection, with a special emphasis on low-dose spiral computed tomography (CT).

II. LUNG CANCER SCREENING: A HISTORICAL PERSPECTIVE

Screening studies for lung cancer date to the 1950s and 1960s when several studies were undertaken using a variety of screening protocols that combined chest radiography and sputum analysis. The protocols employed different screening time intervals and the study design was either uncontrolled or controlled but nonrandomized. The most widely publicized study was the Philadelphia Pulmonary Neoplasm Research Project, in which only 6 of 94 patients with lung cancer detected at screening survived more than 5 years [4]. No study showed an advantage for lung cancer screening.

The subsequent development of more sophisticated techniques of chest radiography and sputum analysis in the 1960s and the methodologic limitations of the early studies led to the concept that lung cancer screening might prove efficacious if a more rigorous study design was used. In that context, three large randomized controlled studies (National Cancer Institute Cooperative Early Lung Cancer Group) were initiated among male smokers in the 1970s at the Mayo Clinic, Memorial Sloan–Kettering Cancer Center, and the Johns Hopkins Medical Institutions.

In the Mayo Lung Project, 10,933 men who were 45 years of age or older and who smoked more than a pack of cigarettes daily were assessed with chest radiographs and sputum cytology [5]. Lung cancers found in these patients were designated as ''prevalence cases.'' The 9,211 men with negative chest radiographs and sputum cytology were randomized into two groups. The control group of 4,593 patients was given the standard Mayo Clinic recommendation at that time, a yearly chest radiograph and sputum cytologic examination, but no individualized follow-up was pursued. The study group of 4,618 patients was scheduled once every four months for a chest radiograph and a sputum container was sent to collect a 3-day pooled sputum sample, which was returned to the Mayo Clinic. All patients were contacted yearly to assess their status. Approximately 75% of men in the study group complied with the every-4-month protocol.

When the study ended in 1983, lung cancer had been detected in 206 patients in the study group and 160 patients in the control group [5]. Resectability was higher in the study group than in the control group (46% vs. 32%) but this advantage was not reflected in mortality rates. The death rates in the two groups were statistically similar: 3.2 per 1000 person-years in the study group compared to 3.0 per 1000 person-years in the control group.

A closer analysis of the data reveals that the every-4-month screening protocol detected a higher proportion of lung cancer at an early stage (42%) than in the control group (25%) and a corresponding 5-year survival benefit was found [6]. However, despite these apparent advantages, no mortality benefit was demonstrated from screening.

Several explanations for the difference between the survival and mortality data have been postulated, including lead-time bias, overdiagnosis, and control-group contamination [3]. Lead-time bias occurs if the lung cancer is detected at an early stage in its natural history but the ultimate time of death is unchanged. In the Mayo Clinic study, the lung cancers in the screened population were detected at an earlier stage than in the control group, resulting in longer survival and apparent 5-year survival benefit. However, assuming the eventual time of death remained unchanged, no mortality benefit would be observed.

Overdiagnosis occurs if cancers that are indolent are disproportionately detected by lung cancer screening. Patients with slow-growing tumors would have a prolonged disease course that would favorably affect 5-year-survival data. Indolent cancers would not be as likely to be detected in the control group because they would remain asymptomatic for an extended period of time and the patient might succumb to other illness. If such indolent cancers were disproportionately found in the screened population, a survival advantage but no mortality benefit would be shown for this population. Length time bias is a related bias but describes detection of indolent cancer over a more limited time frame than overdiagnosis.

Prostate cancer is an example of a disease in which overdiagnosis might occur. Two-thirds of men over 60 years of age that die of other causes have undiagnosed, presumably indolent prostate cancer at autopsy. As for prostate cancer, it was suggested that overdiagnosis of lung cancer might account for the difference between survival and mortality data [3].

Contamination of the control group may also have been problematic in the Mayo Clinic study [5]. Investigators estimated that approximately 50% of control patients in fact underwent chest radiography during the course of the study and thus took on some characteristics of the screened population (contamination). One-third of the lung cancer in the control group was detected as a result of such ''nonstudy'' chest radiographs.

The Memorial Sloan–Kettering Cancer Center and the Johns Hopkins Medical Institutions studies used similar protocols that were substantively different than that of the Mayo Clinic project [7,8]. These studies were designed to determine any advantage gained by the addition of yearly sputum samples to annual chest radiographs. Because chest radiography was used in both the study and the control populations, the trials were not useful to evaluate the efficacy of annual chest radiographs.

The Memorial Sloan–Kettering Cancer Center study consisted of 10,040 men over 45 years of age that smoked at least one pack of cigarettes [7]. Patients were randomly assigned to two groups. The control group, composed of 5,072 men, underwent annual chest radiography. The screened population of 4,985 received an annual chest radiograph and pooled sputum cytology every 4 months. The 288 lung cancers found in these groups were evenly split between the two groups. There was no significant difference in the operability, 5-year survival, or mortality between the screened and control populations.

The Johns Hopkins study employed a protocol that was nearly identical to that of the Memorial Sloan–Kettering Cancer Center study [8]. Similar numbers of lung cancers were detected in the screened and control populations and the survival and mortality data were not significantly different in the two groups. Thus, neither study demonstrated an advantage for annual screening sputum cytology.

Two other studies have been reported from Europe that assessed the screening potential of chest radiography for lung cancer [9–11]. A randomized controlled study from Czechoslovakia reported in the mid-1980s evaluated 6364 male smokers between the ages of 40 and 64 [9,10]. Both screened and control groups were followed over a 3-year period. The screened group ($n = 3172$) underwent both a chest radiograph and sputum cytology every 6 months for the duration of the study. The control group ($n = 3174$) received only a chest radiograph at the end of the 3-year period. Thirty-nine cancers were detected in the screened group compared to 27 in the control group. However, no clear advantage in mortality was demonstrated in the screened group.

A case-controlled study reported from Germany in the late 1980s assessed the rate of lung cancer detection among patients who had undergone biannual surveillance for tuberculosis with chest radiography [11]. The 130 men in this screening program who died of lung cancer were matched with an aged-match control group consisting of men from the same district. No mortality benefit was found for the patients who participated in the screening program.

The failure of these studies to demonstrate a mortality advantage for lung cancer screening with either chest radiography or sputum cytology led most organizations to recommend that routine screening not be undertaken. The American Cancer Society noted that "the Society did not feel it would be responsible to advocate screening for a large group of people . . . without better evidence that they would derive some benefit" [12]. Based on the evidence, the view that "screening for lung cancer . . . is not recommended" has been widely professed [3]. At present, no major organization advocates routine screening for lung cancer.

Over the past several years, several investigators have proposed a reassessment of the data from the four randomized lung cancer trials [13,14]. Strauss et al. noted that although the Johns Hopkins Institute and Memorial Sloan–Kettering Cancer Center studies were not designed specifically to assess the efficacy of chest radiographic screening, both control and screened populations achieved survival rates approximately three times greater than prevailing norms. They suggested that the use of an annual chest radiographic screening protocol might have led to an improved outcome even if a mortality benefit was not shown [13].

Strauss et al. also contended that the improved resectability, lower stage, and better survival in the Mayo and Czech studies could not be adequately explained on the basis of lead-time bias or overdiagnosis. With respect to overdiagnosis, they cited evidence from an autopsy study that suggests indolent lung cancer occurs only rarely [15]. Based on evaluation of the Mayo Lung Project data, they also noted that patients in that trial with early lung cancer who either were medically unsuitable or refused surgical resection had a much lower rate of survival than those who underwent surgical treatment (10% vs. 70%) [16]. Strauss et al. suggested that the behavior of lung cancer is almost always aggressive even when detected at an early stage and, thus, overdiagnosis is unlikely to be a substantial confounding factor [13]. In the view of the authors, the increases in survival and other parameters of the screened group in the Mayo and Czech studies could not be explained by study design biases. They speculated that the screening protocol itself might have led to a better outcome. They recommended a reappraisal of the role of chest radiographs in early lung cancer detection.

Other methodologic criticisms of the Mayo Lung Project have been raised. The contamination that occurred because 50% of the patients in the control group underwent chest radiographs decreased the distinctiveness of the screened and control group, leading to greater difficulty in detecting a difference between populations. A larger trial might, therefore, be required to show a difference [14].

Miettinen has suggested that the nine-year period over which cumulative mortality rate was calculated in the Mayo Lung Project is excessive [17]. He has stated that this period of time likely underestimated the maximum effect of screening. Based on his analysis of the data, the time between 3 and 7 years after completion of prevalence screening is optimal because it ''represents a compromise between one that is narrow enough to address the full effect, and one that is wide enough to show a meaningful number of deaths from the disease.'' He believes that if the more appropriate timing of cumulative mortality rates is used, the Mayo Lung data cannot be interpreted as providing direct evidence against screening.

The lingering questions with respect to the major lung cancer screening trials of the 1970s and 1980s in combination with the development of potent new imaging and nonimaging techniques engendered renewed interest in lung cancer screening throughout the 1990s. The remainder of this chapter describes early results using these newer technologies.

III. LUNG CANCER SCREENING: ANOTHER LOOK WITH NEW LENSES

In recent years, a wealth of new technologies has emerged that are capable of detecting lung cancer at an early, potentially treatable stage. These technologies include low-dose spiral CT (LDCT), digital radiography, advanced sputum analysis, and autofluorescence and virtual bronchoscopy. In the following paragraphs, the potential contributions and challenges of these emerging technologies are discussed, with a special emphasis on LDCT.

A. Low-Dose Spiral Computed Tomography

Computed tomography plays an established role in the assessment of patients with clinically suspected and proven bronchogenic carcinoma. Recently, LDCT has been explored as a tool for detecting early lung cancer in asymptomatic individuals at risk for this disease, with encouraging preliminary results [18–20].

The first large-scale LDCT screening studies that were published in the English literature were performed by Kaneko et al. [18] and Sone et al. [19]. Both of these studies were performed in Japan, a country with a rich history of cancer screening. More recently, Henschke et al. [20] reported their experience with LDCT screening at two large teaching hospitals in New York. The promising results of these preliminary studies have led many researchers, clinicians, health care policy officials and lung cancer patient advocates to revisit the topic of lung cancer screening [21].

In 1996, Kaneko et al. reported the use of biannual chest radiographs and spiral CT scans in screening 1369 Japanese adults at high risk for developing lung cancer [18]. Peripheral lung cancer was detected in 15 (1%) subjects by CT but in only 4 (0.3%) by chest radiography. A vast majority (93%) of detected cancers was classified as Stage I.

In 1998, Sone et al. published their experience in screening 5483 Japanese adults between the ages of 40 and 74 years, including smokers and nonsmokers, using LDCT and miniature fluorophotography [19]. Nineteen patients (prevalence 0.48%) were diagnosed with lung cancer, including 84% with Stage I disease. Miniature fluorophotography was interpreted as negative for malignancy in 18 of the 19 patients with lung cancer. In retrospect, however, judgement errors were present in 3 cases, in which positive findings were erroneously attributed to benign etiologies. Conventional chest radiographs obtained prior to surgery showed no evidence of a lung mass in 10 of 19 patients. There was one false-negative CT scan in a patient with an endobronchial lesion.

In 1999, Henschke et al. reported the results of baseline screening using LDCT and chest radiography in the Early Lung Cancer Action Project (ELCAP), which began in 1993 [20]. In this study, 1000 asymptomatic patients greater than 60 years of age with a positive smoking history (>10 pack-years) underwent screening with both LDCT and chest radiography. LDCT was performed with the following parameters: single breathhold, spiral acquisition; 140 kilovolt peaks (kVp), 40 mA; 10-mm collimation; 2:1 pitch; 5-mm reconstruction interval; and high-resolution (bone) algorithm. Only the lung windows (width 1500, level −650) were provided for interpretation, and each study was interpreted separately by two board-certified radiologists, with a third expert radiologist available for cases that lacked consensus readings.

In order to guide the evaluation of noncalcified pulmonary nodules that were detected in the ELCAP study, the following algorithm was proposed: nodules <5 mm in diameter (average of length and width) were followed by serial CT scans to assess for interval growth over a 2-year period (3, 6, 12, and 24 months), nodules between 5 and 10 mm in diameter were either followed or biopsied, and nodules >10 mm in diameter were biopsied. Patients with more than six noncalcified nodules, diffuse bronchiectasis, ground-glass opacities,

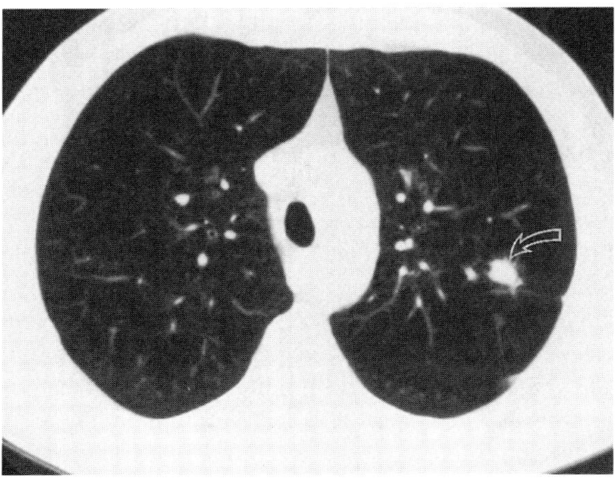

Figure 1 Early lung cancer detection by CT. Computed tomography image (lung windows) reveals an approximately 1.5-cm-diameter spiculated peripheral lung nodule (arrow) in the left upper lobe, which proved to represent an adenocarcinoma. This is the typical size of a lung cancer detected with screening spiral CT scans in the Japanese experience. Also note the presence of centrilobular emphysema.

or any combinations of these features were classified as having diffuse disease and were not evaluated by this algorithm.

In this study, 27 of 1000 (2.7%) subjects were found to have lung cancer by LDCT versus 7 (0.7%) by chest radiography. With regard to the cancers detected by CT, 26 (96%) were resectable and 23 (85%) were Stage I neoplasms. In contrast, chest radiography detected only 4 (17%) of 23 cases of Stage I disease.

The results of the Japanese and ELCAP studies clearly show that LDCT is superior to conventional chest radiography in the detection of early lung cancer. Indeed, a review of the Japanese experience with screening by Kaneko et al. [22] reports that the average peripheral lesion detected by chest radiography was 3.0 cm compared to 1.6 cm for spiral CT (Figs. 1 and 2). These studies also demonstrate the consistent ability of LDCT to detect lung cancer at an early, potentially curable stage (Table 1). Although it may seem intuitive that early detection should result in a decrease in lung cancer mortality, it is important to note that the impact of LDCT on disease-specific mortality has yet to be determined. Unlike other outcome measures (such as patient survival), mortality is not affected by several biases, including lead-time bias, length-time bias, and overdiagnosis [21,23,24]. Mortality is thus considered the ulti-

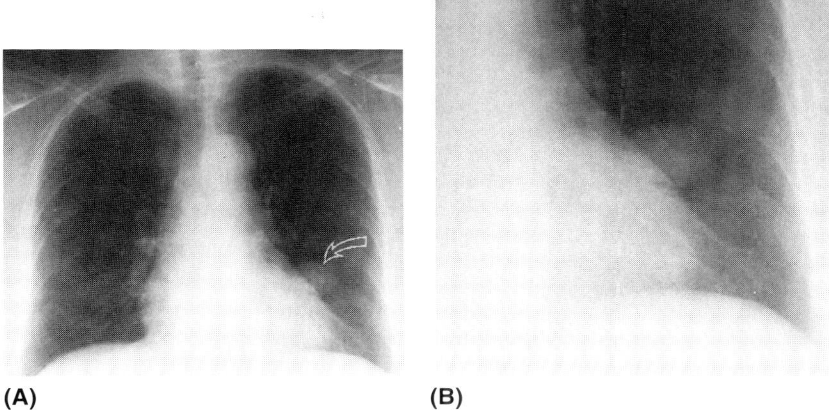

(A) (B)

Figure 2 Lung cancer detection by chest radiography. PA chest radiograph (A) reveals an approximately 3-cm-diameter left lower lobe lung nodule (arrow), which proved to represent an adenocarcinoma. The nodule is seen in better detail on the coned-down image of the left lower lobe in B. This is the typical size of a lung cancer detected with screening chest radiographs in the Japanese experience.

Table 1 LDCT Screening Studies[a]

Study	Screening population	Lung cancer prevalence	%Resectable	%Stage I
Henschke et al. [20]	n = 1000 >10 pk-yrs >60 y/o	27 (2.7%)	96	85
Sone et al. [19]	n = 5483 ± smoking 40–74 y/o	19 (0.48%)	84	84
Kaneko et al. [18]	n = 1369 >20 pk-yrs[b] >50 y/o[b]	15 (1%)	93	93

[a] Abbreviations: LDCT, low-dose spiral CT; Pk-yrs, pack-years of cigarette smoking; y/o, years old.

[b] Most but not all patients met these criteria.

mate outcome measure of a screening study, and a significant reduction in disease-specific mortality is widely regarded as a requisite for a screening study to be adopted as standard care [21,23,24].

Despite the very promising results of these early studies, one should be aware that there are currently several important potential limitations of LDCT (Table 2). First, it is important to note the relatively high false-positive rate of the initial baseline LDCT in the ELCAP study [20]. At baseline screening, 233 of 1000 patients (23.3%) were found to have 1 to 6 noncalcified nodules at LDCT, but only 27 of these nodules proved to be malignant. Notably, however, by following the prescribed guidelines for nodule assessment, only 28 nodules required biopsy. Of these nodules, nearly all (27) were proven malignant.

Although the lack of excessive invasive procedures is reassuring, the potential costs of performing serial follow-up CT scans in such a high percentage of patients has important financial implications for using LDCT as a mass screening tool [21]. For example, a conservative cost estimate ($300.00 per scan) for a false-positive nodule that requires a series of follow-up CT scans to confirm 2-year stability is approximately $1800.00 ($300.00 each for an

Table 2 Current Challenges of LDCT[a]

Current challenges	Potential solutions
Relatively high false-positive rate	Expected decrease at annual repeat screen
High cost for follow-up CT scans of false positives	Additional noninvasive imaging methods (PET, C+CT) may decrease the number of follow-up studies Further study of malignant growth rates of small nodules may allow for fewer follow-up studies
Difficulty in detecting malignant growth rate in small nodules	Computer-aided volumetric measurements will be more accurate
Bias toward detecting adenocarcinomas	Combine LDCT with advanced sputum analysis in order to detect more squamous cell lesions
Potential for ''overdiagnosis''	Further study of this subject is required

[a] Abbreviations: LDCT, low-dose spiral CT; PET, positron emission tomography; C+CT, CT nodule contrast enhancement.

initial screening study, immediate follow-up diagnostic scan, and subsequent follow-up scans at 3, 6, 12, and 24 months). Moreover, there are also psychological costs to consider for patients with false-positive nodules. Such patients must wait 2 years before receiving a final assurance that a nodule is benign. It is likely that some patients are better suited to a ''watch and wait'' approach than others. Thus, before undergoing this procedure, patients should be aware of the potential need for undergoing several follow-up CT scans.

One would expect the false-positive rates of LDCT screening to be greater in areas where there is a high prevalence of granulomatous infections. Indeed, preliminary data from the baseline screening LDCT study at the Mayo Clinic shows that 782 of 1520 screened patients (51%) demonstrated one or more noncalcified nodules (T. Hartman, personal communication, 2000). Although the high prevalence of granulomatous infections is likely the primary reason for the high percentage of patients with lung nodules in this study, technical factors may have also played a role in improved detection of nodules. Technical differences from the ELCAP study included use of a multidetector CT scanner, narrower collimation (5 mm vs. 10 mm), and cineviewing rather than film viewing. The prevalence of lung cancer in this study was below 1%, and 4 patients (0.3%) underwent resection for benign, granulomatous infection. Thus, there may be important geographical barriers to LDCT screening in areas where granulomatous infections are endemic [21].

Compared to baseline prevalence screening, one would anticipate a lower false-positive rate at repeat yearly screening [21]. Recently, Henschke et al. reported their findings from the first annual repeat LDCT exam in the ELCAP screening population [25]. At annual repeat screening, 31 of 623 patients (5%) had truly new or growing nodules compared to baseline screening LDCT. Nine of these nodules proved to be negative or demonstrated benign calcifications on additional high-resolution CT imaging. Of the remaining nodules, 8 were larger than 5 mm in diameter and were biopsied and 7 of these nodules were proven malignant. The overall detection rate of non-small-cell lung cancer on first annual repeat spiral CT was 1%, and 83% were Stage IA neoplasms.

A second potential limitation of LDCT relates to the difficulty of reliably detecting a malignant growth rate in small <1-cm nodules [26]. For example, if a 5-mm nodule doubles in volume over a 6-month period, its diameter will increase by only 1.25 to 6.25 mm [26], a difference that may be difficult to accurately detect using conventional methods of measurement (Fig. 3). More sophisticated methods of nodule measurement will be required to meet the challenge of accurately measuring growth of small nodules. Re-

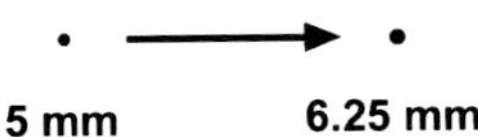

Figure 3 Difficulty in measuring growth of small nodules. Doubling the volume of a 5-mm-diameter nodule results in a diameter increase of only 1.25 mm, a difference that may be difficult to detect with conventional methods of measurement on axial CT images.

cently, there has been promising work in the area of computer-aided three-dimensional nodule measurement using sophisticated software programs (Fig. 4) [27–29]. Once such methods become more widely accessible and less labor intensive, they will likely play an important role in determining growth of small nodules.

A third potential limitation of LDCT screening is its bias toward detecting adenocarcinomas, which comprise the vast majority of peripheral lung cancers [21,30]. In the ELCAP baseline study, over 90% of neoplasms were characterized as an adenocarcinoma cell type; a majority were pure adenocarcinomas and a minority were bronchoalveolar cell carcinomas and adenosquamous subtypes [16]. This bias could be reduced by pairing LDCT with a complementary tool for detecting central neoplasms such as advanced sputum analysis techniques [21]. These techniques are discussed below.

A fourth potential limitation of LDCT concerns the possible ''overdiagnosis'' of lung cancer [21]. With regard to lung cancer screening, the detection of bronchioloalveolar cell adenomas, a benign lesion that may have malignant potential [31,32], is an example of potential overdiagnosis. This is a controversial subject that requires further study.

Finally, as with any screening study, there will be false-negative cases. Kakinuma et al. [33] recently reported seven cases of lung cancer that were initially missed at screening LDCT and subsequently detected on repeat LDCT screening studies performed 6 to 18 months later. Missed nodules were retrospectively categorized as either conspicuous (mean diameter = 11 mm; n = 3) or inconspicuous (mean diameter = 6 mm; n = 4). In order to reduce the number of false-negative cases, these authors emphasize the importance of examining noncalcified nodules with thin-section CT, even when adjacent lesions of prior tuberculosis exist. They also caution that one should carefully inspect pulmonary vessels in order to distinguish them from small pulmonary nodules. Despite an initial ''missed'' diagnosis, six of seven lesions were Stage I neoplasms at the time of diagnosis.

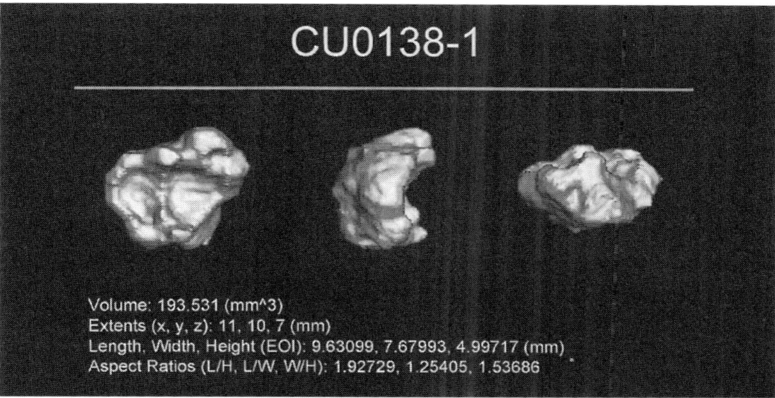

(A)

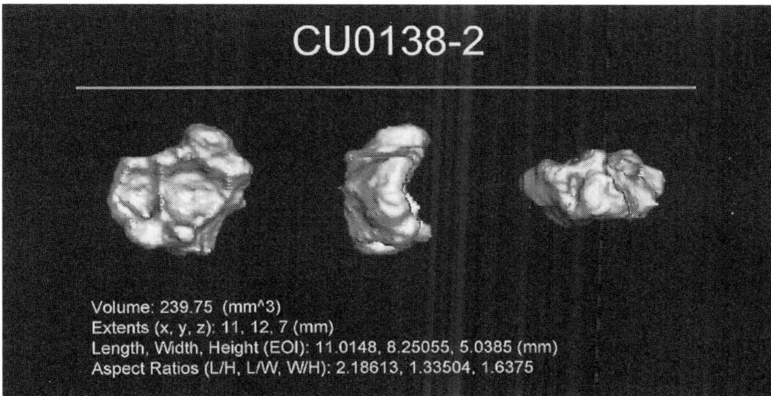

(B)

Figure 4 Three-dimensional volumetric analysis of lung nodule showing early detection of malignant growth rate in proven non-small-cell lung cancer. (A) Three-dimensional volumetric reconstruction images of a small left apical lung nodule with a volume measurement of 193.531 mm^3. (B) Follow-up 3D volumetric reconstruction images of the same nodule performed 4 months later reveals interval increase in volume to 239.75 mm^3. Interval growth of the nodule was not readily apparent on axial high-resolution CT images. (Courtesy of David Yankelevitz, New York Presbyterian Hospital/Weil Cornell Medical Center, New York, New York; from Ref. 65.)

The ELCAP investigators recently reported an analysis of missed lung nodules on screening LDCT that were subsequently identified on followup diagnostic CT scans [34]. Among the 163 patients who underwent diagnostic CT imaging, 36 (22%) had additional nodules which were not detected on LDCT. The majority (85%) of missed nodules measured 5 mm in diameter or less and none were greater than 10 mm in diameter. Thus, small size appears to be the most important factor related to missed nodules on LDCT. Interestingly, a majority of missed nodules were located peripherally.

Recent advances in technology will likely improve the ability of LDCT to detect and accurately characterize lung nodules [27–29,35–38]. These advances include the use of multidetector CT scanners, cine-based viewing, computerized detection methods, and three-dimensional reconstruction methods. Moreover, the addition of more specific noninvasive methods of imaging evaluation such as CT nodule enhancement [39] and ^{18}F-labeled 2-deoxy-D-glucose positron emission tomography imaging (FDG PET) [40–43] may help to reduce the number of cases requiring close follow-up or biopsy [21]. These techniques are discussed further in Chapter 2.

With regard to the use of LDCT for mass screening of lung cancer, future studies are necessary to determine: (1) the reproducibility of the promising preliminary results of LDCT screening when it is applied at other institutions, (2) the effect of LDCT screening upon lung cancer mortality, (3) the cost-effectiveness of LDCT screening, (4) the subgroups of present and former smokers who are most likely to benefit from this screening tool, and (5) the optimal complementary screening method(s) to combine with LDCT in order to detect the full spectrum of lung cancer cell types [21].

The Society of Thoracic Radiology has recently constructed a consensus statement on the topic of screening for lung cancer with LDCT (www.thoracicrad.org). Excerpts from this statement are provided in Table 3.

B. Digital Chest Radiography

The results of the LDCT studies described in the previous section have clearly shown the limited ability of conventional chest radiography to detect early lung cancer. Emerging technological advancements in digital chest radiography, including computer-aided diagnosis, temporal subtraction, and dual energy subtraction methods, may significantly improve the ability of chest radiography to detect small lung nodules [44–46]. These techniques are described in further detail in Chapter 13. Once this technology matures, future studies will be necessary to address the ability of digital chest radiography to detect early lung cancer [21].

Table 3 Excerpts from the Consensus Statement of the Society of Thoracic Radiology

Subject selection

For the general population, an age range should be established. We believe that this should be between 50 and 80 years, depending on the subjects' general health. In high-risk groups such as those occupationally exposed to carcinogens or with a previous NSCLC, selection criteria may vary. Cigarette smoking should be at least 10 or 20 pack-years.

Periodicity

Lacking definitive information, the general trend is to perform annual CT scanning. It has to be understood that some lung cancers will become clinically evident in the periods between screening studies, although how many is yet to be determined.

Screening protocols

Screening protocols will vary with the available imaging technology. It is our opinion that screening be performed with a multirow detector CT so that high-resolution scans can be reformatted retrospectively, without the need to use additional radiation.

The entire thorax should be included in the scan field, preferably in a single breathhold. A helical (spiral) mode of operation should be used. Two sample techniques are given below.

Multislice protocol

Table feed: 30 mm/sec

120–140 kVp

Pitch 3 to 6

20–60 mA

1- to 2.5-mm collimation; with a 1- to 2.5-mm reconstruction interval.

Single-slice spiral scanner protocol

Helical mode, 0.8-sec scan time (the shortest possible)

120 kVp

Pitch 2 to 1

80 mA

3- to 7-mm collimation; with 2.5- to 3.5-mm reconstruction interval.

It is advisable to train technologists or other observers to detect nodules and calcifications at the time of scanning so that high-resolution 1- to 1.25-mm helical images can be performed through any noncalcified nodules at the same time as the primary screening study. This can obviate the need for a repeat study.

Radiation dose

The effective radiation dose associated with the low-dose screening examination is 0.65 mSv (mRem). The approximate dose for "conventional" CT is 5.8 mSv (26). Eliminating the scanogram for the screening CT study can reduce dose. These doses include no high-resolution or follow-up CT studies.

Table 3 Continued

Indeterminate nodules

Indeterminate nodules are solid, smooth-edged, and do not show ''benign calcifications,'' air bronchograms, or converging vessels. They are not spiculated and are of unknown chronicity. The follow-up interval for indeterminate nodules is often dictated by the individual subject and their physician. Sites experienced in lung cancer screening have adopted the following strategy based on the diameter of the nodule:

- <5 mm: high-resolution CT at 3 and/or 6, 12, and 24 months. Consider biopsy/removal for nodules that increase in size (1% malignant in prevalence studies)
- 5–10 mm: high-resolution CT at 3, 6, 12, and 24 months. Biopsy/removal of nodules that increase in size (25–30% malignant)
- >10 mm: consider biopsy of all of these nodules (30–80% malignant). Alternatively, they may be studied with PET scanning or with CT contrast enhancement [27,28].

Physician responsibility

Screening-imposed obligations on the radiologist (similar to mammography) to (1) warn the subject that a negative screen does not preclude the subsequent development of lung cancer, even between scans; (2) ensure the subject knows that some lung cancers may not be amenable to detection by CT screening; (3) ensure that the subject is contacted with results of the CT screening; (4) ensure that appropriate physicians are available to council and treat the patient with a positive result; (5) ensure that patients understand the problem of the number of small lung nodules that are benign and the implications thereof.

To ensure the answer to the question of the efficacy of CT screening for NSCLC is made available as soon as possible, it is recommended that all subjects being screened with CT for lung cancer are done as part of a prospective study. Comparable protocols should be used and the recording of results standardized.

Summary of current recommendations

Lung cancer screening with low-dose CT is a complex subject. It is clear that a standard of care cannot be based on currently published prevalence data. However, there are ongoing studies that are generating prevalence data. The appropriate studies which address lung cancer mortality and cure rates need to be performed and the data analyzed and validated before the true utility of this test can be determined. Thus we do not recommend mass screening for lung cancer at this time, but strongly encourage appropriate subjects to participate in trials so that the true effectiveness of lung cancer screening with low-dose helical CT can be determined at the earliest possible time.

Source: www.thoracicrad.org.

C. Sputum Cytology and Advanced Sputum Analysis Techniques

In screening studies, the sensitivity of sputum cytology for detecting lung cancer is approximately 20 to 30% and the specificity is approximately 98% [6,47,53]. Improvement in sensitivity can be achieved by adherence to proper techniques for collection, processing, and interpretation of samples [48]. Sputum cytology demonstrates the highest sensitivity for squamous cell carcinoma and the lowest yield for adenocarcinoma [21].

In recent years, there have been several exciting advances in sputum analysis techniques, most notably the development of automated analysis of sputum specimens for biomarkers [49,50–56]. This technology capitalizes on advances in our understanding of the molecular events that lead to lung cancer. In the future, it is likely that a panel of biomarkers (Table 4) will be used to identify the early clonal phase of lung cancer, thus allowing detection of lung cancers at a very early stage [52]. Importantly, biomarker characterization may also allow for targeted treatment of early lung cancer [52].

D. Conventional, Autofluorescence, and Virtual Bronchoscopy

Conventional bronchoscopy is a valuable technique for localizing preinvasive lung cancer within the airways. In general, conventional bronchoscopy can detect nodular or polypoid lesions >2 mm in size and flat or superficially spreading lesions >2 cm in diameter [21,57]. With regard to carcinoma in situ, 75% of lesions are superficial or flat and 25% are nodular or polypoid [21,56].

Table 4 Biomarkers

Biomarker	Analysis	Biological role	Application
HnRNP A2/B1	Protein I in sputum cells	mRNA processing	Early detection/ monitoring
K-ras	DNA in sputum homogenates	Cell-cycle regulation	Early detection/ risk assessment
Genomic instability	DNA in sputum homogenates	Chromosomal integrity	Early detection/ risk assessment

Source: Ref 52.

Autofluorescence bronchoscopy (AF) is a recently developed optical imaging method that is designed to improve the detection of small preinvasive lesions that are not visible by conventional, ''white light'' bronchoscopy [53, 56–60]. AF involves illuminating the bronchial surface with violet or blue light (400 to 440 nm) in order to distinguish normal from abnormal tissues. Upon such illumination, dysplastic lesions and carcinoma in situ will show a diminution in the intensity of autofluorescence.

The light-induced fluorescence endoscopy (LIFE) device, which was designed to capitalize on differences in autofluorescence properties in order to aid in the detection and localization of preinvasive lung cancer, has been approved by the FDA for the detection of early lung cancer [56,57]. Except for differences in the illuminating light and the addition of a special camera, the LIFE device is similar to conventional bronchoscopy [56,57]. In the hands of a bronchoscopist who has received extensive training in using this device, it adds only a few minutes to a conventional bronchoscopic procedure. A recent multicenter trial using LIFE showed that it improved the detection rate of preinvasive lung cancer by severalfold compared to conventional fiberoptic bronchoscopy alone [57].

Because of its invasive nature and high cost, screening with AF should currently be reserved for patients with a very high pretest probability of lung cancer [21]. For widespread screening, AF should ideally be coupled with a noninvasive, first-line study that selects patients with a high pretest probability of harboring early lung cancer [21]. For example, a recent study by Phillips et al. describes the use of a breathalyzer to identify volatile organic compounds that may serve as potential markers for lung cancer [61]. Future studies are needed to determine the precise role of this exciting new technology in the detection of early lung cancer.

Virtual bronchoscopy (VB) is a novel noninvasive method for assessing the airways which combines helical computed tomography data and virtual reality computing in order to create three-dimensional endobronchial simulations (Fig. 5) [62–64]. This technique is described in detail in Chapter 9. A recent preliminary investigation by Summers et al. assessed the computer-assisted detection of polypoid airway lesions on virtual bronchoscopy images [63]. This technique was associated with a relatively high sensitivity (90%) for lesions >5 mm in diameter, but was limited by a poor specificity.

Current limitations of VB include its labor-intensive nature, the limited experience of most radiologists with this technique, and its inability to differentiate malignant from benign lesions [21,62–64]. Future technological advances will hopefully overcome many of these obstacles.

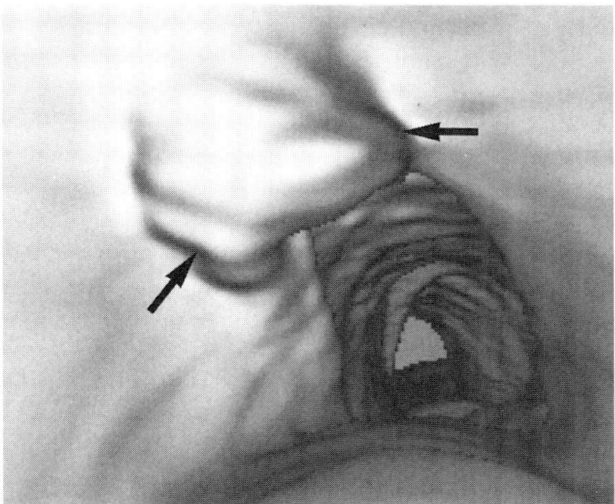

Figure 5 Virtual airway imaging. Virtual bronchoscopic image (internal rendering) reconstructed from a helical CT data set (2.5-mm collimation; 1.25-mm reconstruction interval) reveals an endoluminal lesion anteriorly (arrows), which proved to represent a benign polyp. The limited ability of virtual bronchoscopy to distinguish benign from malignant lesions is a current limitation of this technology.

IV. LUNG CANCER SCREENING: FUTURE DIRECTIONS

The current wealth of emerging technologies for the early detection of lung cancer provides hope that we may be able to reduce the burden of this 20th century disease in the early 21st century [21]. To date, LDCT and advanced sputum analysis techniques appear to be the most promising emerging technologies for lung cancer screening, but ongoing advances in other techniques may change this perspective in the near future. Because of their proclivities for different cell types, LDCT and sputum analysis should be considered complementary rather than competitive screening tools.

Important questions to answer before proceeding to mass screening include the effect of screening on lung cancer mortality, the cost-effectiveness of widespread screening, the optimal screening tools to use, and the subsets of present and former smokers who are most likely to benefit from screening. National studies are being planned to answer these questions.

REFERENCES

1. Landis SH, Murray T, Bolden S, Wingo PA. Cancer statistics, 1999. Cancer J Clin 1999; 49:8–31.
2. Mountain CF. Revisions in the international system for staging lung cancer. Chest 1997; 111:1710–1717.
3. Eddy DM. Screening for lung cancer. Ann Intern Med 1989; 111:232–237.
4. Boucot KR, Weiss W. Is curable lung cancer detected by semi-annual screening? J Am Med Assoc 1973; 224:1361–1365.
5. Fontana RS, Sanderson DR, Woolner LB, Taylor WF, Miller WE, Muhm JR. Lung cancer screening: the Mayo program. J Occup Med 1986; 28:746–750.
6. Fontana RS, Sanderson DR, Taylor WF et al. Early lung cancer detection: results of the initial (prevalence) radiologic and cytologic screening in the Mayo Clinic study. Am Rev Resp Dis 1984; 130:561–565.
7. Melamed MR, Flehinger BJ, Zaman MB, Heelan RT, Perchick WA, Martini N. Screening for early lung cancer: results of the Memorial Sloan–Kettering study in New York. Chest 1984; 86:44–53.
8. Tockman MS. Survival and mortality from lung cancer in a screened population: the Johns Hopkins Study. Chest 1986; 89(Suppl):324S–325S.
9. Kubik A, Polak J. Lung cancer detection: results of a randomized prospective study in Czechoslovakia. Cancer 1986; 57:2427–2437.
10. Kubik A, Haerting J. Survival and mortality in a randomized study of lung cancer detection. Neoplasma 1990; 37:467–475.
11. Ebeling K, Nischan P. Screening for lung cancer-results from a case-control study. Int J Cancer 1987; 40:141–144.
12. American Cancer Society. Guidelines for the cancer related check-up. Cancer 1980; 30:199–207.
13. Strauss GM, Gleason RE, Sugarbaker DJ. Chest X-ray screening improves outcome in lung cancer: a reappraisal of randomized trials on lung cancer screening. Chest 1995; 107(Suppl):270–279.
14. Henschke CI, Yankelevitz DF. Screening for lung cancer. J Thorac Imaging 2000;15:21–27.
15. McFarlane MJ, Feinstein AR, Wells CK. Clinical features of lung cancer discovered as a post-mortem ''surprise.'' Chest 1986; 90:520–523.
16. Flehinger BJ, Kimmel M, Melamed MR. The effect of surgical treatment on survival from early lung cancer: implications for screening. Chest 1992; 101: 1013–1018.
17. Miettinen OS. Screening for lung cancer. Radiol Clin North Am 2000; 38:479–486.
18. Kaneko M, Eguchi K, Ohmatsu H, et al. Peripheral lung cancer: screening and detection with low-dose spiral CT versus radiography. Radiology 1996; 201: 798–802.
19. Sone S, Takashima S, Li F, et al. Mass screening for lung cancer with mobile spiral computed tomography scanner. Lancet 1998; 351:1242–1245.

20. Henschke CI, McCauley DI, Yankelevitz DF, et al. Early Lung Cancer Action Project: overall design and findings from baseline screening. Lancet 1999; 54: 99–105.
21. Boiselle PM, Ernst A, Karp DD. Lung cancer detection in the 21st century: potential contributions and challenges of emerging technologies. Am J Radiol 2000; 175:1215–1221.
22. Kaneko M. CT scanning for lung cancer in Japan: International Conference on Prevention and Early Diagnosis of Lung Cancer, Varese, Italy, December 9–10, 1998, Cancer 2000; 89:2485–2588.
23. Riegelman RK, Hirsch RP. Screening. In: Riegelman RK, Hirsch RP, eds. Studying a study and testing a test: How to read the health science literature. 3rd ed. Boston, MA: Little, Brown, 1996:183–191.
24. Strauss GM, Gleason RE, Sugarbaker DJ. Screening for lung cancer: another look; a different view. Chest 1997; 111:754–768.
25. Henschke CI, Naidich DP, Yankelevitz DF, et al. Results of Early Lung Cancer Action Program (ELCAP): first-annual repeat low-dose CT screening in high risk subjects (abstract); Radiology 1999; 213:303.
26. Erasmus JF, Connolly JE, McAdams HP, Roggli VL. Solitary pulmonary nodules: part II. Evaluation of the indeterminate nodule. RadioGraphics 2000; 20: 59–66.
27. Wyckoff N, McNitt-Gray MF, Goldin JG, Sayre JW, Aberle DR. The use of contrast-enhancement, texture and three-dimensional size and shape features for classification of solitary pulmonary nodules (abstr). Radiology 1999; 213:172.
28. Zhao B, Yankelevitz DF, Reeves A, Henschke CI. Two-dimensional multi-criterion segmentation of pulmonary nodules on helical CT images. Med Phys 1999; 26(6): 889–895.
29. Yankelevitz DF, Gupta R, Zhao B, Henschke CI. Small pulmonary nodules: evaluation with repeat CT—preliminary experience. Radiology 1999; 212:561–566.
30. Jett J, Feins R, Kvale P, et al. Pretreatment evaluation of non-small-cell lung cancer. Am J Respir Crit Care Med 1997; 156:320–322.
31. Logan PM, Miller RR, Evans K, Müller NL. Bronchogenic carcinoma and coexistent bronchioloalveolar cell adenomas: assessment of radiology detection and follow-up in 28 patients. Chest 1996; 109:713–717.
32. Miller RR. Bronchioloalveolar cell adenoma. Am J Surg Pathol 1990; 14:904–912.
33. Kakinuma R, Ohmatsu, H, Kaneko M, et al. Detection failures in spiral CT screening for lung cancer: analysis of CT findings. Radiology 1999; 212:61–66.
34. Naidich DP, Yankelevitz DF, McGuinness G, et al. Noncalcified nodules missed on low-dose helical CT (abstr). Radiology 1999; 213(p):303.
35. Liang Y, Kruger RA. Dual-slice versus single-slice spiral scanning: comparison of the physical performance of two computed tomography scanners. Med Phys 1996; 23: 205-220.
36. Seltzer SE, Judy PF, Adams DF, et al. Spiral CT of the chest: comparison of cine and film-based viewing. Radiology 1995; 197:73–78.

37. Tillich M, Kammerhuber F, Reittner P, et al. Detection of pulmonary nodules with helical CT: comparison of cine and film-based viewing. Am J Radiol 1997; 169:1611–1614.
38. Armato SG III, Giger ML, Moran CJ, et al. Computerized detection of pulmonary nodules on CT scans. RadioGraphics 1999; 19:1303–1311.
39. Swensen SJ, Viggiano RW, Midthun DE, et al. Lung nodule enhancement at CT: multicenter study. Radiology 2000; 214:273–280.
40. Al-Sugair A, Coleman RE. Applications of PET in lung cancer. Semin Nucl Med 1998; 28:303–319.
41. Coleman RE. PET in lung cancer. J Nucl Med 1999; 40:814–820.
42. Patz EF, Lowe VJ, Hoffman JM, et al. Focal pulmonary abnormalities: Evaluation with [18F]fluorodeoxyglucose PET scanning. Radiology 1993; 188:487–490.
43. Gupta NC, Maloof J, Gunel E. Probability of malignancy in solitary pulmonary nodules using fluorine-18-FDG and PET. J Nucl Med 1996; 37:943–948.
44. Kobayashi T, Xu XW, MacMahon H, et al. Effect of a computer-aided diagnosis scheme on radiologists' performance in detection of lung nodules on radiographs. Radiology 1996; 199:843–848.
45. Kido S, Ikozoe J, Naito H, et al. Clinical evaluation of pulmonary nodules with single-exposure dual-energy subtraction chest radiography with an iterative noise-reduction algorithm. Radiology 1995; 194:407–412.
46. MacMahon H, Engelmann RM, Behlen FM, et al. Computer-aided diagnosis of pulmonary nodules: results of a large-scale observer test. Radiology 1999; 213: 723–726.
47. Frost JK, Ball WC Jr, Levin ML. Early lung cancer detection: results of the initial (prevalence) radiologic and cytologic screening in the Johns Hopkins study. Am Rev Respir Dis 1984; 130:549–554.
48. Kennedy TC, Proudfoot SP, Franklin WA, et al. Cytopathological analysis of sputum in patients with airflow obstruction and significant smoking histories. Cancer Res, 1996; 56:4673–4768.
49. Field JK. Selection and validation of new lung cancer markers for the molecular-pathological assessment of individuals with a high risk of developing lung cancer. In: Brambilla C, Brambilla E, eds. Lung tumors: fundamental biology and clinical management. New York: Marcel Dekker, 1999:287–302.
50. Tockman MS, Mulshine JL, Piantadosi S, et al. Prospective detection of preclinical lung cancer: results from two studies of heterogeneous nuclear ribonucleoprotein A2/B1 overexpression. Clin Cancer Res 1997; 3:2237–2246.
51. Gazdar AF, Minna JD. Molecular detection of early lung cancer (editorial). J Natl Cancer Inst 1999; 91:299–301.
52. Mulshine JL, Henschke CI. Prospects for lung cancer screening (commentary). Lancet 1999; 355:592–593.
53. Ahrendt SA, Chow JT, Xu LH, et al. Molecular detection of tumor cells in bronchoalveolar lavage fluid from patients with early stage lung cancer. J Natl Cancer Inst 1999; 91:332–339.

54. Hibi K, Westra WH, Borges M, Goodman S, Sidransky D, Jen J. PGP9.5 as a candidate tumor marker for non-small-cell lung cancer. Am J Pathol 1999; 155: 711–715.
55. Payne PW, Sebo TJ, Doudkine A, et al. Sputum screening by quantitative microscopy: reexamination of a portion of the National Cancer Institute cooperative early lung cancer study. Mayo Clin Proc 1997; 72:697–704.
56. Lam S, Shibuya H. Early diagnosis of lung cancer. Clin Chest Med 1999; 20: 53–61.
57. Lam S, Kennedy T, Unger M, et al. Localization of bronchial intraepithelial neoplastic lesions by fluorescence bronchoscopy. Chest 1998; 113:696–702.
58. Vermylen P, Pierard P, Roufosse C, et al. Detection of bronchial preneoplastic lesions and early lung cancer with fluorescence bronchoscopy: a study about its ambulatory feasibility under local anaesthesia. Lung Cancer 1999; 25:161–168.
59. Alexander W. Autofluorescence for bronchial imaging. J Clin Laser Med Surg 1991; 9:331–333.
60. Prakash UBS. Advances in bronchoscopic procedures. Chest 1999; 116:1403–1408.
61. Phillips M, Gleeson K, Hughes JM, et al. Volatile organic compounds in breath as markers of lung cancer: a cross-sectional study. Lancet 1999; 353:1930–1933.
62. Vining DJ, Liu K, Choplin RH, Haaponik EF. Virtual bronchoscopy: relationships of virtual reality endobronchial simulations to actual bronchoscopic findings. Chest 1996; 109:549–553.
63. Summers RM, Selbie WS, Malley JD, et al. Polypoid lesions of airways: early experience with computer-assisted detection by using virtual bronchoscopy and surface curvature. Radiology 1998; 208:331–337.
64. Fleiter R, Merkle EM, Aschoff AJ, et al. Comparison of real-time virtual and fiberoptic bronchoscopy in patients with bronchial carcinoma: opportunities and limitations. Am J Radiol 1997; 169:1591–1595.
65. Henschke CI, Yankelevitz DI. CT screening for lung cancer. Radiol Clin North Am 2000; 38:487–495.

2
Noninvasive Assessment of the Solitary Pulmonary Nodule

Jeremy J. Erasmus
MD Anderson Cancer Center
University of Texas
Houston, Texas

Holman Page McAdams
Duke University Medical Center
Durham, North Carolina

Eric Crotty
Children's Hospital Medical Center
Cincinnati, Ohio

I. INTRODUCTION

Solitary pulmonary nodules (SPN) are commonly defined as well-marginated, round lung opacities with a diameter of 3 cm or less. This definition excludes poorly marginated or irregular opacities that are a common initial manifestation of lung cancer. In order to encompass these abnormalities, this definition is either not strictly adhered to or the term solitary pulmonary nodule is replaced by the more loosely defined term solitary pulmonary opacity. Solitary pulmonary opacities, including SPNs, are a common radiological finding with an estimated 150,000 detected annually [1]. Although most are benign and usually the sequela of pulmonary infections, lung cancer constitutes an important proportion of solitary pulmonary opacities. Although only 20–30% of patients with non-small-cell lung cancer present with a solitary nodule, these patients are potentially curable if surgical resection is performed [2,3]. Unfortunately,

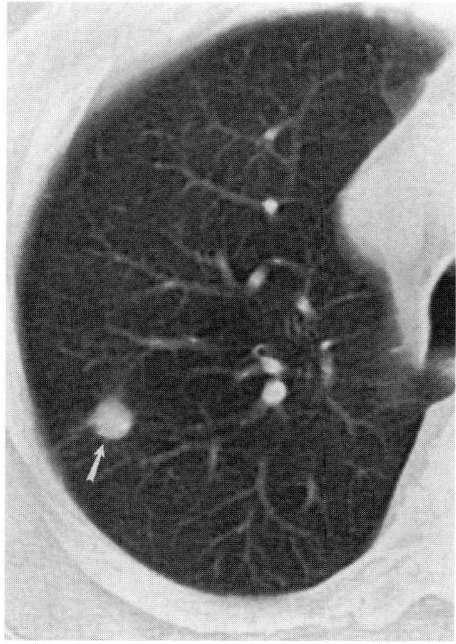

Figure 1 Pulmonary nodule detected on chest radiograph (not shown) in a 61-year-old asymptomatic man with history of cigarette smoking. Computed tomography shows a small, well-circumscribed, noncalcified nodule in right upper lobe (arrow). Because of the high probability of malignancy, the nodule was resected and revealed a noncaseating granuloma.

it can be difficult to prospectively identify these malignant nodules and consequently many resected nodules are benign (Fig. 1). The morbidity and high cost associated with unnecessary resection have provided the impetus to improve noninvasive evaluation of solitary pulmonary opacities. This chapter reviews evaluation strategies and recent advances in imaging that can improve the accuracy of differentiating benign and malignant solitary pulmonary opacities.

II. CLINICAL ASSESSMENT

Clinical features, including presenting symptoms, age, and past medical and smoking history, can provide an indication as to the etiology of a nodule and

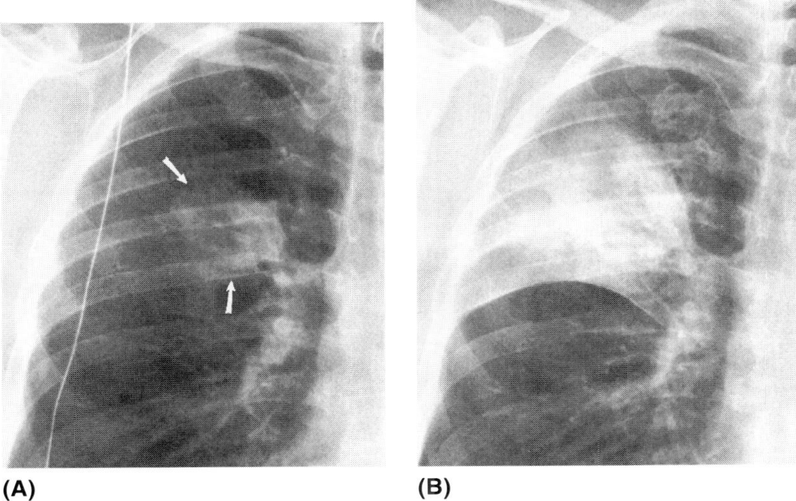

Figure 2 Round pneumonia in woman who presented with fever and cough. (A) Chest radiograph shows poorly marginated opacity in the right upper lobe (arrows). (B) Follow-up radiograph performed 48 hr later shows diffuse consolidation in the right upper lobe. Although more common in children, round pneumonia is occasionally seen in adults [64].

are important in determining patient management. Management of a nodule depends on the likelihood of malignancy and includes observation, resection, and biopsy. Observation is usually undertaken if the probability of malignancy is low or the patient's clinical status either precludes further evaluation or suggests a nonmalignant etiology. For instance, in a patient presenting with a new focal abnormal pulmonary opacity and clinical findings of pneumonia, radiographical reassessment after a short interval may be all that is necessary to exclude malignancy and confirm a diagnosis of round pneumonia (Fig. 2). Surgical resection of a solitary pulmonary opacity is usually performed when the probability of malignancy is high. Thus, if a new nodule is detected in a young adult with a peripheral sarcoma, this is most likely a solitary metastasis and resection is commonly performed. For cases between these two extremes, biopsy is frequently performed, using bronchoscopy, transthoracic needle biopsy, or video-assisted thoracoscopy.

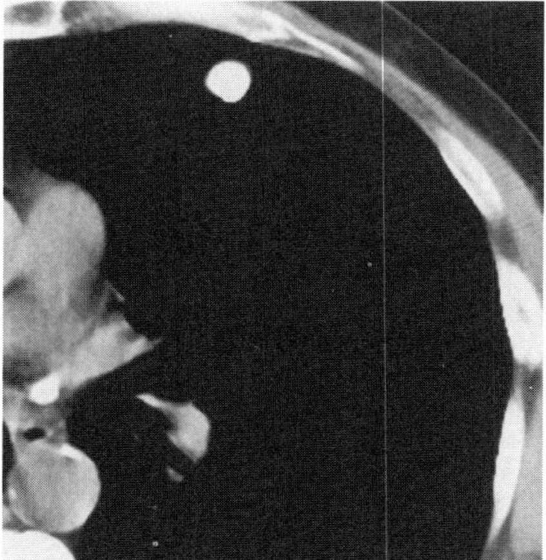

Figure 3 Histoplasmoma. Computed tomography shows diffusely calcified nodule in the left upper lobe. Note small calcified lymph node within mediastinum. Diffuse calcification is indicative of a benign etiology and, in the absence of a primary osteosarcoma, no further evaluation is required.

III. RADIOLOGICAL EVALUATION

Although an increasing number of solitary pulmonary opacities are diagnosed by computed tomography (CT), either incidentally or as part of lung cancer screening studies, many are still initially detected on chest radiographs. If the nodule is diffusely calcified (Fig. 3), or comparison with older radiographs shows stability in size for more than 2 years, the nodule is presumed to be benign and no further evaluation is recommended. Many nodules, however, require further radiological evaluation because (1) it can be difficult to determine whether a small nodule is calcified or stable in size on chest radiographs and (2) preexisting radiographs are often not available for review. Because up to 20% of small or subtle radiographical abnormalities thought to represent nodules are not within the lung, chest fluoroscopy, which is relatively inexpensive, is occasionally performed before CT [4]. Fluoroscopy often enables a determination of whether the opacity is in the lung (Fig. 4) and, by using a lower kilovolt peak (kVp) than conventional radiographical techniques, more optimally demonstrates calcification. However, fluoroscopy does not always enable confident determination of whether a radiographical abnormality is a

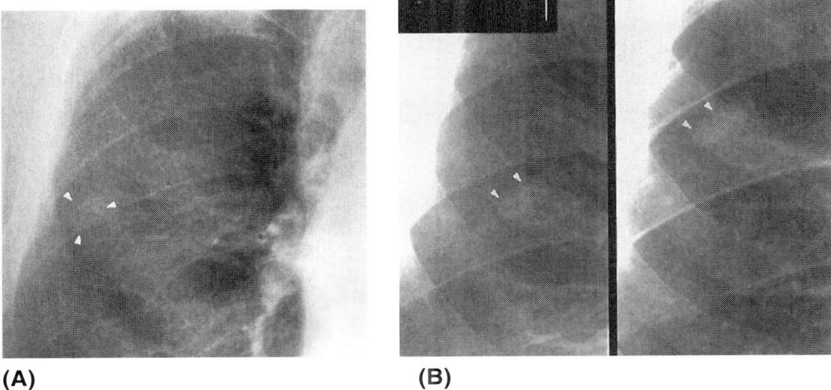

Figure 4 Rib fracture mimicking a pulmonary nodule. (A) Posteroanterior radiograph of right upper lung shows poorly marginated opacity overlying ribs (arrowheads). (B) Fluoroscopic view shows healing fracture of right anterior rib (arrowheads). Fluoroscopy often allows a confident diagnosis, obviating the need for CT evaluation.

pulmonary nodule. CT is often performed to further evaluate these radiographical abnormalities. CT is accurate in determining where the abnormality is located and, if in the lung, optimally evaluates morphological characteristics of the nodule (Fig. 5). CT is also useful in determining if the nodule is truly solitary and assessing for growth on serial studies. Interpretive difficulty, however, also occurs with CT. It can be difficult to determine whether a small opacity is a nodule, a vessel, or a pseudonodule due to partial volume averaging of adjacent intrathoracic structures. This difficulty can often be resolved by either increasing or decreasing the slice collimation. If standard 7-mm-slice collimation has been used, obtaining images through the region of abnormality using a slice collimation of 1 to 3 mm is useful in eliminating partial volume averaging. If 1- to 3-mm-slice collimation has been used (as is common in protocols utilized to evaluate the pulmonary arteries for emboli), the difficulty of differentiating a vessel from a small nodule is often overcome by reconstructing the original data at thicker collimation or by using maximal intensity projection (MIP) images (Fig. 6). Maximal intensity projection images are generated from an axial slab of volumetrical data obtained when spiral CT is performed. By displaying the continuity of vessels, this technique has been shown to improve nodule detection and discrimination from vessels [5]. Cine viewing of axial CT images at a workstation has also been shown to aid nodule detection and distinction of nodules from vessels [6].

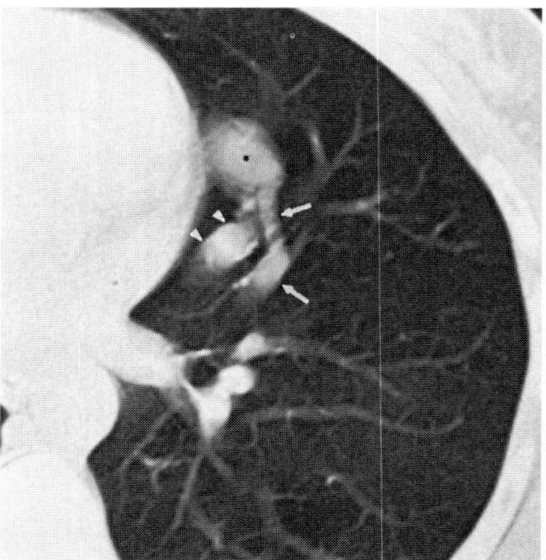

Figure 5 Arteriovenous malformation (AVM) in woman with hereditary hemorrhagic telangiectasia. Chest radiograph (not shown) showed a small solitary nodule in lingula. Computed tomography reveals an enlarged feeding artery (arrows) and an enlarged draining vein (arrowheads) as well as the nidus of the vascular malformation (*). Morphologic characteristics are diagnostic for arteriovenous malformation. Computed tomography also revealed a few smaller AVMs in both lungs (not shown).

A. Nodule Morphology

Evaluation of morphologic features, including size, margins, contour, and density, can be useful in determining whether a nodule is benign or malignant [7,8]. Although the likelihood of malignancy increases with increasing nodule size, widespread use and improvements in CT technology, coupled with a recent interest in CT screening for lung cancer, have resulted in the frequent detection of small nodules (1–5 mm) that are not usually visible on chest radiographs [9–11]. While the majority are most likely benign, recent studies of resected small nodules have shown that a considerable number are either primary or secondary pulmonary malignancies [12,13]. Consequently small nodule size does not exclude malignancy.

Typically, benign nodules have well-defined margins and a smooth contour while malignant nodules have poorly defined or spiculated margins and a lobular or irregular contour (Figs. 7,8, and 9) [7,14–17]. There is, however, considerable overlap between benign and malignant nodules in this regard. For instance, although a spiculated margin with distortion of adjacent vessels (often described as a sunburst or corona radiata appearance) is highly suggestive of malignancy, benign nodules can occasionally have this appearance.

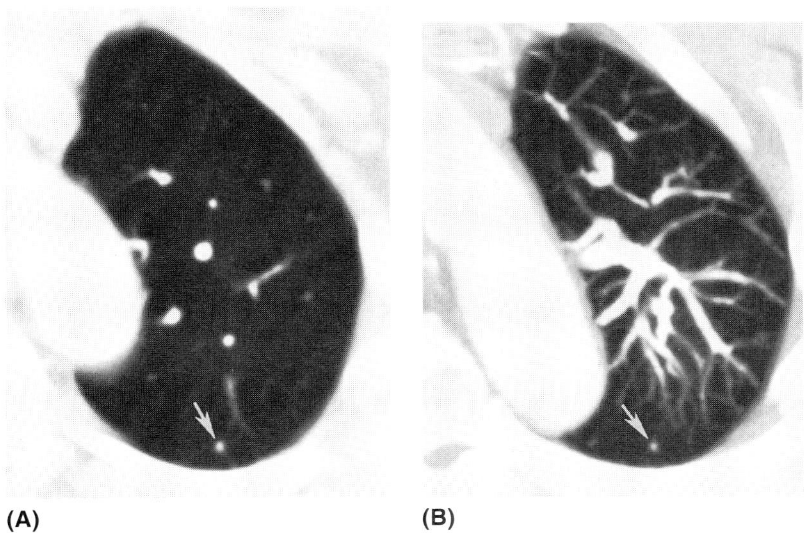

Figure 6 Small nodule visualization using maximal intensity projection (MIP) image. (A) Computed tomography shows small nodular opacity in left lung (arrow). Confident differentiation from pulmonary vessels is difficult. (B) Axial MIP image allows nodule (arrow) to be more easily differentiated from tubular vessels.

Also, up to 20% of malignant nodules have smooth contours and well-defined margins [7,15]. These characteristics are more typically observed in metastatic lesions than in primary lung neoplasms.

Internal morphology of a nodule, with the exception of fat [attenuation of −40 to −120 Hounsfield units (HU)] and calcification, is unreliable in distinguishing a malignant from a benign nodule [7,14,15,18–20]. Fat within a nodule is a characteristic finding of hamartomas and is detected by CT in up to 50% of these neoplasms (Figs. 10 and 11) [19]. While this finding negates further evaluation, hamartomas constitute a very small percentage of SPNs. Calcification of a nodule can be useful in determining benignity, although the majority of benign nodules are not calcified [7,18]. Calcification that is diffusely solid, centrally punctate, laminated, or ''popcornlike'' in appearance is diagnostic of a benign nodule. Occasionally, however, benign-appearing calcification can be seen in metastatic nodules in patients with osteosarcoma (Fig. 12). Furthermore, calcification can be detected histopathologically in up to 14% of lung cancers and is occasionally visible on CT [21,22] (Fig. 13). This calcification is typically stippled, eccentric, or amorphous. De-

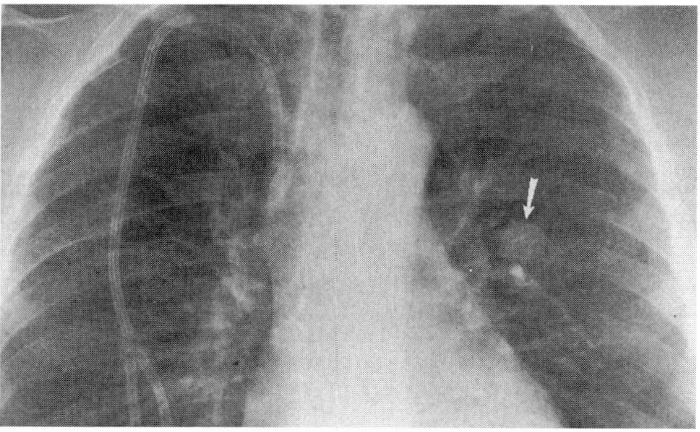

(A)

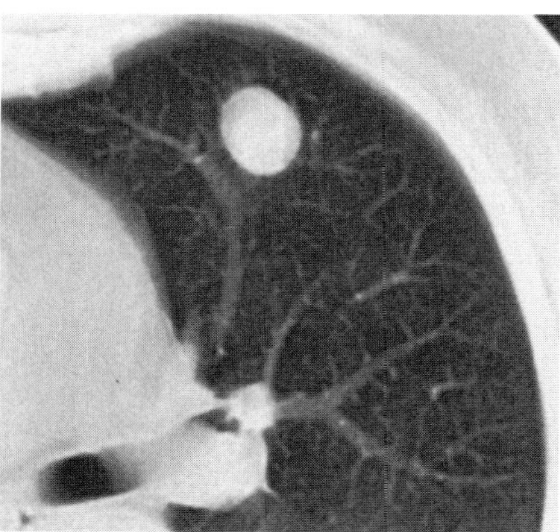

(B)

Figure 7 Mucormycosis manifesting as solitary pulmonary nodule in a patient with multiple myeloma. (A) Chest radiograph shows well-circumscribed pulmonary nodule (arrow). (B) Computed tomography confirms left upper lobe pulmonary nodule. Note well-defined margins and smooth contour, findings suggestive of a benign etiology.

tection of this pattern of calcification suggests a high probability of malignancy, although a similar pattern can occasionally be seen in benign nodules.

Computed tomography is a considerably more sensitive imaging modality for detecting calcification when compared to radiographic evaluation [14,20,23]. Calcification is usually detected visually when thinly collimated slices (1 to 3 mm) are performed through the nodule (Fig. 14). Partial volume

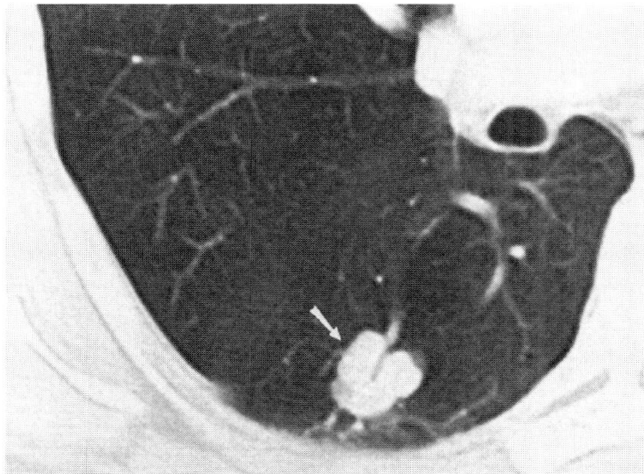

Figure 8 Solitary metastasis from renal cell malignancy. Computed tomography shows nodule (arrow) with lobular contour in right lower lobe. Lobular contour is due to uneven growth, a finding often associated with malignancy.

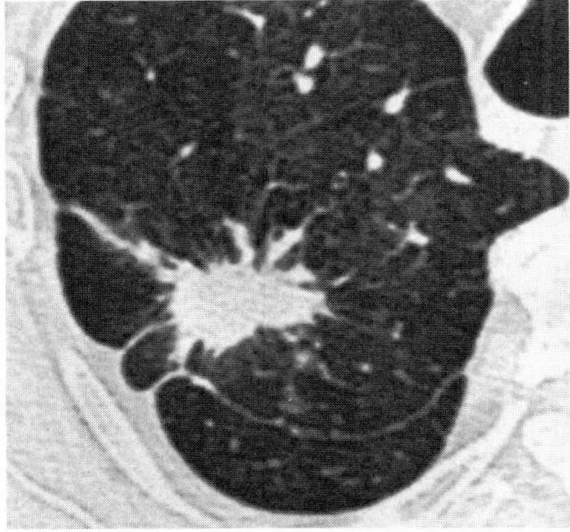

Figure 9 Non-small-cell lung cancer. Computed tomography shows nodule in right upper lobe with irregular contour and spiculated margin. Appearance is highly suggestive for malignancy.

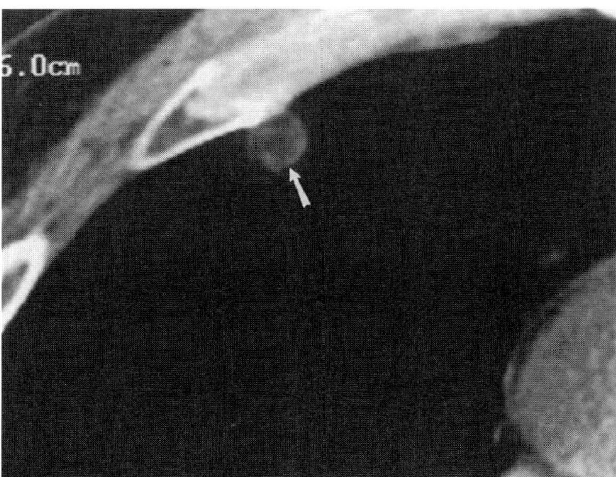

Figure 10 Hamartoma. Computed tomography shows small, peripheral well-circumscribed nodule in right upper lobe (arrow). Low attenuation within nodule (attenuation −106 HU) is consistent with fat and diagnostic of hamartoma.

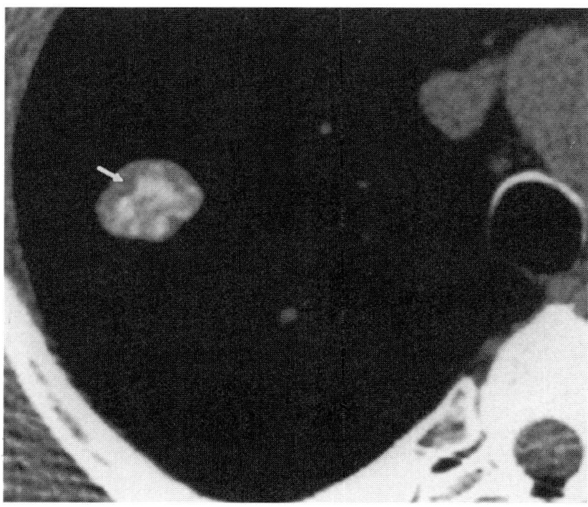

Figure 11 Hamartoma. Computed tomography shows well-circumscribed nodule in right upper lobe. Focal punctate calcifications are suggestive of hamartoma. Similar calcifications can, however, be seen in carcinoid tumors. Small focal areas of fat within the nodule are diagnostic of hamartoma (arrow).

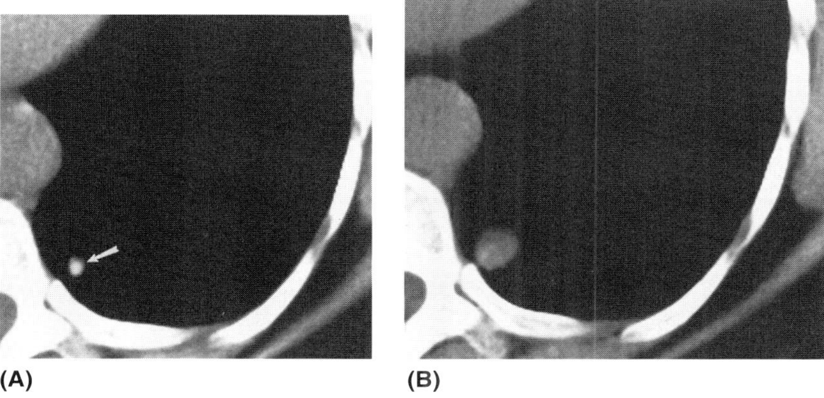

Figure 12 Metastatic osteosarcoma. (A) Computed tomography shows small, high attenuation nodule in lower lobe (arrow). The appearance is suggestive of a benign etiology. (B) Computed tomography obtained 3 months later reveals interval growth of nodule. Resection revealed metastatic osteosarcoma.

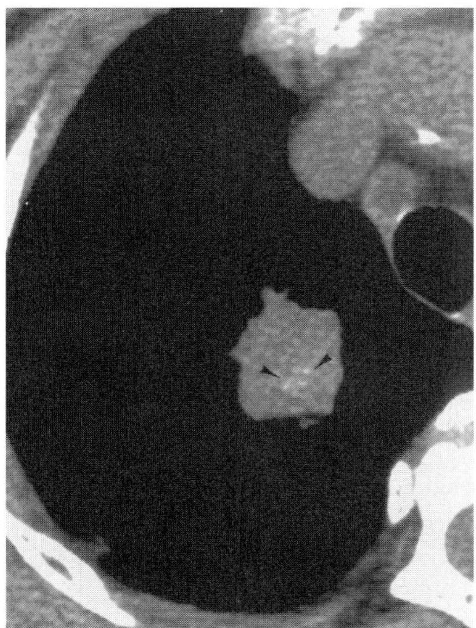

Figure 13 Non-small-cell lung cancer. Computed tomography reveals amorphous calcification in nodule, a pattern typical of malignancy (arrowheads). Adenocarcinoma was confirmed at resection.

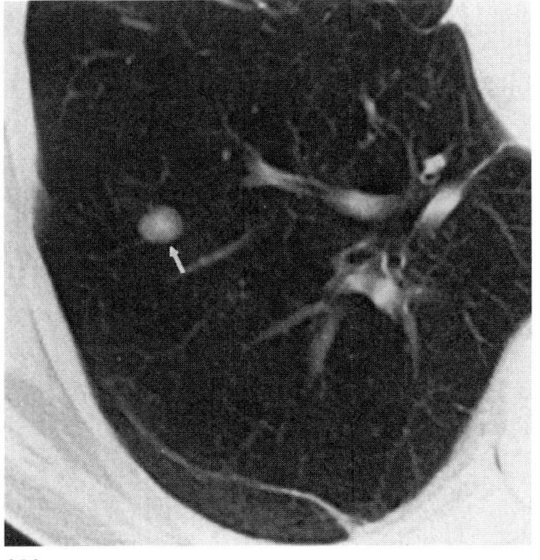

(A)

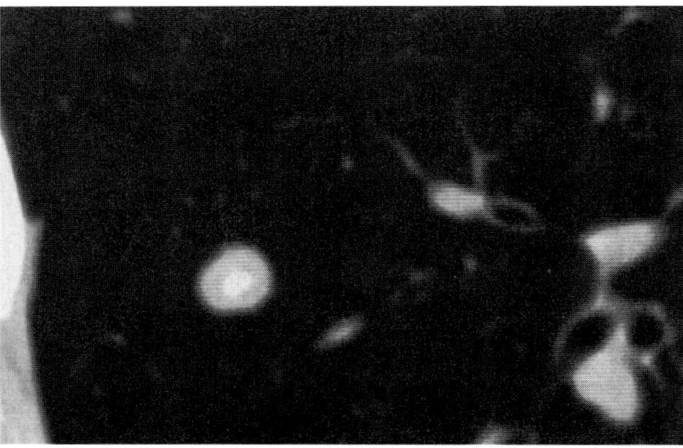

(B)

Figure 14 Postinfectious granuloma. (A) Standard CT (7-mm collimation, lung window) shows nodule (arrow) with possible small, central punctate calcification. (B) Thin-section CT (1.5-mm collimation) better demonstrates the central punctate calcification in nodule and is diagnostic of a benign etiology.

averaging can make calcification within a small nodule visually inapparent when thicker collimated slices (7 to 10 mm) are obtained. It has recently been shown that calcification can be inferred when a 3- to 7-mm nodule is visible on standard mediastinal images (level 25, window 350) obtained using 10-mm collimation [24]. Although this method can be used if it is not possible to repeat the study, in most cases reimaging with thinner collimated slices is preferable. Measurement of CT attenuation values (CT densitometry) can also be used to infer the presence of calcium within a nodule [14,20,25,26]. The use of this technique is, however, inappropriate if the nodule is spiculated or if the opacity is greater than 3 cm in diameter. A CT attenuation value of 200 Hounsfield units is usually used to distinguish between calcified and non-calcified nodules. If the density of the nodule is in the benign range (>200 HU), serial radiological observation is performed at 3, 6, 12, 18, and 24 months to confirm absence of growth. The sensitivity and specificity of this technique for benign disease is not optimal, and the popularity of CT densitometry for discriminating benign from malignant nodules has declined since its inception in the early 1980s [27,28]. More recently, it has been proposed that measurement of CT attenuation values obtained at different kilovolt peaks may be useful in detecting visually inapparent amounts of calcium in a nodule [29,30]. Dual-energy CT compares the attenuation of a nodule imaged at 140 kVp to the attenuation of the nodule imaged at 80 kVp. This technique is based on increased photon absorption by calcium as the beam energy is decreased. Theoretically, this results in an increase in the CT attenuation number of a calcified nodule as the kVp decreases. A recent multi-institutional trial, however, has shown that dual-energy CT is unreliable for distinguishing benign from malignant nodules [31].

Cavitation occurs in benign and malignant nodules. Malignant cavities typically have thick, irregular walls, while benign cavities have smooth, thin walls (Figs. 15, 16, and 17) [15,32,33]. For instance, 97% of cavitary nodules with a wall thickness greater than 16 mm are malignant and 93% with a wall thickness less than 4 mm are benign [32,33]. Although these measurements can be of some value in nodule evaluation, cavity wall thickness cannot be used to confidently differentiate benign and malignant nodules Fig. 17).

B. Nodule Growth

Evaluation of growth is performed by reviewing preexisting chest radiographs or CTs. The majority of malignant nodules double in volume between 30 and 400 days [34]. Nodular opacities that double in volume more rapidly than 30 days are usually infectious or inflammatory in origin (Fig. 18), whereas those that double in volume more slowly than 400 days are usually benign pul-

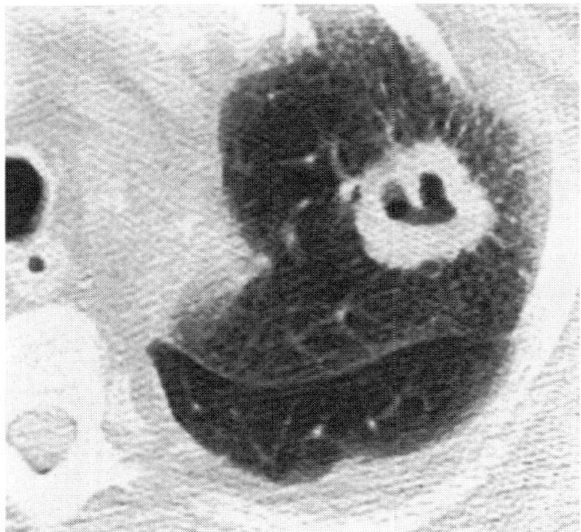

Figure 15 Squamous-cell lung cancer. Computed tomography shows thick-walled cavitary nodule in left upper lobe. Thick walls and eccentric cavitation are suggestive, but not diagnostic, of malignancy.

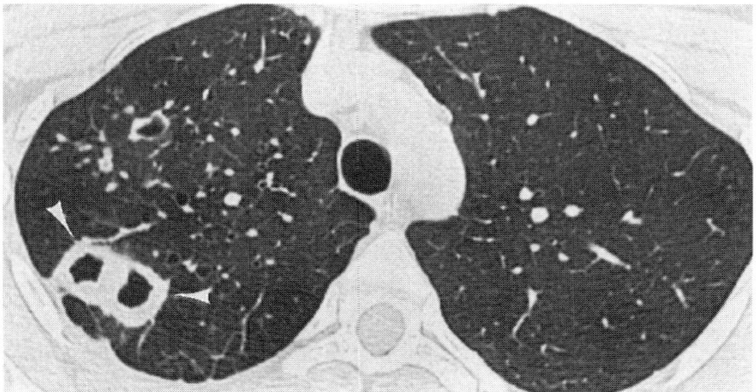

Figure 16 Nontuberculous mycobacterium infection (*Mycobacterium avium intracellulare*). Computed tomography shows well-circumscribed, cavitary nodule (arrowheads) with thick walls in right upper lobe. Note bronchiectasis and scattered branching tubular opacities, findings often associated with *M. avium intracellulare* infection.

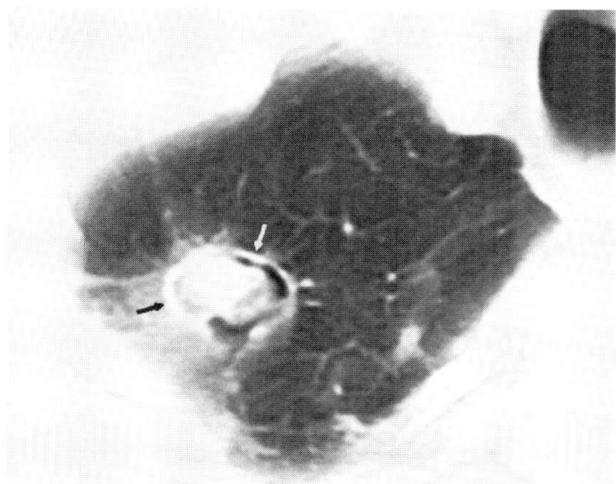

Figure 17 Squamous-cell lung cancer. Computed tomography shows thin-walled cavitary nodule in right upper lobe (arrows). Soft tissue within nodule is due to necrotic lung. Extensive necrosis can occasionally result in thin walls and erroneously suggest a benign etiology.

monary neoplasms or sequelae of prior pulmonary infections. An absence of visible growth over a 2-year period is generally reliable in determining benignity [1,35,36]. Recently, the use of these criteria to infer benignity has been questioned [37]. These concerns are particularly important when the accuracy of growth assessment in small nodules is considered. To detect growth on a radiograph requires a nodule to change in diameter by 3 to 5 mm [37,38]. The small change in diameter (approximately 25%) that occurs when a small nodule doubles in volume makes it difficult to assess interval growth in these nodules. For example, a 4-mm nodule will increase to only 5 mm in diameter after doubling in volume and, consequently, will appear stable on the chest radiograph. Although this change in diameter can theoretically be detected by CT, slight differences in the level at which the image is obtained occurs commonly from study to study and makes the confident detection of a small diameter change difficult. The use of CT does, however, in most cases allow an accurate assessment of growth and it has been recently reported that growth can be detected in lung cancers as small as 5 mm when CT imaging is repeated within 30 days [39]. Furthermore, the measurement of serial volumes, rather than diameters, of small nodules has been suggested to be an accurate and potentially useful method to assess growth [40]. Presently, however, there is no consensus as to what parameters should be measured, when the first and subsequent serial CTs should be performed, or the

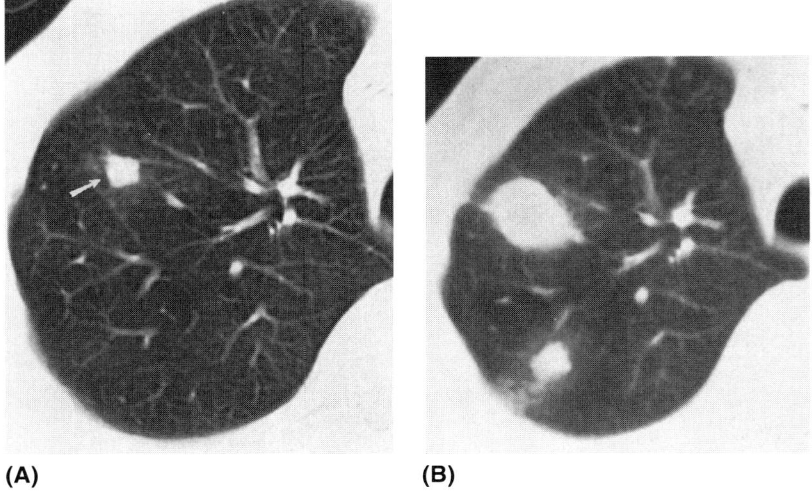

(A) (B)

Figure 18 Nocardia infection in heart transplant recipient. (A) Computed tomography shows small, well-circumscribed right upper lobe nodule (arrow). (B) Computed tomography 1 week later shows marked increase in size of right upper lobe nodule and interval development of smaller right upper lobe pulmonary nodules. Transthoracic needle aspiration biopsy confirmed diagnosis of *Nocardia* infection. Rapid growth is indicative of a benign, in this case infectious, etiology.

period of time required to ascertain that a small nodule is benign based on absence of growth.

C. Nodule Enhancement and Metabolism

Perfusion and metabolism of malignant pulmonary nodules is qualitatively and quantitatively different from that of benign nodules. Contrast-enhanced CT can be used to differentiate between benign and malignant nodules because the intensity of enhancement is directly related to the vascularity of the nodule and therefore to the likelihood of malignancy [41–43]. This technique has recently been shown in a multi-institutional prospective trial to be useful for evaluation of nodules that are indeterminate in etiology after standard radiological evaluation [43]. Three-millimeter collimation images of the nodule are obtained before and after the intravenous administration of contrast (2 mL/sec; 300 mg iodine/mm; 420 mg iodine/kg). Serial 5-sec spiral acquisitions (3-mm collimation scans with 2-mm reconstruction intervals; 120 kVp, 280 mA, pitch of 1:1; standard reconstruction algorithm;

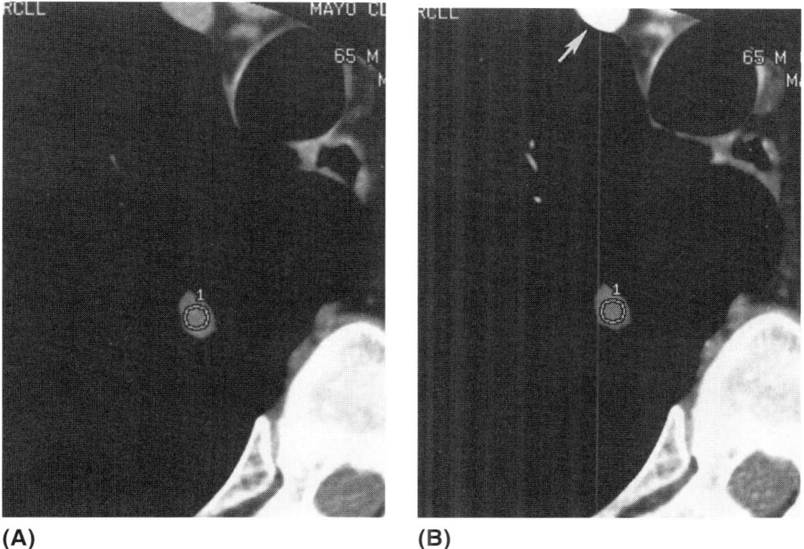

Figure 19 Benign pulmonary nodule. (A) Noncontrast computed tomography shows right lung nodule with attenuation value of 28 HU. (B) Contrast computed tomography shows no visual enhancement of nodule. Attenuation value measured 33 HU. The findings are consistent with a benign diagnosis. Note contrast in mediastinal vessels (arrow). (Courtesy of Tom Hartman, Mayo Clinic, Rochester, Minnesota.)

15-cm field of view) are performed at 1, 2, 3, and 4 min after the administration of contrast. Enhancement is determined by subtracting the precontrast attenuation of the nodule from the maximal nodule attenuation after contrast administration. Typically, malignant nodules enhance more than 20 HU, while benign nodules enhance less than 15 HU [43] (Fig. 19). There are, however, several potential limitations to clinical application of this technique. Many nodules do not fulfill the selection criteria used in this study. For instance, nodules smaller than 5 mm in diameter and nodules that were not relatively spherical were excluded. Also, in some cases, it can be difficult to consistently reimage the nodule after contrast administration because of differences in the depth of inspiration. The technique does, however, have clinical utility: A nodule that enhances less than 15 HU is almost certainly benign (sensitivity 98%, specificity 58%, accuracy 77%) and can be managed conservatively with serial radiologic assessment. While the use of contrast-enhanced CT may reduce the number of benign nodules resected, a significant proportion of benign nodules will enhance. Such nodules remain indeterminate in etiology and require additional radiologic evaluation, biopsy, or resection.

The use of CT nodule enhancement requires important attention to technical details. First, it is important to carefully follow the imaging protocol as outlined above. Second, with regard to obtaining region of interest (ROI) measurements, the circular or oval region of interest is centered on the image closest to the nodule equator and should comprise roughly 70% of the diameter of a nodule. All ROI measurements should be made on mediastinal window settings in order to to ensure that partial volume averaging is minimized. Careful inspection of the bronchovascular structures adjacent to the nodule will allow one to obtain ROI measurements at similar levels in the z axis of the nodule on serial scans. Third, this technique should only be performed on nodules that are relatively homogeneous in attenuation, without evidence of fat, calcification, cavitation, or necrosis. Finally, patients considered for this technique should be able to perform reproducible breath holds. In order to aid patients in performing reproducible breath holds, it is suggested to instruct them to "take a small breath in and hold it" (rather than a deep breath).

Positron emission tomography (PET) imaging is an alternative to contrast-enhanced CT. Metabolism of glucose is typically increased in malignant nodules compared to benign nodules. PET, using the D-glucose analog ^{18}F-labeled 2-deoxy-D-glucose (FDG), can be used to image this increase in glucose metabolism, allowing differentiation of malignant from benign nodules (Fig. 20) [44–48]. Sensitivity, specificity, and accuracy for detection of malignancy in nodules 10 mm or greater in diameter is 96, 88, and 94%, respectively, with FDG PET imaging [44,47–53]. Because the probability of malignancy is high when a nodule has increased FDG uptake, these nodules should be either biopsied or resected. When FDG uptake by a nodule 10 mm or greater in diameter is low, it will almost certainly be benign. False-negative results are uncommon, but can occur with some carcinoid tumors and bronchioloalveolar cell carcinomas (Fig. 21) [54,55]. Limitations in spatial resolution can also result in false-negative studies when lesions smaller than 10 mm in diameter are evaluated [56]. The use of FDG PET as a single test has, however, been reported to be a better predictor of malignancy than standard clinical and morphologic criteria used in Bayesian analysis [51]. In an attempt to detect the small percentage of malignant nodules falsely designated benign after FDG PET imaging, serial radiological assessment for 2 years is performed on all nodules with low FDG uptake that are not biopsied or resected. Although the high specificity of PET imaging for benign lesions can substantially reduce the number of benign nodules resected, benign neoplasms and nodules due to

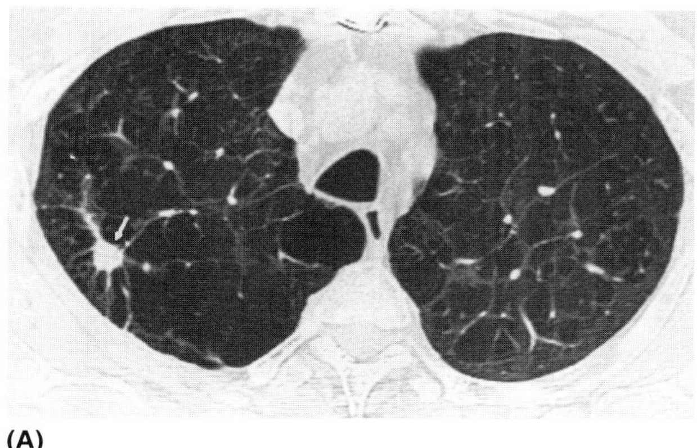

(A)

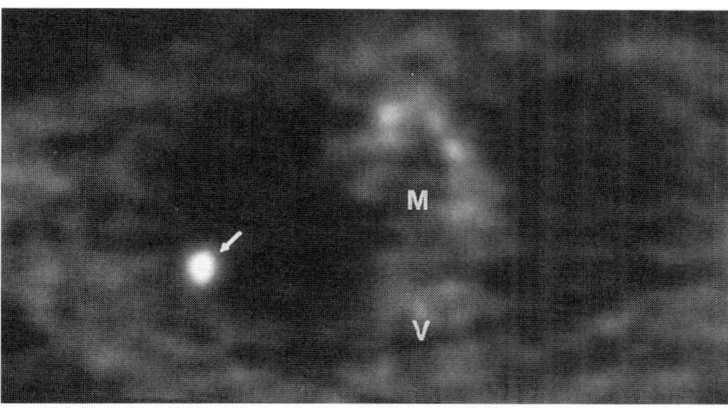

(B)

Figure 20 Non-small-cell lung cancer manifesting as hypermetabolic nodule on [^{18}F] fluorodeoxyglucose (FDG) positron emission tomographic scan. (A) Computed tomography shows small nodule in right upper lobe (arrow). Note marked emphysematous lung disease. (B) Axial positron emission tomographic image with [^{18}F] fluorodeoxyglucose shows increased FDG uptake within nodule (arrow) when compared to mediastinum. The findings are suggestive of malignancy and resection revealed lung cancer. M, mediastinum; V, vertebral body.

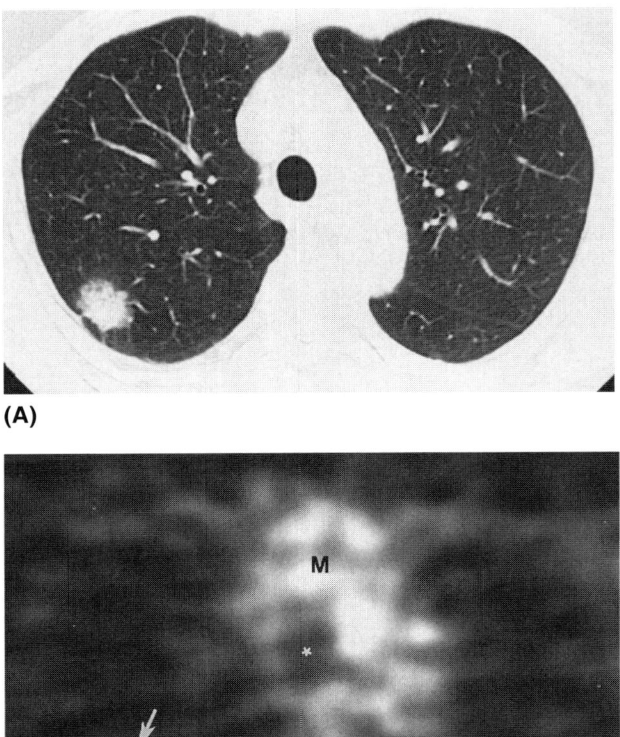

Figure 21 Bronchioloalveolar cell cancer manifesting as hypometabolic nodule on [^{18}F] fluorodeoxyglucose (FDG) positron emission tomographic scan. (A) Computed tomography shows a poorly marginated right upper lobe nodule containing small focal lucencies. Appearance is suspicious for bronchioloalveolar cell cancer. (B) Axial positron emission tomographic image with [^{18}F] fluorodeoxyglucose shows minimal FDG uptake within nodule (arrow) when compared to mediastinum. Findings are suggestive of benignity. Transthoracic needle aspiration biopsy was performed because of CT appearance and revealed bronchioloalveolar cell cancer. M, mediastinum; *, trachea. (From Ref. 65.)

infection and inflammation (tuberculosis, histoplasmosis, rheumatoid arthritis, etc.) can result in false-positive diagnoses (Fig. 22).

IV. PREDICTIVE MODELS AND DECISION ANALYSIS

Many nodules remain indeterminate in etiology after comprehensive noninvasive radiological assessment. At this point, a decision to observe, biopsy, or resect the nodule is made. This decision is usually made based on the subjective perception of probability of malignacy using clinical parameters such as patient age and cigarette-smoking history as well as the radiologic features of the nodule [57]. Unfortunately, clinical judgment incorrectly classifies a high proportion of malignant nodules as benign [57,58]. Accordingly, there have been ongoing attempts to develop more accurate, objective methods to optimize decision making in this regard.

Computer-assisted decision analytical models may improve the management of patients with indeterminate nodules. These techniques factor in risks of biopsy and surgical resection, accuracy of biopsy results, morbidity-adjusted life expectancies of patients, and cost data to predict the optimal management strategy for an indeterminate nodule based on estimates of probability of malignancy [59–61]. Such techniques have been used to compare three different management strategies: radiological observation, immediate resection, and transthoracic needle aspiration biopsy. These studies suggest that the most cost-effective strategy is observation when the probability of cancer is low ($p\text{Ca} < 0.05$), surgical resection when the probability of cancer is high ($p\text{Ca} > 0.60$), and biopsy when the probability of cancer is between 0.05 and 0.6 [34,38,62,63].

In patients with an indeterminate nodule, decision making can also be assisted by such methodologies as Bayesian analysis, artificial neural network analysis, or multivariate logistic-regression models [7,57,62–64]. When these methods are used to predict the likelihood of malignancy for a given nodule, they typically perform slightly better than human observers given the same clinical and radiologic information. However, the clinical utility and applicability of this slight degree of improvement remains to be shown.

V. SUMMARY

Solitary pulmonary opacities, including SPNs, are a common radiological abnormality that are often detected incidentally. Although the majority are benign, lung cancer constitutes an important proportion of solitary pulmonary nodules. The goal of management is to correctly differentiate these malignan-

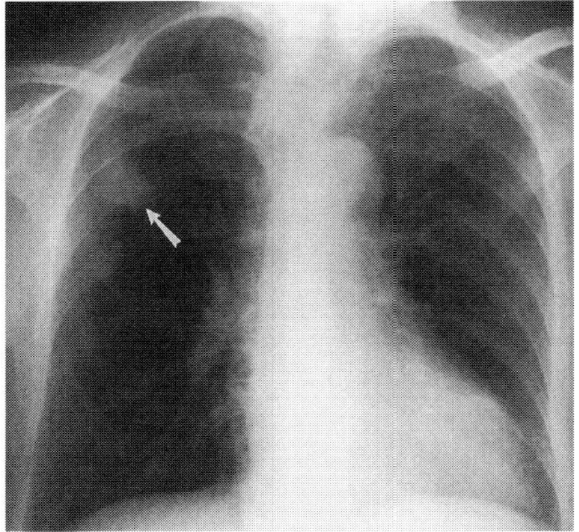

(A)

(B)

Figure 22 *Mycobacterium tuberculosis* infection manifesting as hypermetabolic nodule on [^{18}F] fluorodeoxyglucose (FDG) positron emission tomographic scan. (A) Posteroanterior radiograph shows poorly marginated nodule in right upper lobe. (B) Coronal positron emission tomographic image with [^{18}F] fluorodeoxyglucose shows marked FDG uptake within nodule (arrow) when compared to mediastinum. Findings are suggestive of malignancy. Transthoracic needle aspiration biopsy was negative for malignancy; culture was positive for *M. tuberculosis*. Radiograph following antituberculous therapy showed complete resolution of tuberculoma. M, mediastinum; L, liver.

cies from benign nodules so that appropriate treatment can be initiated. The detection of specific patterns of calcification and stability in size for 2 years or more have historically been the only reliable findings useful for determining nodule benignity. More recently, the ability to distinguish benign and malignant SPNs has improved with assessment of nodule perfusion and metabolism using contrast-enhanced CT and FDG PET imaging, respectively. Together with transthoracic needle aspiration biopsy, these new imaging modalities have dramatically improved preoperative identification of benign nodules and reduced the number surgically resected. Many nodules still, however, remain indeterminate in etiology after extensive radiological evaluation. Thus, research efforts continue toward development of entirely new or at least improved imaging and analytical techniques for evaluation of these nodules.

REFERENCES

1. Lillington GA. Disease-a-Month. 37 ed. St. Louis, MO: Mosby Year Book, 1991.
2. Viggiano RW, Swensen SJ, Rosenow III EC. Evaluation and management of solitary and multiple pulmonary nodules. Clin Chest Med 1992; 13:83–95.
3. Mountain CF. Revisions in the international system for staging lung cancer. Chest 1997; 111:1710–1717.
4. Khouri NF, Meziane MA, Zerhouni EA, Fishman EK, Siegelman SS. The solitary pulmonary nodule. Chest 1987; 91:128–133.
5. Coakley FV, Cohen MD, Johnson MS, Gonin R, Hanbna MP. Maximum intensity projection images in the detection of simulated pulmonary nodules by spiral CT. Br J Radiol 1998; 71:135–140.
6. Selzer SE, Judy PF, Adams DF, et al. Spiral CT of the chest: comparison of cine and film-based viewing. Radiology 1995; 197:773–787.
7. Gurney JW. Determining the likelihood of malignancy in solitary pulmonary nodules with Bayesian analysis. Radiology 1993; 186:405–413.
8. Seemann MD, Staebler A, Beinert T, Dienemann H, Obst B, Matzko M, Pistitsch C, Reiser MF. Usefulness of morphological chracteristics for the differentiation of benign from malignant solitary pulmonary lesions using HRCT. Eur Radiol 1999; 9:409–417.
9. Henschke CI, McCauley DI, Yankelevitz DF, Naidich DP, McGuinness G, Miettinen OS, Libby DM, Pasmantier MW, Koizumi J, Altorki NK, Smith JP. Early lung cancer action project: overall design and findings from baseline screening. Lancet 1999; 354:99–105.
10. Kaneko M, Eguchi K, Ohmatsu H, Kakinuma R, Naruke T, Suemasu K, Moriyama N. Peripheral lung cancer: screening and detection with low-dose spiral CT versus radiography. Radiology 1996; 201:798–802.
11. Sone S, Takashima S, Li F, Yang Z, Honda T, Maruyama Y, Hasegawa M, Yamanda T, Kubo K, Hanamura K, Asakura K. Mass screening for lung cancer with mobile spiral computed tomography scanning. Lancet 1998; 351:1242–1245.

12. Munden RF, Pugatch RD, Liptay MJ, Sugarbaker DJ, Le LU. Small pulmonary lesions detected at CT: clinical importance. Radiology 1997; 202:105–110.
13. Ginsberg MS, Griff SK, Go BD, Yoo H-H, Schwartz LH, Panicek DM. Pulmonary nodules resected at video-assisted thoracoscopic surgery: etiology in 426 patients. Radiology 1999; 213:277–282.
14. Zerhouni EA, Stitik FP, Siegelman SS, Proto AV, Muhn JR, Walsh JW, Martinez CR, Heelan RT et al. CT of the pulmonary nodule: a cooperative study. Radiology 1986; 160:319–327.
15. Zwirewich CV, Vedal S, Miller RR, Müller NL. Solitary pulmonary nodule: high-resolution CT and radiologic-pathologic correlation. Radiology 1991; 179: 469–476.
16. Sider L. Radiographic manifestations of primary bronchogenic carcinoma. Radiol Clin North Am 1990; 28:583–597.
17. Theros EG. Varying manifestations of peripheral pulmonary neoplasms: a radiologic-pathologic correlative study. Am J Radiol 1977; 128:893–914.
18. O'Keefe ME Jr, Good CA, McDonald JR. Calcification in solitary nodules of the lungs. Am J Radiol 1957; 77:1023–1033.
19. Siegelman SS, Khouri NF, Scott Jr WW, Leo FP, Hamper UM, Fishman EK, Zerhouni EA. Pulmonary hamartoma: CT findings. Radiology 1986; 160:313–317.
20. Siegelman SS, Khouri MF, Leo FP, Fishman EK, Braverman RM, Zerhouni EA. Solitary pulmonary nodules: CT assessment. Radiology 1986; 160:307–312.
21. O'Keefe ME, Good CA, McDonald JR. Calcification in solitary nodules of the lung. Am J Radiol 1957; 77:1023–1033.
22. Mahoney MC, Shipley RT, Corcoran HL, Dickson BA. CT demonstration of calcification in carcinoma of the lung. Am J Radiol 1990; 154:255–258.
23. Siegelman SS, Zerhouni EA, Leo FP, Khouri NF, Stitik FP. CT of the solitary pulmonary nodule. Am J Radiol 1980; 135:1–13.
24. Yankelevitz DF, Henschke CI. Derivation for relating calcification and size in small pulmonary nodules. Clin Imaging 1998; 22:1–6.
25. Zerhouni EA, Boukadoum M, Siddiky M, Newbold JM, Stone DC, Shirey MP, Spivey JF, Hesselman CW, Leo FP, Stitik FP et al. A standard phantom for quantitative CT analysis of pulmonary nodules. Radiology 1983; 149:767–773.
26. Huston JI, Muhm JR. Solitary pulmonary nodules: evaluation with a CT reference phantom. Radiology 1989; 170:653–656.
27. Midthun DE, Swensen SJ, Jett JR. Approach to the solitary pulmonary nodule. Mayo Clin Proc 1993; 68:378–385.
28. Swensen SJ, Harms GF, Morin RL, Meyers JL. CT evaluation of solitary pulmonary nodules: value of 185-H reference phantom. Am J Radiol 1991; 156:925–929.
29. Higashi Y, Nakamura H, Matsumoto T, Nakanishi T. Dual-energy computed tomographic diagnosis of pulmonary nodules. J Thorac Imaging 1994; 9:31–34.
30. Bhalla M, Shepard JO, Nakamura K, Kazerooni EA. Dual kV CT to detect calcification in solitary pulmonary nodule. J Comput Assist Tomogr 1995; 19:44–47.
31. Swensen SJ, Yamashita K, McCollough CH, Viggiano RW, Midthun DE, Patz EF Jr, Muhm JR, Weaver AL. Lung nodules: Dual-kilovolt peak analysis with CT-multicenter study. Radiology 2000; 214:81–85.

32. Woodring JH, Fried AM. Significance of wall thickness in solitary cavities of the lung: a follow-up study. Am J Radiol 1983; 140:473–474.
33. Woodring JH, Fried AM, Chuang VP. Solitary cavities of the lung: diagnostic implications of cavity wall thickness. Am J Radiol 1980; 135:1269–1271.
34. Lillington GA, Caskey CI. Evaluation and management of solitary multiple pulmonary nodules. Clin Chest Med 1993; 14:111–119.
35. Good CA, Wilson TW. The solitary circumscribed pulmonary nodule. J Am Med Assoc 1958; 166:210–215.
36. Good CA. Management of patient with solitary mass in lung. Chic Med Soc Bull 1953; 55:893–896.
37. Yankelevitz DF, Henschke CI. Does 2-year stability imply that pulmonary nodules are benign? Am J Radiol 1997; 168:325–328.
38. Cummings SR, Lillington GA, Richard RJ. Managing solitary pulmonary nodules. Am Rev Respir Dis 1986; 134:453–460.
39. Yankelevitz DF, Gupta R, Zhao B, Henschke CI. Small pulmonary nodules: evaluation with repeat CT—preliminary experience. Radiol 1999; 212:561–566.
40. Yankelevitz DF, Reeves AP, Kostis WJ, Zhao B, Henschke CI. Determination of malignancy in small pulmonary nodules based on volumetrically determined growth rates. Radiology 1998; 209(suppl):375.
41. Yamashita K, Matsunobe S, Tsuda T, Nemoto T, Matsumoto K, Miki H, Konishi J. Solitary pulmonary nodule: preliminary study of evaluation with incremental dynamic CT. Radiology 1995; 194:399–405.
42. Zhang M, Kono M. Solitary pulmonary nodules: evaluation of blood flow patterns with dynamic CT. Radiology 1997; 205:471–478.
43. Swensen SJ, Viggiano RW, Midthun DE, Müller NL, Sherrick A, Yamashita K, Naidich DP, Patz EF, Hartman TE, Muhn JR, Weaver AL. Lung nodule enhancement at CT: multicenter study. Radiology 2000; 214:73–80.
44. Patz EF Jr, Lowe VJ, Hoffman JM, Paine SS, Burrowes P, Coleman RE, Goodman PC. Focal pulmonary abnormalities: evaluation with F-18 fluorodeoxyglucose PET scanning. Radiology 1993; 188:487–490.
45. Gupta NC, Frank AR, Dewan NA, Redepenning LS, Rothberg ML, Mailliard JA, Phalen JJ, Sunderland JJ, Frick MP. Solitary pulmonary nodules: detection of malignancy with PET with 2-[F-18]-fluoro-2-deoxy-D-glucose. Radiology 1992; 184:441–444.
46. Dewan NA, Gupta NC, Redepenning LS, Phalen JJ, Frick MP. Diagnostic efficacy of PET-FDG imaging in solitary pulmonary nodules. Chest 1993; 104:997–1002.
47. Knight SB, Delbeke D, Stewart JR, Sandler MP. Evaluation of pulmonary lesions with FDG-PET. Chest 1996; 109:982-988.
48. Valk PE, Pounds TR, Hopkins DM, Haseman MK, Hofer GA, Greiss HB, Myers RW, Lutrin CL. Staging non-small cell lung cancer by whole-body positron emission tomographic imaging. Ann Thorac Surg 1995; 60:1573–1582.
49. Scott WJ, Schwabe JL, Gupta NC, Dewan NA, Reeb SD, Sugimoto JT. Positron emission tomography of lung tumors and mediastinal lymph nodes using [18F] fluorodeoxyglucose. Ann Thorac Surg 1994; 58:698–703.
50. Conti PS, Lilien DL, Hawley K, Keppler J, Grafton ST, Bading JR. PET and [^{18}F]-FDG in Oncology: a clinical update. Nucl Med Biol 1996; 23:717–735.

51. Gupta NC, Maloof J, Gunel E. Probability of malignancy in solitary pulmonary nodules using fluorine-18-FDG and PET. J Nucl Med 1996; 37:943–948.
52. Hübner KF, Buonocore E, Gould HR, Thie J, Smith GT, Stephens S, Dickey J. Differentiating benign from malignant lung lesions using ''quantitative'' parameters of FDG PET images. Clin Nucl Med 1996; 21:941–949.
53. Lewis P, Griffin S, Marsden P, Gee T, Nunan T, Malsey M, Dussek J. Whole-body ^{18}F-fluorodeoxyglucose positron emission tomography in preoperative evaluation of lung cancer. Lancet 1994; 344:1265–1266.
54. Erasmus JJ, McAdams HP, Patz EF Jr, Coleman RE, Ahuja V, Goodman PC. Evaluation of primary pulmonary carcinoid tumors using FDG PET. Am J Radiol 1998; 170:1369–1373.
55. Higashi K, Ueda Y, Seki H, Yuasa K, Oguchi M, Noguchi T, Taniguchi M, Tonami H, Okimura T, Yamamoto I. Fluorine-18-FDG PET is negative in bronchioloalveolar lung carcinoma. J Nucl Med 1998; 39:1016–1020.
56. Lowe VJ, Fletcher JW, Gobar L, Lawson M, Kirchner P, Valk P, Karis J, Hubner K, Delbeke D, Heiberg EV, Patz EF, Coleman RE. Prospective investigation of PET in lung nodules (PIOPILN). J Clin Oncol 1998; 16:1075–1084.
57. Gurney JW, Lyddon DM, McKay JA. Determining the likelihood of malignancy in solitary pulmonary nodules with Bayesian analysis. Part II. Application. Radiology 1993; 186:415–422.
58. Edwards WM, Cox RS Jr, Garland LH. The solitary nodule (coin lesion) of the lung: an analysis of 52 consecutive cases treated by thoracotomy and a study of preoperative diagnostic accuracy. Am J Radiol 1962; 88:1020–1042.
59. Kunstaetter R, Wolkove N, Kreisman H, Cohen C, Frank H. The solitary pulmonary nodule. Med Decis Making 1985; 5:61–75.
60. Lillington GA, Cummings SR. Decision analysis approaches in solitary pulmonary nodules. Semin Respir Med 1989; 10:227–231.
61. Gambhir SS, Shepherd JE, Shah BD, Hart E, Hoh CK, Valk PE, Emi T, Phelps ME. Analytical decision model for the cost-effective management of solitary pulmonary nodules. J Clin Oncol 1998; 16:2113–2125.
62. Henschke CI, Yankelevitz DF, Mateescu I, Brettle DW, Rainey TG, Weingard FS. Neural networks for the analysis of small pulmonary nodules. Clin Imaging 1997; 21:390-399.
63. Swensen SJ, Silverstein MD, Edell ES, Traastek VF, Aughenbaugh GL, Ilstrup DM et al. Solitary pulmonary nodules: clinical prediction model versus physicians. Mayo Clin Proc 1999; 74:319–329.
64. Nakamura K, Yoshida H, Engelmann R, MacMahon H, Katsuragawa S, Ishida T, Ashizawa K, Doi K. Computerized analysis of the likelihood of malignancy in solitary pulmonary nodules with use of artificial neural networks. Radiology 2000; 214:823–830.
65. Wagner AL, Szabunio M, Hazelett KS, Wagner SG. Radiologic manifestations of round pneumonia in adults. Am J Radiol 1998; 170:723–726.
66. Erasmas JJ, McAdams PH, Patz EF Jr. Non-small cell lung cancer: FDG-PET imaging. J Thorac Imaging 1999; 14:247-256.

3

State-of-the-Art Thoracic Lymph Node Imaging

Phillip M. Boiselle
Harvard Medical School and
Beth Israel Deaconess Medical Center
Boston, Massachusetts

I. INTRODUCTION

The nodal status (N) is an integral part of the tumor/node/metastasis (TNM) staging system (Tables 1 and 2) for non-small-cell lung cancer (NSCLC) and provides important information for determining prognosis and planning appropriate therapy [1–3]. For example, a patient with a T1 or T2 lesion and no evidence of metastatic nodal disease (N0) or distant metastases (M0) has a relatively favorable prognosis (approximately 65% 5-year survival) following surgical resection [1]. On the other hand, a patient with a T1 or T2 lesion with metastatic disease to contralateral mediastinal lymph nodes (N3) but no distant metastases (M0) has a poor prognosis (less than 10% 5-year survival rate) and is considered inoperable [1].

The assessment of thoracic lymph nodes is thus an important aspect of staging patients with NSCLC. Traditionally, imaging evaluation of thoracic lymph nodes has relied on anatomic features, principally nodal size, in order to distinguish benign from malignant lymph nodes. However, this strategy has been limited by a poor sensitivity and specificity. In recent years, physiologic imaging techniques, most notably ^{18}F-labeled 2-deoxy-D-glucose positron emission tomography (FDG PET), have been applied with greater success.

In this chapter, we illustrate and review the state-of-the-art in thoracic lymph node imaging with anatomic and physiologic imaging techniques. An

Table 1 TNM Descriptors

Primary tumor (T)	
TX	Primary tumor cannot be assessed or tumor proven by the presence of malignant cells in sputum or bronchial washings but not visualized by imaging or bronchoscopy
T0	No evidence of primary tumor
Tis	Carcinoma in situ
T1	Tumor ≤3 cm in greatest dimension, surrounded by lung or visceral pleura, without bronchoscopic evidence of invasion more proximal than the lobar bronchus[a] (*i.e.*, not in the main bronchus)
T2	Tumor with any of the following features of size or extent: >3 cm in greatest dimension Involves main bronchus, ≥2 cm distal to the carina Invades the visceral pleura Associated with atelectasis or obstructive pneumonitis that extends to the hilar region but does not involve the entire lung
T3	Tumor of any size that directly invades any of the following: chest wall (including superior sulcus tumors), diaphragm, mediastinal pleura, parietal pericardium; or tumor in the main bronchus <2 cm distal to the carina, but without involvement of the carina; or associated atelectasis or obstructive pneumonitis of the entire lung
T4	Tumor of any size that invades any of the following: mediastinum, heart, great vessels, trachea, esophagus, vertebral body, carina; or tumor with a malignant pleural or pericardial effusion,[b] or with satellite tumor nodule(s) within the ipsilateral primary-tumor lobe of the lung
Regional lymph nodes (N)	
NX	Regional lymph nodes cannot be assessed
N0	No regional lymph node metastasis
N1	Metastasis to ipsilateral peribronchial and or ipsilateral hilar lymph nodes and intrapulmonary nodes involved by direct extension of the primary tumor
N2	Metastasis to ipsilateral mediastinal and/or subcarinal lymph node(s)
N3	Metastasis to contralateral mediastinal, contralateral hilar, ipsilateral or contralateral scalene, or supraclavicular lymph node(s)
Distant metastasis (M)	
MX	Presence of distant metastasis cannot be assessed
M0	No distant metastasis
M1	Distant metastasis present[c]

Source: Ref. 1.

[a] The uncommon superficial tumor of any size with its invasive component limited to the bronchial wall, which may extend proximal to the main bronchus, is also classified T1.

[b] Most pleural effusions associated with lung cancer are due to tumor. However, there are a few patients in whom multiple cytopathologic examinations of pleural fluid show no tumor. In these cases, the fluid is nonbloody and is not an exudate. When these elements and clinical judgment dictate that the effusion is not related to the tumor, the effusion should be excluded as a staging element and the patient's disease should be staged T1, T2, or T3. Pericardial effusion is classified according to the same rules.

[c] Separate metastatic tumor nodule(s) in the ipsilateral nonprimary–primary lobe(s) of the lung also are classified M1.

Table 2 Stage Grouping—TNM Subjects[a]

Stage	TNM Subject
0	Carcinoma in situ
IA	T1NOM0
IB	T2NOM0
IIA	T1N1M0
IIB	T2N1M0
	T3N0M0
IIIA	T3N1M0
	T1N2M0
	T2N2M0
	T3N2M0
IIIB	T4N0M0
	T4N1M0
	T4N2M0
	T1N3M0
	T2N3M0
	T3N3M0
	T4N3M0
IV	Any T Any N M1

Source: Ref. 1.
[a] Staging is not relevant for occult carcinoma, designated TXN0M0.

emphasis is placed on the role of imaging in evaluating nodal status in patients with NSCLC.

II. ANATOMIC IMAGING

A. Computed Tomography

Computed tomography is the most widely utilized cross-sectional imaging modality for staging patients with bronchogenic carcinoma. With regard to the assessment of lymph nodes, CT relies on anatomic features, most notably lymph node size, in order to distinguish between benign and malignant lymph nodes.

Although very early investigations with CT suggested sensitivities and specificities comparable to mediastinoscopy, subsequent studies performed with more thorough nodal sampling have shown that the accuracy of CT is significantly lower. For example, in a study that employed extensive nodal sampling and correlation with CT imaging of nodal stations, McLoud et al. [4] reported a sensitivity of 62% and a specificity of 64% for CT, using 1 cm as the upper limits of normal size for short axis of lymph nodes. These results emphasize the limitations of using nodal size to determine nodal status: Enlarged nodes may be hyperplastic rather than neoplastic (Fig. 1), and small nodes may harbor foci of metastatic disease [3].

Because of the low specificity of CT, enlarged nodes must be biopsied for accurate staging [2,3]. Indeed, benign nodes as large as 4 cm in diameter have been described in association with bronchogenic carcinoma [2]. Such nodes are most often seen in the setting of postobstructive pneumonitis.

Despite its limitations, CT still plays several important roles in the assessment of nodal status in patients with NSCLC [3]. First, by accurately identifying and localizing enlarged lymph nodes, CT provides important information that aids the selection of the most appropriate procedure (mediastinoscopy, mediastinotomy, thoracoscopy, transbronchial needle aspiration, or percutaneous CT-guided biopsy) for biopsy (Table 3) [5–10]. For example,

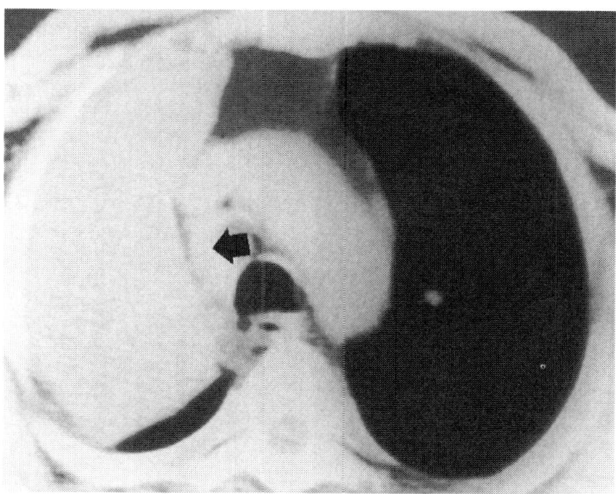

Figure 1 Enlarged, hyperplastic mediastinal node in a patient with an obstructing bronchogenic carcinoma in the right upper lobe. Contrast-enhanced CT at the level of the aortic arch reveals a 2.5-cm short-axis-diameter right paratracheal node, which was shown to be hyperplastic at mediastinoscopy. (From Ref. 3).

Table 3 Staging Procedures and Accessible Lymph Node Stations (AJCC-UICC Classifications)[a]

Procedure	Accessible nodal stations
Cervical mediastinoscopy	Highest mediastinal (1) Upper (2) and lower (4) paratracheal Subcarinal-anterior and superior (7)
Anterior or parasternal mediastinotomy	Subaortic (5) Paraaortic (6)
Thoracoscopy and video-assisted thoracoscopic surgery (VATS)	In the right hemithorax Upper (2R) and lower paratracheal (4R) Prevascular and retrotracheal (3) Subcarinal-posterior & inferior (7) Paraesophageal (8) Pulmonary ligament (9R) Hilar (10R) In the left hemithorax Subaortic (5) Paraaortic (6) Pulmonary ligament (9L) Hilar (10L)
Transbronchial needle aspiration biopsy (TBNA)	Lower (4) paratracheal Subcarinal (7) Hilar (10) Interlobar (11)
Percutaneous CT-guided biopsy	Upper (2R) and lower (4R) right paratracheal Subaortic (5) Paraaortic (6) Subcarinal (7) Paraesophageal (8) Hilar (10)

Source: Refs. 5–10.

[a] AJCC, American Joint Committee on Cancer; UICC, Union Internationale Contre le Cancer. Numbers in parentheses correspond to AJCC-UICC node classifications

aorticopulmonary window lymph nodes are not accessible by cervical mediastinoscopy and thus require another method of biopsy such as anterior or parasternal mediastinotomy or thoracoscopy.

Second, CT can be used to guide nodal biopsies, either indirectly or directly. For example, the techniques of virtual bronchoscopy and CT fluoros-

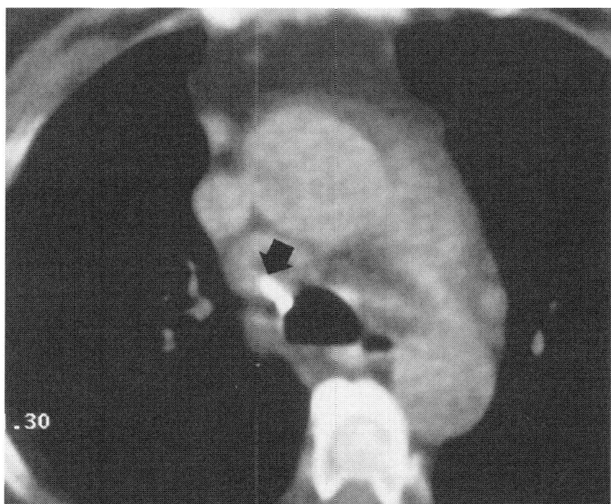

Figure 2 Computed tomography fluoroscopic guidance of transbronchial needle aspiration biopsy (TBNA). Noncontrast CT image at the level of the aorticopulmonary window demonstrates satisfactory positioning of needle tip (arrow) within enlarged lower right paratracheal lymph node, which was proven malignant at biopsy. (Courtesy of N. Goldberg, Beth Israel Deaconess Medical Center, Boston, Massachusetts.)

copy can be used to guide transbronchial needle aspiration (TBNA) procedures (Figure 2). Such guidance has been shown to improve the accuracy and reduce the time of this procedure [6,7]. In certain cases, CT-guided percutaneous biopsy of lymph nodes may also play a role in nodal staging [10].

An emerging role of CT involves the provision of complementary anatomic information for correlation with physiologic FDG PET studies. Combined anatomic and physiologic imaging is described below.

Similar to its limitations for evaluating mediastinal lymph nodes, CT has also been shown to have a low sensitivity and specificity for assessing hilar lymph node metastases [4,11]. The evaluation of hilar lymph nodes has become an important factor in the selection of patients with early lung cancer (T1, N0, M0) and poor pulmonary reserve for minimal resection procedures such as segmentectomy and wedge resection [11].

It has recently been suggested that hilar nodal contour may be a more accurate predictor of metastatic involvement than nodal size. In a study that assessed the ability of CT to detect hilar nodal metastases, Shimoyama et al. [12] classified lymph nodes with straight or concave margins to the lung as benign and those with convex margins as malignant. Using this criterion, these investigators reported a relatively high sensitivity (87%) and specificity (88%) for detecting hilar nodal metastases. Future studies involving larger numbers of patients are necessary to confirm these promising results.

B. Magnetic Resonance Imaging

There was an initial expectation that magnetic resonance (MR) imaging would provide a more accurate assessment of nodal status than CT. Unfortunately, however, studies have shown that signal characteristics and relaxation times do not reliably distinguish between malignant and benign lymph nodes [13–15]. Similarly to CT, MR relies predominantly on size criteria for determining nodal status. Thus, it is not surprising that MR and CT have been shown to have comparable accuracy in the assessment of mediastinal nodal metastases in patients with NSCLC (Fig. 3) [16].

Despite similar accuracy, there are several relative advantages and disadvantages of MR compared to CT [3,11,15]. The multiplanar capability of MR provides superior assessment of the aorticopulmonary window and subcarinal nodal stations, regions that are often difficult to evaluate on axial images (Fig. 4). The ease with which MR differentiates lymph nodes from vascular structures provides another potential advantage of this technique, particularly in the assessment of hilar lymph nodes (Fig. 3). For this reason, MR is more accurate than CT in the assessment of hilar nodes, especially when vascular enhancement is suboptimal or absent on CT scans [17]. Thus, MR may be helpful as a problem-solving tool for inconclusive CT cases.

Two relative disadvantages of MR should be noted [3,11,15]. First, calcification within lymph nodes may be overlooked at MR imaging, thus potentially resulting in the misdiagnosis of a benign, calcified lymph node as concerning for metastatic disease. Second, because of the poorer spatial resolution of MR compared to CT, a group of discrete, adjacent normal-sized lymph nodes may occasionally blur together on MR images and appear as a single large nodal mass, which may be erroneously diagnosed as metastatic disease.

Due to the limited ability of CT and MR to accurately characterize lymph nodes on the basis of anatomic criteria, there has been growing interest in physiologic methods of nodal assessment. The next section of this chapter describes recent advances in physiologic imaging of lymph nodes with MR and FDG PET.

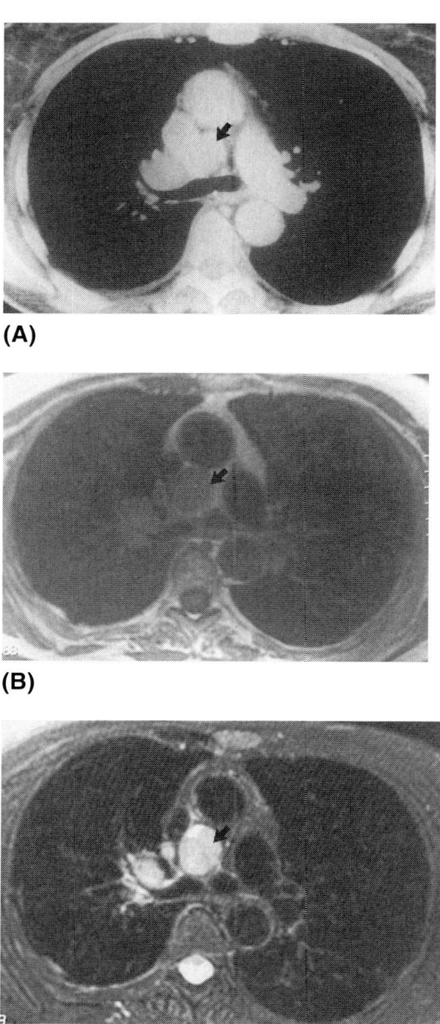

Figure 3 Anatomic imaging of mediastinal nodes with CT and MR. (A) Contrast-enhanced CT image shows an enlarged, 2.5-cm short-axis-diameter, precarinal lymph node (arrow). At biopsy, this lymph node was proven malignant. (B) T1-weighted axial MR image shows enlarged precarinal lymph node (arrow) and enlarged right hilar nodes, with signal intensity similar to skeletal muscle. Note improved visibility of hilar nodes on MR compared to CT. (C) T2-weighted axial MR image shows enlarged precarinal lymph node (arrow) and right hilar nodes, both of which are characterized by bright signal intensity. The MR signal intensity characteristics do not reliably distinguish benign and maligrant lymph nodes. (From Ref. 11.)

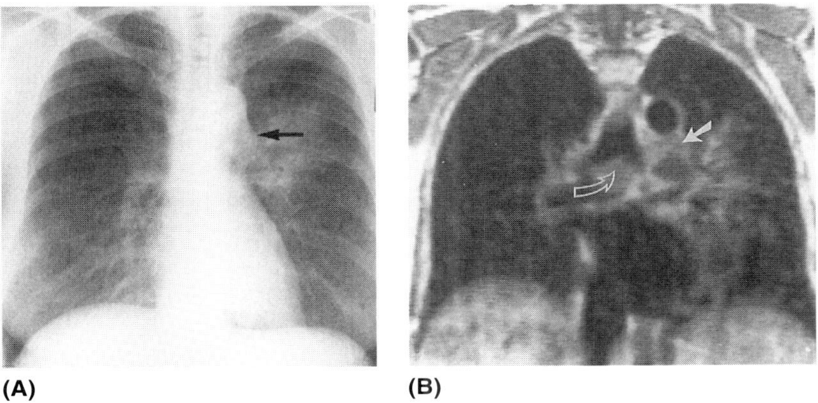

Figure 4 Assessment of mediastinal nodes in coronal plane with MR imaging. (A) Posteroanterior (PA) chest radiograph reveals a poorly defined left upper lobe mass and an abnormal convex contour of the aorticopulmonary window (arrow). (B) Coronal T1-weighted MR image of the thorax demonstrates enlarged lymph nodes in the aorticopulmonary window (closed arrow) as well as within the subcarinal region (open arrow). (From Ref. 3.)

III. PHYSIOLOGIC IMAGING

A. Magnetic Resonance Imaging

The addition of contrast agents to MR imaging provides an opportunity to characterize lymph nodes in functional terms. With regard to conventional MR contrast agents, a preliminary investigation by Laissey et al. [18] assessed the use of dynamic gadolinium-enhanced MR imaging in the assessment of mediastinal lymph nodes in patients with NSCLC. In this small series (n = 9 patients), neoplastic lymph nodes showed a peak enhancement at 60 to 80 sec, whereas benign nodes demonstrated only slight enhancement and no peak. These preliminary findings should be confirmed in a larger series of patients.

More recently, there have been exciting developments in the area of novel MR contrast agents, including superparamagnetic ultrasmall iron oxide particles [3,11,19–25]. Magnetic resonance lymphography, which refers to the use of this novel agent to assess lymph nodes, involves imaging acquisition (gradient-echo and T2- and T2*-weighted sequences) before and 24 to 48 hr following intravenous administration of ultrasmall iron oxide particles [3,11].

Magnetic resonance lymphography is based on the principle that different cell types exhibit varying degrees of uptake of iron oxide [3,11]. For example, normal macrophages demonstrate avid uptake of iron oxide. Importantly, the number of functional macrophages per unit volume of tissue varies between normal and neoplastic nodes. For this reason, normal lymph nodes will demonstrate a decrease in signal intensity on T2- and T2*-weighted sequences following iron oxide administration, whereas such a decrease in signal is often absent or less marked in neoplastic nodes (Figs. 5 and 6) [3,11]. Thus, MR lymphography provides an opportunity to differentiate neoplastic and benign nodes on the basis of differing signal intensity following adminstration of iron oxide (Figs. 5 and 6).

Preliminary clinical investigations have shown this method to be valuable for distinguishing benign and malignant nodes in patients with head and neck cancer [19,20] and urologic and pelvic malignancies [21,25]. With regard to its role in assessing mediastinal lymph nodes in patients with NSCLC, Kernstine et al. [26] recently compared this technique to CT and FDG PET imaging

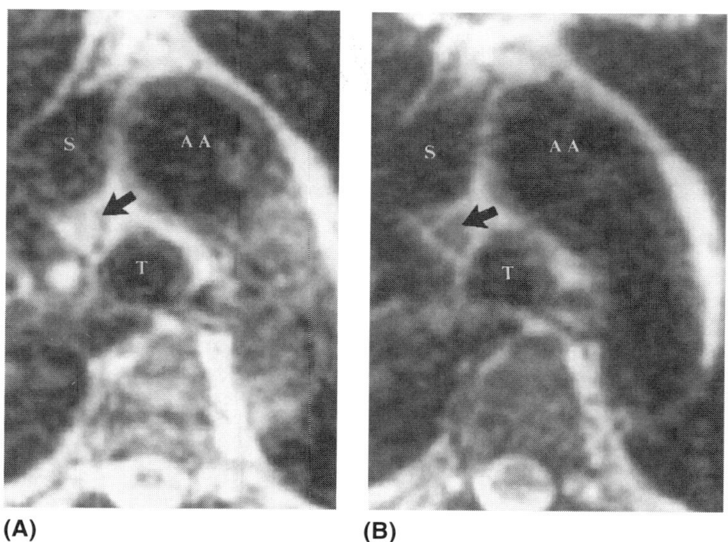

Figure 5 Magnetic resonance lymphography of a benign lymph node. (A) Predose T2-weighted fast spin-echo axial image at the level of the aortic arch reveals a 10-mm-diameter right paratracheal lymph node (arrow), which demonstrates a homogeneous bright signal intensity. (B) Postdose T2-weighted fast spin-echo axial image demonstrates a homogeneous decrease in signal intensity in the right paratracheal lymph node. At biopsy, there was no evidence of malignancy. S, superior vena cava; AA, aortic arch; T, trachea. (From Ref. 3.)

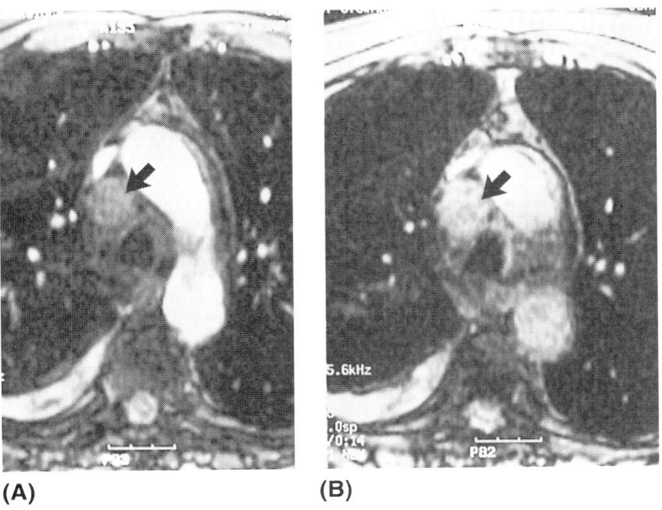

Figure 6 Magnetic resonance lymphography of a malignant lymph node. Predose (A) and postdose (B) gradient-echo axial images show an enlarged right paratracheal lymph node (arrow) which does not decrease in signal intensity following adminstration of iron oxide. At biopsy, this lymph node was proven malignant. (From Ref. 11.)

in the assessment of mediastinal lymph nodes in a cohort of NSCLC patients. These investigators found MR lymphography to be slightly more accurate than CT and slightly less accurate than PET. Although statistically significant, the differences in accuracy were quite small and considered clinically irrelevant by the investigators. Of note, this study is limited by the small number of patients ($n = 9$) who were imaged with all three modalities compared to a larger number ($n = 64$) who were imaged with both PET and CT.

Less promising results with MR lymphography were reported by Bluemke et al. [22]. These authors performed a preliminary investigation of the role of MR lymphography in directing TBNA of mediastinal lymph nodes and reported a sensitivity of 100% and a specificity of only 38%. This study was limited by a small number of patients ($n = 12$) and a small number of sampled lymph nodes ($n = 12$).

The results of ongoing multicenter trials are necessary to determine the true sensitivity and specificity of MR lymphography in the assessment of nodal status in patients with NSCLC. Hopefully, optimization of imaging parameters and contrast agent dose will result in improved sensitivity and specificity.

B. FDG PET Imaging

Positron emission tomography imaging is based on the long-recognized principle that neoplastic cells exhibit increased glucose metabolism compared to normal tissues and most benign processes [3,11]. In recent years, these metabolic alterations have been successfully imaged with PET by using radiolabeled glucose analogs [27]. ^{18}F-labeled 2-deoxy-D-glycose, which is a D-glucose analog labeled with a positron-emitting fluorine-18 substituted for a hydroxy group at the carbon-12 position, is the most commonly used PET agent for imaging thoracic neoplasms [27]. FDG PET is highly accurate for distinguishing between benign and malignant pulmonary nodules [28]. Because regional and distant metastases demonstrate abnormal metabolic activity similar to the primary neoplasm, this technique can also be used to assess for nodal and distant metastases (Fig. 7) [27].

With regard to its role in assessing nodal status, several studies have shown that FDG PET is significantly more accurate than CT for this purpose [29–38]. For example, in a study that employed extensive lymph node sampling, Steinert et al. [30] reported a sensitivity of 89% and a specificity of 99% for FDG PET. Dwamena et al. [37] recently reported a meta-analysis comparison of mediastinal staging studies performed using FDG PET (14 studies, 514 patients) and CT (29 studies, 2226 patients) in the 1990s. Not surprisingly, they found that PET was significantly more accurate than CT for demonstrating nodal metastases. Mean sensitivity and specificity were 79 and 91% for PET, compared to 60 and 77% for CT. It is important to note the smaller number of patients enrolled in PET studies ($n = 514$) than CT studies ($n = 2226$) in this meta-analysis.

Gupta et al. [34] recently compared the efficacy of FDG PET and CT imaging for evaluating small (<1 cm), intermediate (1 to 3 cm), and large (>3 cm) mediastinal lymph nodes. In this study, FDG PET was significantly more accurate than CT for evaluating all lymph node sizes (94% vs. 61%) and individual nodal size groups. FDG PET was equally reliable and accurate for detecting disease in small and large lymph node lesions. Remarkably, the sensitivity, specificity, and accuracy for detecting malignancy in nodes <1 cm in diameter were 97, 82, and 95%, respectively.

Farrell et al. [38] recently studied the role of FDG PET in nodal staging of 84 patients with CT evidence of Stage I NSCLC and compared PET staging to histopathologic staging. The disease was accurately staged in 86% of patients with PET, understaged in 2%, and overstaged in 12%. For all nodal disease levels (N1–N3), FDG PET demonstrated sensitivity, specificity, and negative predictive values of 82, 86, and 97%. The sensitivity was greater for

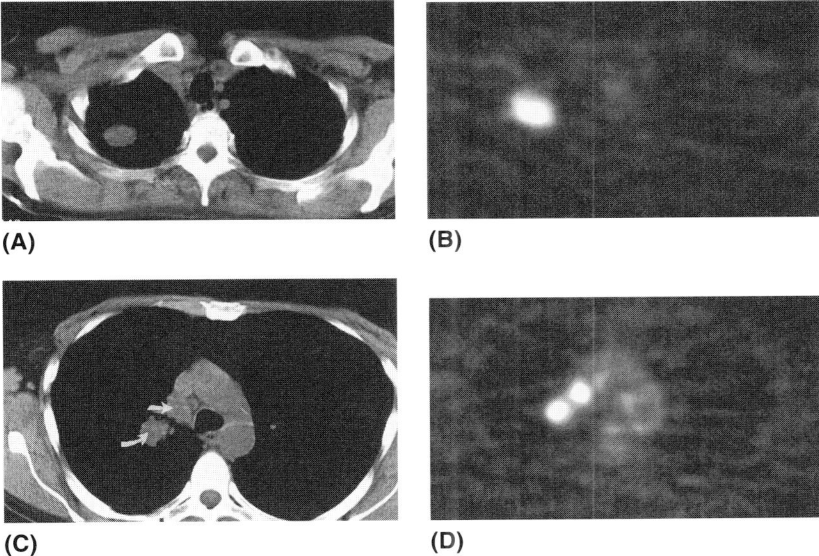

Figure 7 Assessment of primary neoplasm and nodal metastases using FDG PET imaging. (A) Axial CT image at lung apex reveals a 2-cm-diameter right upper lobe nodule. (B) Axial PET image at similar level to A shows that the nodule is hypermetabolic, consistent with a malignant neoplasm. (C) Axial CT scan at the level of the aortic arch demonstrates enlarged right paratracheal straight arrow) and hilar nodes (curved arrow). (D) Axial PET image at similar level to C reveals increased activity in right paratracheal and hilar nodes, consistent with metastatic disease, which was proven at mediastinoscopy. (From Ref. 3.)

N2 and N3 disease (100%) than for N1 disease (71%), but specificity and negative predictive value levels were similar for all nodal stages. Based on the high sensitivity of FDG PET for detecting N2 and N3 disease and the high negative predictive value of this technique, these authors suggest that patients with T1 or T2 primary lesions with negative nodes on both CT and FDG PET imaging may not require mediastinoscopy prior to thoracotomy.

At present, the main limitation of FDG PET imaging is the limited number of hospitals and radiology practices with access to dedicated PET scanners [3]. The increased availability of FDG through regional distribution centers has generated interest in FDG imaging using less expensive and more widely available devices [39]. The rate-limiting factor of nondedicated PET FDG imaging is its limited intrinsic detector efficiency. This factor results in low

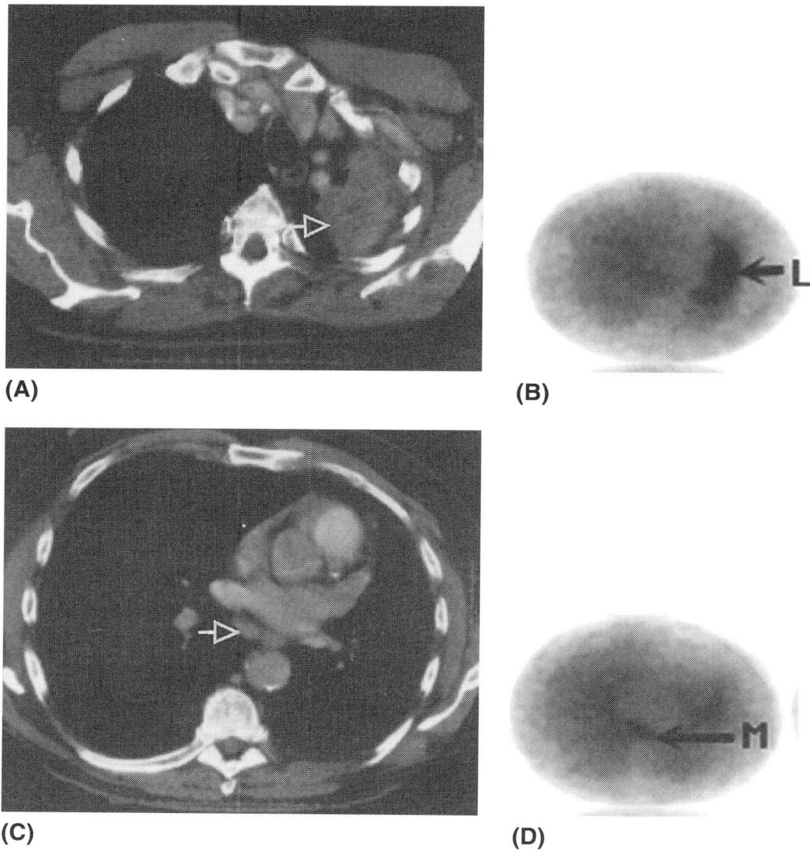

Figure 8 Assessment of primary neoplasm and nodal metastases using FDG with dual-head single-photon-emission computed tomographic (SPECT) Anger camera coincidence mode imaging. (A) Axial CT image of lung apex reveals a large left apical mass (arrow), which was proven to represent non-small-cell lung cancer. (B) Axial SPECT FDG image at similar level demonstrates increased metabolic activity in left apex (L) corresponding to site of neoplastic mass. (C) Axial CT image at level of inferior pulmonary veins reveals an enlarged, contralateral paraesophageal lymph node (arrow). (D) Axial SPECT FDG image at similar level to (C) demonstrates increased metabolic activity within the node (M), consistent with metastatic disease. (Courtesy of A. Parker, Beth Israel Deaconess Medical Center, Boston, Massachusetts.)

counts, which decreases lesion detectability. Fortunately, however, the low background activity of the lungs maximizes visibility of lung nodules and paratracheal and hilar lymph nodes (Fig. 8) [39]. In contrast, in areas where background activity is higher (e.g., the abdomen), there is poorer lesion visibility, particularly with small (less than 1.5-cm-diameter) lesions.

A recent study by Shreve et al. [39] compared the performance of a dual-head single photon emission computed tomographic (SPECT) Anger camera operated in coincidence mode (nondedicated PET FDG imaging) with a dedicated PET scanner in the imaging of 31 oncology patients with malignant involvement of a variety of organ systems. Of the thoracic lesions depicted with dedicated PET imaging, nondedicated PET FDG imaging was able to detect 13 (93%) of 14 lung lesions and 20 (65%) of 31 mediastinal lymph nodes. For lymph nodes greater than 1.5 cm in diameter, 15 (94%) of 16 were detected with nondedicated PET FDG imaging. Future studies in larger numbers of patients are necessary in order to determine the true sensitivity and specificity of nondedicated PET FDG imaging in NSCLC patients.

Although physiologic imaging with FDG PET imaging represents a marked improvement over anatomic imaging techniques, it is not without limitations. For example, false-positive results may be encountered in active granulomatous infections such as tuberculosis and false-negative results may be seen in the setting of microscopic foci of metastatic disease within small lymph nodes [3]. Thus, one would expect the specificity of FDG PET imaging to be lower in areas with a high prevalence of active granulomatous infections.

IV. COMBINED ANATOMIC AND PHYSIOLOGIC IMAGING

Several recent studies suggest that combined anatomic and physiologic imaging using CT and FDG PET is more accurate than PET imaging alone [31–33,35,36]. For example, Vansteenkiste et al. [31] prospectively compared the accuracy of CT scanning, FDG PET imaging blinded to CT, and FDG PET visually correlated with CT in the detection of N2 metastatic mediastinal lymph nodes in patients with NSCLC. Although FDG PET blinded to CT was significantly more accurate than CT alone, a combined approach resulted in even higher accuracy. Similarly, Gupta et al. [33], Magnani et al. [35], and Albes et al. [36] have found that combined CT and FDG PET interpretation is more accurate than either technique alone. Thus, CT and FDG PET should be considered as complementary rather than competitive imaging techniques.

Combined anatomic and physiologic imaging can be performed by either visual correlation or image fusion techniques. Vansteenkiste et al. [32] recently compared these two methods of analysis and found an added benefit of image fusion over visual correlation in only 1 of 56 cases (overall accuracy 73% vs. 71%). Thus, it seems likely that the more practical approach of visual correlation will suffice in most cases.

Importantly, a combined strategy of CT and FDG PET imaging has been shown to be cost-effective. Using a conservative decision-tree analysis, Gambhir et al. [40] demonstrated that such an approach resulted in a savings of roughly $1100.00 per patient compared to CT imaging alone. Moreover, this strategy was associated with a slightly increased life expectancy.

V. SUMMARY

The assessment of nodal status is an important aspect of staging patients with NSCLC. Anatomic imaging techniques such as CT and MR, which rely primarily upon nodal size, are limited by poor sensitivity and specificity. Recent advances in physiologic imaging with FDG PET have resulted in improved accuracy, which can be further enhanced by correlation with CT images. At present, a combined anatomic and physiologic approach using CT and FDG PET is the most accurate and cost-effective imaging method for determining nodal status in NSCLC patients.

REFERENCES

1. Mountain CF. Revisions in the international system for staging lung cancer. Chest 1997; 111:1710–1717.
2. Jett J, Feins R, Kvale P, et al. Pretreatment evaluation of non-small cell lung cancer: official statement of the American Thoracic Society and the European Respiratory Society. Am J Respir Crit Care Med 1997; 156:320–332.
3. Boiselle PM, Patz EF, Vining DJ, et al. Imaging of mediastinal lymph nodes: CT, MR, and FDG PET. RadioGraphics 1998; 18:1061–1069.
4. McLoud TC, Bourgoin PM, Greenberg RW, et al. Bronchogenic carcinoma: analysis of staging in the mediastinum with CT by correlative lymph node mapping and sampling. Radiology 1992; 182:319–323.
5. Mentzer SJ, Swanson SJ, DeCamp MM, et al. Mediastinoscopy, thoracoscopy, and video-assisted thoracic surgery in the diagnosis and staging of lung cancer. Chest 1997; 112(suppl):239S–241S.
6. Vining DJ, Liu K, Choplin RH, et al. Virtual bronchoscopy: Relationships of

virtual reality endobronchial simulations to actual bronchoscopic findings. Chest 1996; 109:549–553.
7. Goldberg SN, Raptopoulous V, Boiselle PM, et al. Improved diagnostic yield for transbronchial mediastinal lymph node biopsy using CT-fluoroscopic guidance. Radiology 2000; 216:764–767.
8. Harki TJ, Wang K. Broncoscopic needle aspiration of mediastinal and hilar lymph nodes. J Bronchol 1997; 4:238–249.
9. Cymbalista M, Waysberg A, Zacharias C, et al. CT demonstration of the 1996 AJCC-UICC regional lymph node classification for lung cancer staging. RadioGraphics 1999; 19:899–900.
10. Protopapas Z, Westcott JL. Transthoracic needle biopsy of mediastinal lymph nodes for staging lung and other cancers. Radiology 1997; 199:489–496.
11. Boiselle PM. MR imaging of thoracic lymph nodes: a comparison of computed tomography and positron emission tomography. MRI Clinics of North America 2000; 8:33–41.
12. Shimoyama K, Murata K, Takahashi M, et al. Pulmonary hilar lymph node metastases from lung cancer: evaluation based on morphology at thin-section incremental, dynamic CT. Radiology 1997; 203:187–195.
13. Dooms GC, Hricak H, Moseley ME, et al. Characterization of lymphadenopathy by magnetic resonance relaxation times: Preliminary results. Radiology 1985; 155:691–697.
14. Glazer GM, Orringer MB, Chenevert TL, et al. Imaging of mediastinal lymph nodes: relaxation time/pathologic correlation with implications in staging of lung cancer with MR imaging. Radiology 1988; 168:429–431.
15. Quint LE, Francis IR, Wahl RL, et al. Preoperative staging of non-small cell carcinoma of the lung: imaging methods. Am J Roentgenol 1995; 164:1349–1359.
16. Webb WR, Gatsonis C, Zerhouni EA, et al. CT and MR imaging in staging non-small cell bronchogenic carcinoma: Report of the Radiologic Diagnostic Oncology Group. Radiology 1991; 178:705–713.
17. Naidich DP, Zerhouni EA, Siegelman SS, eds. Lung cancer. In: Computed Tomography and Magnetic Resonance Imaging of the Thorax. 2d ed. New York: Raven Press, 1991:275–302.
18. Laissy JP, Gay-Depassier P, Soyer P, et al. Enlarged mediastinal lymph nodes in bronchogenic carcinoma: assessment with dynamic contrast-enhanced MR imaging [work in progress]. Radiology 1994; 191:263–267.
19. Anzai Y, Prince MR. Iron oxide-enhanced MR lymphangiography: the evaluation of cervical lymph node metastases in head and neck cancer. J Magn Reson Imaging 1997; 7:75–81.
20. Anzai Y, Blackwell K, Hirschowitz SL, et al. Initial clinical experience with Dextran-coated superparamagnetic iron oxide for detection of lymph node metastases in patients with head and neck cancer. Radiology 1998; 207: 799–808.
21. Bellin MF, Roy C, Kinkel K, et al. Lymph node metastases: safety and effectiveness of MR imaging with ultrasmall superparamagnetic iron oxide particles—initial clinical experience. Radiology 1998; 207:799–808.

22. Bluemke DA, Borman RN, Wang K. MR lymph node contrast agent (Combidex®): use in directing bronchoscopic fine needle aspiration of mediastinal nodes [abstract 1041]. Radiology 1998; 209(suppl):375.
23. Weissleder R, Elizondo G, Wittenberg J, et al. Ultrasmall superparamagnetic iron oxide: an intravenous contrast agent for assessing lymph nodes with MR imaging. Radiology 1990; 175:494–498.
24. Weissleder R, Hui-Cheng H, Bogdanova A. Bogdonov A. Magnetically labeled cells can be detected by MR imaging. J Magn Reson Imaging 1997; 7:258–263.
25. Harisinghani MG, Saini S, Slater GJ, et al. MR imaging of pelvic lymph nodes in primary pelvic carcinoma with ultrasmall superparamagnetic iron oxide (Combidex): Preliminary observations. J Magn Reson Imaging 1997; 7:161–163.
26. Kernstine KH, Stanford W, Mullan BF, et al. PET, CT, and MRI with Combidex for mediastinal staging in non-small cell lung carcinoma. Ann Thorac Surg 1999; 68:1022–1028.
27. Patz EF, Goodman PC. Positron emission tomography imaging of the thorax. Radiol Clin North Am 1994; 32:811–823.
28. Patz EF, Lowe VJ, Hoffman JM, et al. Focal pulmonary abnormalities: evaluation with F-18 fluorodeoxyglucose PET scanning. Radiology 1993; 188:487–490.
29. Wahl RL, Quint LE, Greenough RL, et al. Staging of mediastinal non-small cell lung cancer with FDG PET, CT, and fusion images: preliminary prospective evaluation. Radiology 1994; 191:371–377.
30. Steinert HC, Hauser M, Allemann F, et al. Non-small cell lung cancer: nodal staging with FDG PET versus CT with correlative lymph node mapping and sampling. Radiology 1997; 202:441–446.
31. Vansteenkiste JF, Stroobants SG, De Leyn PR, et al. Mediastinal lymph node staging with FDG-PET scan in patients with potentially operative non-small cell lung cancer: a prospective analysis of 50 cases. Chest 1997; 112:1480–1486.
32. Vansteenkiste JF, Stroobants SG, Dupont PJ, et al. FDG-PET scan in potentially operable non-small cell lung cancer: Do anatometabolic PET-CT fusion images improve localisation of regional lymph node metastases? Eur J Nucl Med 1998; 25:1495–1501.
33. Gupta NC, Graeber GM, Rogers JS, 2nd ed. Comparative efficacy of positron emission tomography FDG and computed tomographic scanning in preoperative staging of non-small cell lung cancer. Ann Surg 1999; 229:286–291.
34. Gupta NC, Graeber GM, Bishop HA: Comparative efficacy of positron emission tomography with fluorodeoxyglucose in evaluation of small (<1 cm), intermediate (1 to 3 cm) and large (>3 cm) lymph node lesions. Chest 2000; 117:773–778.
35. Magnani P, Carretta A, Rizzo G, et al. FDG/PET and spiral CT image fusion for mediastinal lymph node assessment of non-small cell lung cancer patients. J Cardiovas Surg 1999; 40:741–748.
36. Albes JS, Leitzenmayer R, Schott U, et al. Improvement of non-small-cell lung cancer staging by positron emission tomography. Thorac Cardiovas Surg 1999; 47:42–47.

37. Dwamena BA, Sonnad SS, Angobaldo JO, Wahl RL. Metastases from non-small cell lung cancer: mediastinal staging in the 1990s—meta-analytic comparison of PET and CT. Radiology 1999; 213:530–536.
38. Farrell MA, McAdams HP, Herndon JE, Patz EF. Non-small cell lung cancer: FDG PET for nodal staging in patients with stage I disease. Radiology 2000; 215:886–890.
39. Shreve PD, Steventon RS, Deters EC, et al. Oncologic diagnosis with 2-[Fluorine-18]Fluoro-2-deoxy-D-glucose imaging: dual-head coincidence gamma camera versus positron emission tomographic scanner. Radiology 1998; 207:431–437.
40. Gambhir SS, Hoh CK, Phelps ME, et al. Decision tree sensitivity analysis for cost-effectiveness of FDG-PET in the staging and management of non-small-cell lung carcinoma. J Nucl Med 1996; 37:1428–1436.

4
Multidetector Helical CT

J. Richard Choi
United States Army Medical Corps and
Walter Reed Army Medical Center
Washington, DC

Phillip M. Boiselle
Harvard Medical School and
Beth Israel Deaconess Medical Center
Boston, Massachusetts

I. INTRODUCTION

The clinical introduction of helical computed tomography (CT) in 1991 represented an important advance over conventional, incremental CT scanners. By producing a single volumetric data set of the thorax within one breath hold, helical CT effectively eliminated respiratory misregistration, significantly reduced respiratory and cardiac motion, decreased contrast volumes, and markedly improved the quality of multiplanar reconstruction images [1–2].

Approximately 1 decade later, multidetector helical CT (MHCT) is the latest technological breakthrough in CT scanners [3–8]. In place of a single detector array, MHCT scanners contain multiple detector arrays arranged as a matrix of multiple detector rows. Each row contains 500–900 elements, and many rows together form a curved array containing thousands of detector elements [7]. These, together with super-high-heat-capacity X-ray tubes, allow tremendous flexibility in how a scan is obtained. In comparison to single-detector CT, MHCT can be used to decrease scan time, increase spatial resolution, increase signal-to-noise ratio, or to combine all three. Moreover, MHCT

Table 1 Comparison of Existing Detector Designs

Manufacturer	No. of elements	Type of array	Detector widths (mm)
GE[a]	16	Equal-width	16 × 1.25
Marconi[b]	8	Unequal-width	2 × 1.0., 2 × 1.5, 2 × 2.5, 2 × 5.0
Siemens[c]	8	Unequal-width	2 × 1.0., 2 × 1.5, 2 × 2.5, 2 × 5.0
Toshiba[d]	34	Unequal-width	4 × 0.5, 30 × 1.0

Source: Ref. 7.
[a] GE Medical Systems (Milwaukee, WI).
[b] Marconi Medical Systems (Cleveland, OH).
[c] Siemens Medical Systems (Iselin, NJ).
[d] Toshiba Medical Systems (Tustin, CA).

offers the unique opportunity to create thin and thick section images from the same data set.

In this chapter, we describe the technical aspects of MHCT scanning, with a special emphasis on thoracic imaging applications. The purpose is to review the basic principles of this technique rather than to describe specific protocols for imaging. Our clinical experience with MHCT has been with the Lightspeed QXi CT scanner (General Electric, Milwaukee, WI). Although there are technical differences among MHCT scanners produced by various manufacturers (Table 1), the fundamental scanning principles are similar.

II. TECHNICAL DIFFERENCES BETWEEN SINGLE-AND MULTIDETECTOR HELICAL COMPUTED TOMOGRAPHY

A. Single-Detector Helical Computed Tomography Scanners

Single-detector helical CT uses an X-ray tube coupled with a single-detector array (Fig. 1). The X-ray beam is collimated prior to reaching the patient using a multistep prepatient collimator. Scan parameters for a single-detector helical CT scanner are determined by beam energy and dose (in kilovolts and milliamperes), collimation, table speed, and gantry rotation speed. The amount of collimation is determined prospectively by the operator and determines the effective image slice thickness. Due to scatter and continuous table motion during helical scanning, actual slice thickness can vary slightly depending on

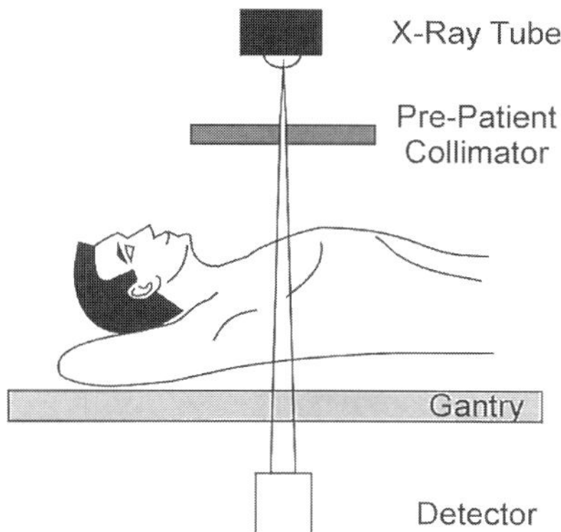

Figure 1 Single-detector helical CT. An X-ray beam is collimated by a prepatient collimator prior to entering a single-detector array. Slice thickness is mainly determined by collimator setting.

table speed and pitch. Pitch is defined as table feed per 360° gantry rotation divided by image slice thickness. Higher pitch results in faster scan time, but also can result in image reconstruction artifacts. Normally, pitch is kept between 1 and 2 for most studies. Gantry rotation speed varies between 0.7 and 1 sec/360° rotation.

B. Multidetector Helical Computed Tomography Scanners

In MHCT, the X-ray beam is still collimated, but image slice thickness is a function of detector matrix selection. By choosing the number of active detector rows, one can select from a variety of slice widths. Depending upon which detector configuration is chosen, the beam is collimated to include all active detectors simultaneously (Fig. 2). Because multiple detectors are used to collect data simultaneously, the traditional concept of pitch is not applicable in MHCT. Rather, a parameter called an effective pitch is sometimes substituted to indicate a comparable value to the pitch used in single-detector helical CT. An effective pitch is defined as table feed per 360° gantry rotation divided by image slice thickness divided by number of active detectors.

Because of the complexity of pitch values in MHCT, it is important to be aware of which pitches are optimal for a particular brand of scanner. For example, with the Lightspeed scanner, two discrete pitch modes have been

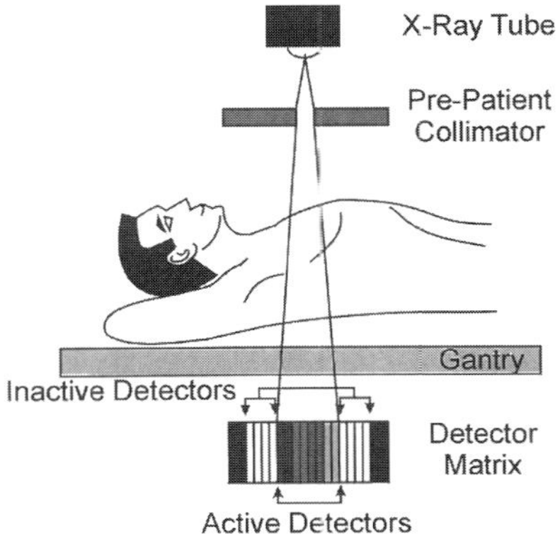

Figure 2 Multidetector helical CT. An X-ray beam is still collimated by a prepatient collimator prior to entering multiple-detector arrays. Slice thickness is determined by active detector selection.

selected as the preferred values for clinical scanning: 3.0, also referred to as HiQuality (effective pitch of 0.75); and 6.0, also referred to as HiSpeed (effective pitch of 1.5).

Use of Matrix Array

MHCT derives its name from its use of multiple detector arrays rather than a single detector array (Fig. 2). These are usually arranged next to one another in a row and form a matrix of multiple detector rows. The detectors can be selected individually or as a group of two to four to increase effective detector thickness. Each detector group is then connected via its own signal-processing unit to a central computer. The central computer then calculates individual image slices through a complex algorithm incorporating data from all active detectors. Current technology in computer- and data-analysis capabilities limits simultaneous detector use to a maximum of four channels. Each channel may contain the output of a single detector or the sum of outputs of neighboring detectors, which can be combined to create images of varying slice thickness. For example, with the Lightspeed scanner, there are 16 detectors of 1.25 mm. The information from these detector rows can be combined into four channels of information, providing nominal slice thickness values of 1.25, 2.5, 3.75, 5.0, 7.5, and 10 mm (Fig. 3).

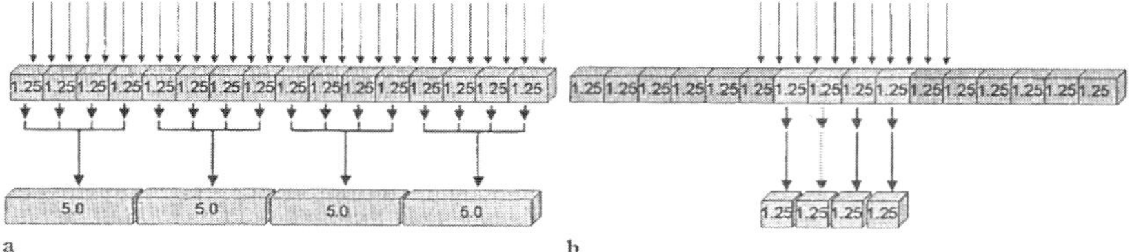

Figure 3 Cross-sectional profile of an equal-width detector design (Lightspeed, GE, Milwaukee, Wisconsin). (A) To acquire four 5-mm thick sections, all 16 detectors are activated. The signals from adjacent groups of four detectors are combined into one channel, creating a virtual detector with a section thickness of 5 mm. (B) To acquire four 1.25-mm-thick sections, only the central four detectors are activated. (From Ref. 7.)

Rapid advances in technology will soon allow for the acquisition of greater than four channels of data simultaneously. Indeed, MHCT scanners will be able to simultaneously detect eight or more channels by the time of this publication.

Interleaved Slices

Single-detector CT uses data from a single helical rotation to reconstruct individual image slices. In contrast, MHCT uses data from all active channels to reconstruct each individual slice. This means that adjacent detector elements collect a different segment of each individual slice. Using a simplified example, in a four-detector configuration with an effective pitch of 1, each image is reconstructed from data gathered by detector 1 from the first 90° gantry rotation, detector 2 from the second 90° gantry rotation, detector 3 from the third 90° gantry rotation, and detector 4 from the fourth 90° gantry rotation (Fig. 4). Therefore, after a single gantry rotation, data are obtained for four complete image slices. With increased pitch, the missing data are interpolated from adjacent slices just as in single-detector helical CT scanners. Of course, in actual use, the scanner obtains volumetric data over the scanned range and uses a complex mathematical algorithm to reconstruct each image. By use of interpolation, images can be reconstructed at any table position. Furthermore, some scanners allow retroactive decoupling of scan acquisition data from multiple detectors. This allows retrospective reconstruction of thinner or thicker slices from the original data set. The allowable slice thickness that can be reconstructed is dependent on the detector configuration at the time of original

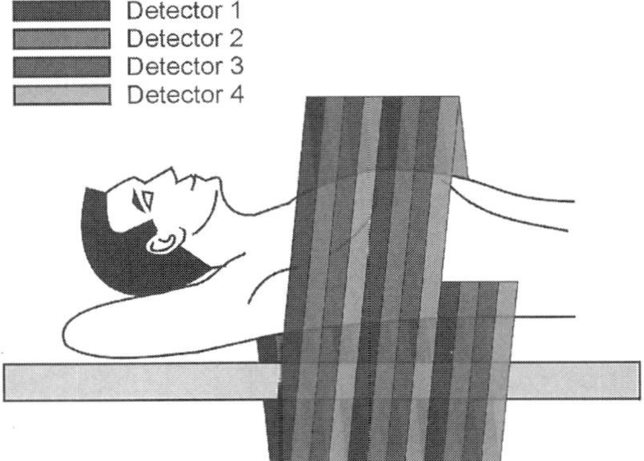

Figure 4 Multidetector helical CT and matrix array. With four active detectors, single gantry rotation results in four simultaneous slice acquisitions.

data acquisition. Retrospective reconstruction into thinner slices can be useful for further characterization of small lung nodules or interstitial lung disease and may preclude the need for additional image acquisitions in many cases. It may also aid in obtaining optimal slice thickness for multiplanar reconstructions.

III. FUNDAMENTAL ADVANTAGES OF MULTIDETECTOR HELICAL COMPUTED TOMOGRAPHY

The main advantages of MHCT relate to its increased speed compared to that of single-detector helical CT. MHCT can be used to enhance CT imaging in a number of different ways, e.g., to reduce scan time, improve resolution, increase the signal-to-noise ratio, or to combine these factors. An additional advantage is the ability to retrospectively create thin or thick sections from the same raw data.

A. Shorter Scan Time

MHCT can be used to decrease overall scan time by increasing table speed and using simultaneous data acquisition with multiple detectors. Using

MHCT, speed is dependent on two major factors: the number of detectors simultaneously sampled and the gantry rotation period [9]. With a similar collimation and gantry rotation time, a four-channel MHCT scanner will reduce scanning time by a factor of 4. Reduction of gantry rotation time to 0.5 sec has recently been introduced. Compared to a single detector scanner with a 1-sec gantry rotation time, a four-channel MHCT scanner with a 0.5-sec gantry rotation time will result in scanning 8 times faster. Thus, depending on technical parameters, a MHCT scanner may allow scanning at a rate 4 to 8 times faster than that of a typical single-detector scanner.

Faster scanning time allows for several advantages over single-detector scanners as follows: increased length of coverage during a single breath hold, use of less intravenous contrast volume, improved consistency in phase of enhancement throughout the imaging volume, and decreased respiratory and cardiac motion.

These advantages will likely have their greatest impact in the area of CT angiography (Fig. 5). Indeed, the advantages of MHCT angiography over

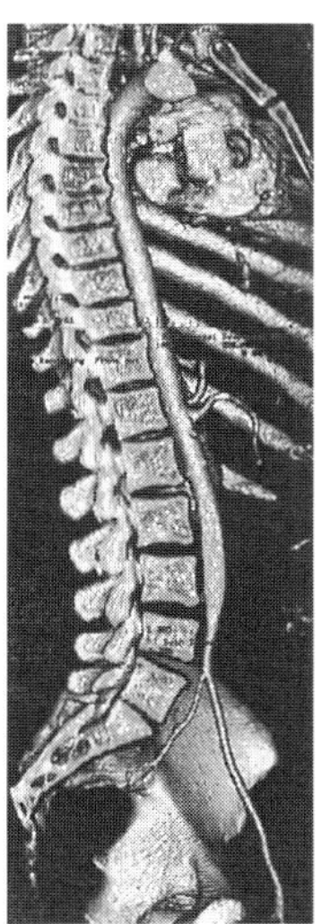

Figure 5 MHCT angiography of thoracic and abdominal aorta. Sagittal oblique 3D volume-rendered image of the thoracic and abdominal aorta demonstrates ability of MHCT to image the entire aorta and its major branches during a single imaging acquisition. Note lack of significant stairstep artifact. (Courtesy of V. Raptopoulos, Beth Israel Deaconess Medical Center, Boston, Massachusetts.)

single-detector CT angiography have been nicely demonstrated in a recent study by Rubin et al. [9]. In this study, the authors compared single- versus four-channel helical CT angiography in the assessment of 48 patients with aortic aneurysm or dissection. In comparison to single-detector CT, four-channel MHCT was 2.6 times faster, resulted in a scanning efficiency that was 4.1 times greater, and was associated with a contrast efficiency that was 2.5 times greater. MHCT also allowed for a 57% decrease in contrast volume without a significant change in aortic enhancement. Despite a roughly 60% shorter scanning duration, MHCT still allowed for a mean reduction in slice thickness of 40%. These authors found no advantage of single-detector CT aortography over MHCT aortography.

MHCT has expanded the capabilities of CT angiography to include vascular structures previously not well imaged by single-detector helical CT, such as the coronary arteries (Fig. 6) and subsegmental pulmonary arteries (Fig. 7). With regard to cardiac imaging, MHCT scanners with a 0.5-sec gantry

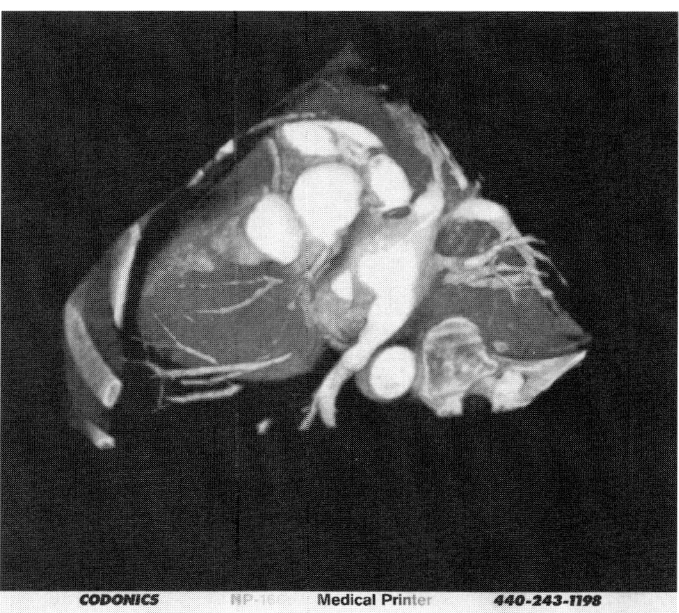

Figure 6 MHCT of coronary arteries. Coronal oblique 3D volume rendering of heart shows ability of MHCT to image coronary arteries. (Courtesy of P. Costello, Brigham and Women's Hospital, Boston, Massachusetts.)

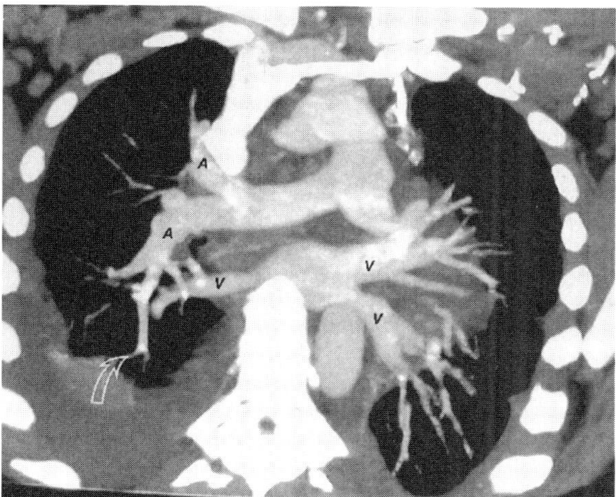

Figure 7 MHCT pulmonary angiography. Rotational (''paddlewheel'') 2D reconstruction [21] image shows ability of MHCT to image subsegmental pulmonary arteries (arrow). Also note ability to connect peripheral and central vessels as well as the ease with which to distinguish pulmonary arteries (A) from veins (V) using this reconstruction method. Small pleural effusions are present.

rotation period and a 180° reconstruction algorithm currently provide a temporal resolution of 0.3 sec [4,10]. Such fast scanning, coupled with EKG gating, allows for coronary artery evaluation [4,10], a technique that was previously limited to electron beam CT scanning. To date, the precise role of MHCT in the evaluation of coronary arteries has yet to be determined.

B. Improved Spatial Resolution

MHCT can be used to improve spatial resolution. This is especially apparent in the z axis (orthogonal plane to slice acquisition plane), where slice thickness determines the z axis resolution, but improved spatial resolution is also visible in the axial plane. By allowing a greater number of images to be acquired in the same amount of time, one can obtain thinner image slices. The spatial resolution advantage in the axial plane is due to reduced amount of partial volume averaging artifacts.

The ability to image the chest in a single breath hold using very narrow collimation will likely have an important impact on CT pulmonary angiography. The use of narrow collimation with this technique has been shown to be an important factor in improving the visibility of subsegmental arteries [11]. A preliminary investigation by Patel et al. [12] compared pulmonary artery visibility in three groups of patients ($n = 20$ in each group) with suspected pulmonary embolus who underwent different CT pulmonary angiography protocols as follows: Group 1: single-detector scanner, 3-mm collimation; Group 2: MHCT scanner, 2.5 mm collimation; and Group 3: MHCT scanner, 1.25-mm collimation. Although visualization of lobar arteries was similar among all groups, visualization of segmental arteries was slightly improved with MHCT scanning. The most notable difference, however, was in the assessment of subsegmental arteries, which were visible in 36% of cases in Group 1, 46% in Group 2, and 68% in Group 3. These data suggest that MHCT is superior to single-detector CT for peripheral pulmonary artery visualization, particularly when narrow (1.25-mm) collimation is employed.

The ability to image the entire chest with thin slices will likely also have an important impact on studies performed for lung nodule detection and assessment of the airways. With regard to lung nodule detection, it has been shown that thin-section images are more sensitive than thick-section images for detecting small, subcentimeter lesions [13]. Thin slices also allow for improved nodule characterization. With regard to airway imaging, the ability to obtain thin-section images over a large anatomical region such as the entire bronchial tree will enhance the ability to perform 2D and 3D renderings of the airway (Fig. 8).

A particular advantage of the MHCT scanner relates to its multiplanar reconstruction capabilities. In the coronal, sagittal, and oblique planes, image resolution is determined mainly by image acquisition slice thickness. Although stairstep artifact can be reduced with thinner reconstruction intervals, one is still limited by partial-volume artifact that causes blurring of the reconstructed image. By allowing thinner images to be acquired during a single-breath-hold scan, image resolution of multiplanar images can be dramatically improved. If volumetric image acquisition is obtained with 1-mm thick slices (also referred to as an isotropic volumetric scan), then image reconstructions can be performed with ~1-mm voxels (three-dimensional pixel with x, y, and z dimensions of 1 mm). This allows any reconstructed image in the oblique plane to have comparable spatial resolution to the original axial image. In the following example (Figs. 9, 10, and 11), a box of fruit (apple, orange, strawberries, grapes, and peach) was scanned with varying image acquisition slice thicknesses of 1, 3, and 5 mm; pitches of 1, 2, and 3; and varying reconstruction intervals of 1, 3, and 5 mm. The coronal reconstructed images demonstrate the best spatial resolution for images that were scanned at 1-mm thickness

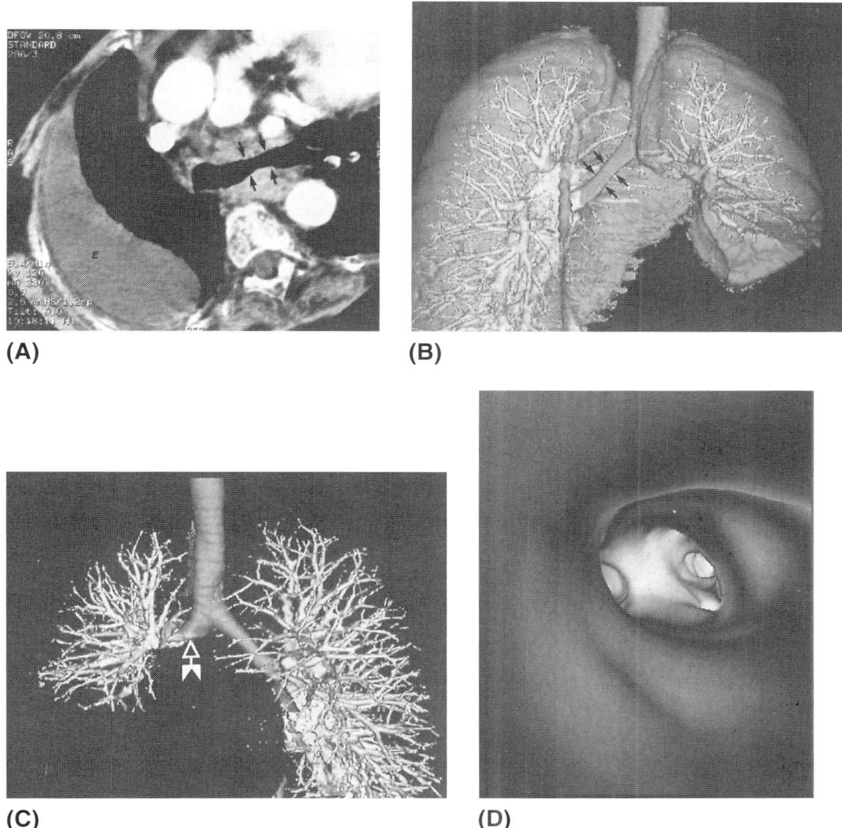

Figure 8 MHCT 2D and 3D reconstruction images of the airway in a patient with non-small-cell lung cancer. All reconstructions were performed from the same CT data set. (A) Two-dimensional curved oblique reconstruction image along axis of left mainstem bronchus shows narrowing (arrows) due to extrinsic compression by adjacent lymph nodes. Note loculated right pleural effusion (E). (B) Volume rendering of airway and lungs (posterior view) shows narrowing of left mainstem bronchus (arrows) as well as obstruction of bronchus intermedius. (C) Bronchus intermedius obstruction (arrow) is seen to better degree on anterior view of volume rendering of airway. (D) Virtual bronchoscopy (internal rendering) image of peripheral airways distal to left mainstem narrowing shows normal appearance of airway lumen.

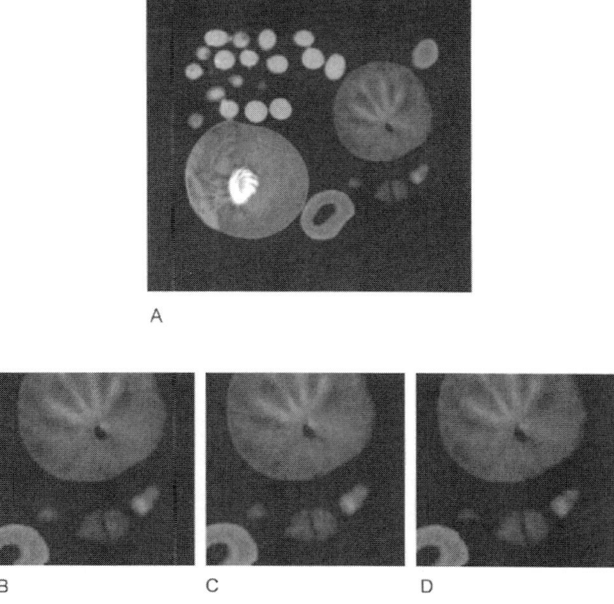

Figure 9 Effect of varying pitch on multiplanar image reconstruction. As pitch increases, image detail is lost, especially along the imaging plane, due to increased interpolation needed for image reconstruction. Note how image detail, especially along the fruit pulp and edges, is degraded with increasing pitch. (A) Coronal reconstruction of a fruit box with pitch of 1 (pitch 1; slice thickness 1 mm; reconstruction interval 1 mm; 5-mm coronal reconstruction). (B) Close-up of coronal reconstruction from Fig. 9A. (C) Close-up of coronal reconstruction of a fruit box with pitch of 2 (pitch 2; slice thickness 1 mm; reconstruction interval 1 mm; 5-mm coronal reconstruction). (D) Close-up of coronal reconstruction of a fruit box with pitch of 3 (pitch 3; slice thickness 1 mm; reconstruction interval 1 mm; 5-mm coronal reconstruction).

regardless of pitch. In contrast, 5-mm-thick slices have the worst spatial resolution, even if they are reconstructed at 1-mm intervals. For most image reconstructions, original image acquisition slice thickness has the greatest effect on image quality, followed by reconstruction intervals and, last, pitch.

Improved quality of reconstructed images with MHCT compared to single-detector CT has been shown in both experimental [14] and clinical studies [15]. In an experimental study, Fleischmann et al. [14] compared stairstep

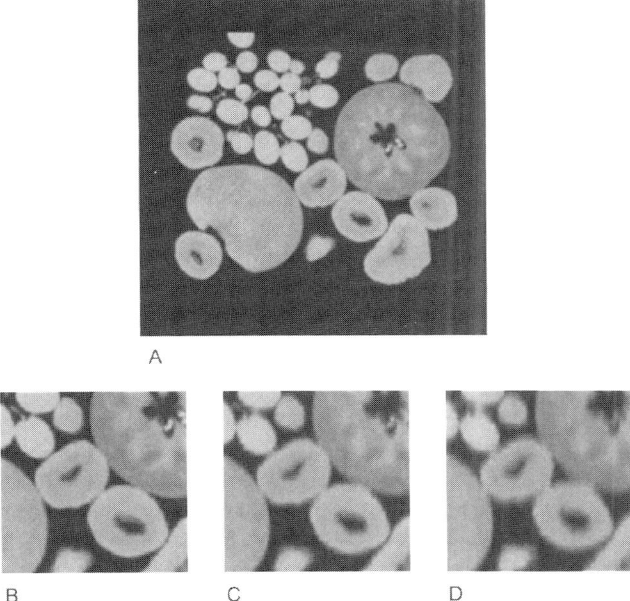

Figure 10 Effect of varying acquisition slice thickness on multiplanar image reconstruction. Resolution is diminished in the reconstructed plane orthogonal to the imaging plane as slice thickness is increased. Orthogonal image resolution is approximately equal to the acquisition slice thickness for most reconstruction techniques. Objects smaller than the acquired slice thickness, such as grape stems or seeds in this example, become blurred, while larger objects are less affected. (A) Coronal reconstruction of a fruit box with acquisition slice thickness of 1 mm (slice thickness 1 mm; pitch 1; reconstruction interval 1 mm; 5-mm coronal reconstruction). (B) Close-up of coronal reconstruction from Fig. 10A. (C) Close-up of coronal reconstruction with acquisition slice thickness of 3 mm (slice thickness 3mm; pitch 1; reconstruction interval 1 mm; 5-mm coronal reconstruction). (D) Close-up of coronal reconstruction with acquisition slice thickness of 5 mm (slice thickness 5 mm; pitch 1; reconstruction interval 1mm, 5-mm coronal reconstruction).

artifacts with MHCT and single-detector CT by imaging an acrylic rod. These investigators found that stairstep artifacts on volume-rendered reconstruction images were quantitatively and qualitatively smaller with MHCT than with single-detector scanners. In a clinical study, Boiselle et al. [15] qualitatively assessed the degree of stairstep artifact for 2D multiplanar reconstruction CT

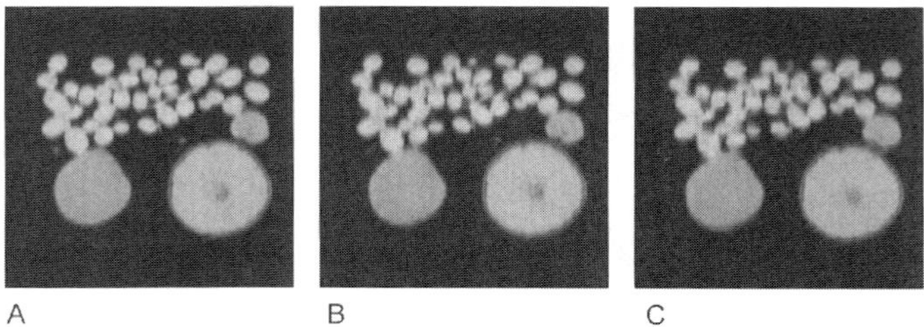

Figure 11 Effect of varying reconstruction interval on multiplanar image reconstruction: With increasing reconstruction intervals, artifacts such as stairstepping become more apparent. Note that a 1-mm reconstruction interval does not equal 1-mm resolution in the reconstructed image shown (maximum resolution for these reconstructions from 5-mm acquired slices is approximately 5 mm). (A) Coronal reconstruction of a fruit box with reconstruction interval of 1 mm (reconstruction interval 1 mm; slice thickness 5mm; pitch 1; 5-mm coronal reconstruction). (B) Coronal reconstruction of a fruit box with reconstruction interval of 3 mm (reconstruction interval 3 mm; slice thickness 5 mm; pitch 1; 5-mm coronal reconstruction). (C) Coronal reconstruction of a fruit box with reconstruction interval of 5 mm (reconstruction interval 5 mm; slice thickness 5 mm; pitch 1; 5-mm coronal reconstruction).

pulmonary angiography images in 40 patients imaged with single-detector CT and 40 patients imaged with MHCT. In this study, images obtained with MHCT were graded as having significantly less stairstep artifact (Fig. 12).

As clinical experience with the use of 2D and 3D reconstructed images increases, the spectrum of indications for such reconstructions will likely broaden. For example, preliminary studies have suggested a potential role for multiplanar reconstruction images in the assessment of diffuse interstitial lung disease [16] and lung nodule detection (Fig. 13) [17].

C. Improved Signal-to-Noise Ratio

By allowing images to be obtained from multiple detectors, MHCT can provide an improved signal-to-noise-ratio. MHCT allows this to happen during both data collection and postprocessing. During initial data collection, if one uses the same table speed and slice thickness as for single-detector helical CT scanning, the effective pitch is reduced to one-fourth of its former value, quadrupling the effective tube current (in milliamperes), resulting in decreased image noise and improved image quality [4]. During postprocessing, if the initial images are deemed to have a poor signal-to-noise ratio due to body

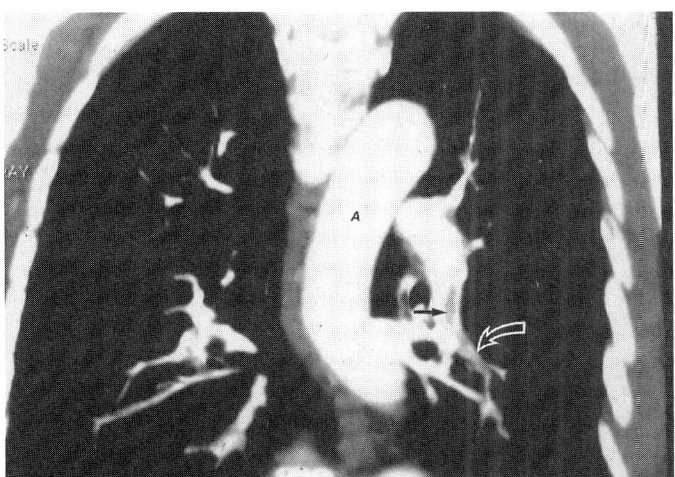

Figure 12 MHCT pulmonary angiography multiplanar reconstruction image. Coronal 2D reconstruction from CT pulmonary angiography study shows nonocclusive intraluminal thrombus within common basilar trunk of left lower lobe pulmonary artery (black arrow) surrounded by contrast. Occlusive thrombus is seen more distally within the lateral basilar segmental and subsegmental branches (curved white arrow). Note absence of significant stairstep artifacts. A, aorta.

habitus or inadequate kilovolt and milliampere settings, one has the option to combine data from additional detectors to improve the image quality. For example, if the initial images are difficult to interpret due to streak artifact from hardware or foreign body, reconstructing these images with data from adjacent detectors will decrease the amount of artifact observed.

D. Retrospective Selection of Thinner or Thicker Slices

MHCT scanners allow retrospective image reconstruction to thinner or thicker image slices after the scan has been completed, as long as the original acquisition data is intact. In thoracic imaging, the ability to retrospectively obtain thin section images through lung nodules detected on routine scans is likely the most important application for this feature.

Importantly, this feature also allows one to obtain high-quality 2D and 3D reconstructions from scans performed in routine clinical practice by retro-

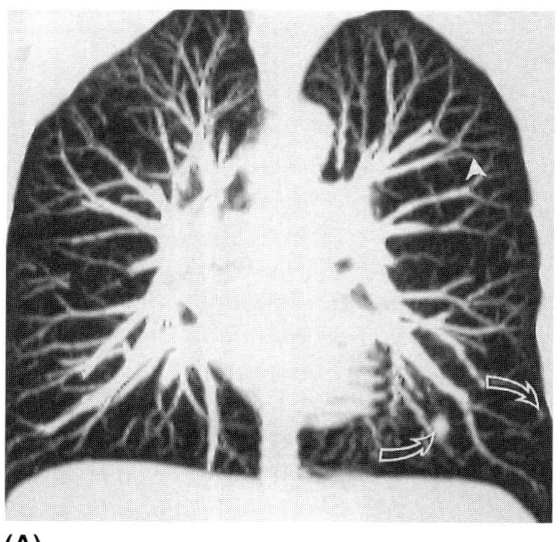

(A)

(B)

Figure 13 Value of 2D multiplanar reconstruction images in lung nodule detection. (A) Coronal reconstruction maximal intensity projection image shows two small lung nodules in left lower lobe (curved open arrows). Note excellent visibility of peripheral vessels (arrowhead) and lack of significant artifact except for pulsation artifacts adjacent to left heart border. (B) Axial image from original CT dataset shows the larger of the two left lower lobe lung nodules (curved open arrow). This nodule was initially overlooked on the axial image but was readily detected on the reconstructed images.

spectively choosing appropriately thin collimation images from the original dataset (Fig. 14). In contrast, with single-detector CT, high-quality reconstructions require prospective use of thin collimation or additional imaging acquisitions with thin collimation images. The latter results in increased scan time and additional radiation exposure.

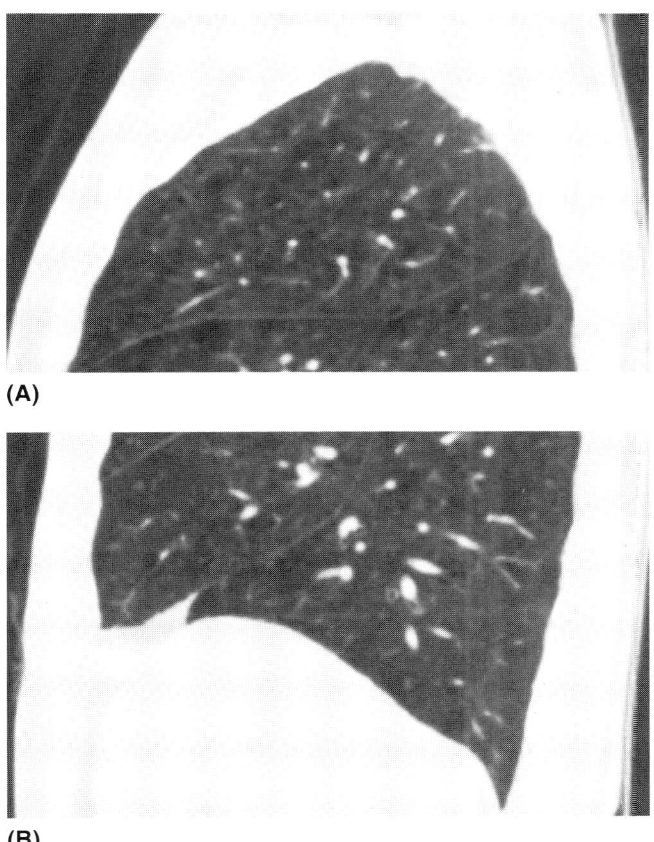

Figure 14 Sagittal reconstruction images of the right lung in an emphysema patient with marked dyspnea. Scanning was performed in two separate acquisitions (A and B) due to patient's very limited breath-hold ability. The use of 1.25-mm collimation (a nearly isotropic volumetric scan) results in multiplanar reconstruction images with comparable spatial resolution to the original axial images (not shown). Note the presence of diffuse centrilobular emphysema and focal apical scarring posteriorly.

At present, the range of benefits of this feature are just beginning to be explored. For example, preliminary data suggest a role in the assessment of patients with suspected diffuse lung disease, who are traditionally imaged exclusively with noncontiguous high-resolution CT images. For example, Mastora et al. [18] recently employed simultaneous reconstruction of contiguous 5-mm and noncontiguous 1-mm (high-resolution) images in the assessment of 86 patients undergoing MHCT evaluation for diffuse lung disease. These authors found that the contiguous 5-mm-thick sections provided additional diagnostic information in 13% of cases, most often by detecting lung nodules that were not evident on the high-resolution CT study.

E. Combining the Strengths of Multidetector Helical Computed Tomography: Increased Flexibility of Imaging

MHCT allows for considerable flexibility in CT imaging. One can combine the various strengths of MHCT in any number of ways to yield varying combinations of improved speed, resolution, and signal-to-noise ratio. For example, in a given case, one can simultaneously decrease the slice width by 50% (improved spatial resolution), increase the table speed by 50% (improved speed), and increase the milliamperes by 30% (decreased image noise) [4].

IV. LIMITATIONS OF MULTIDETECTOR HELICAL COMPUTED TOMOGRAPHY

Despite the many advantages of MHCT, one should be aware of the relative limitations of this emerging technology. The combination of narrow collimation and a large area of coverage (e.g., CT angiography studies) can result in very large data sets that are not practical to view on standard films. Such data sets are ideally viewed in a ''filmless'' environment with cineviewing at a workstation. Moreover, the cost of filming such large data sets can be prohibitive. Subsequently, many departments have chosen either to only film selected images or to completely forego producing hardcopy images. Even in a ''filmless'' PACS environment, however, this new technology may create challenges regarding how best to manipulate and store the large amount of data generated by MHCT studies. Rubin has recently proposed several alternative visualization techniques in order to tackle the ''data explosion'' produced by MHCT studies [19]. Before such alternative techniques can be introduced into daily practice, we will have to await the development of substantial improvements in automated processing, processing speed, and user interface [19].

Other relative limitations of MHCT include the increased complexity of imaging protocols, the increased importance of proper timing for optimal enhancement in vascular studies, and the potential to increase the radiation dose, depending on the specific scanning parameters employed. With regard to radiation exposure, if MHCT is performed with equal slice thickness to single-detector CT, MHCT actually results in a slightly decreased dose to the patient due to better dose efficiency of the detector; however, this advantage is lost or reversed if thinner slices are routinely employed with MHCT [6]. Importantly, preliminary investigations suggest that one may perform MHCT of the lungs with a ''low-dose'' technique for some clinical indications [20]. Future research in this area is necessary.

V. CONCLUSION

MHCT is an important advancement in helical CT technology and provides increased capability and flexibility of thoracic imaging with CT. Compared to single-detector helical CT, MHCT offers the opportunity to increase scanning speed, improve spatial resolution, improve signal-to-noise ratio, simultaneously create thin and thick sections, and perform higher quality reconstruction images. By fully understanding the principles of MHCT, one can tailor CT individual examinations in order to optimize image quality. To date, the greatest advantage of MHCT is in the area of CT angiography. However, this emerging technology will likely improve all aspects of thoracic CT imaging.

REFERENCES

1. Leung AN. Spiral CT of the thorax in daily practice: optimization of technique. J Thoracic Imag 1997; 12: 2–10.
2. Kalender WA, Seissler W, Klotz E, Vock P. Spiral volumetric CT with single-breath-hold technique, continuous transport, and continuous scanner rotation. Radiology 1990; 176:181–183.
3. Hu H, He HD, Foley WD, et al. Four multidetector-row helical CT: image quality and volume coverage speed. Radiology 2000; 215:55–62.
4. Kopecky KK, Buckwalter KA, Sokiranski R. Multi-slice CT spirals past single-slice CT in diagnostic efficacy. Diag Imag 1999; 4:36–42.
5. Klingenbeck-Regn K, Schaller S, Flohr T, et al. Subsecond multi-slice computed tomography: basics and applications. Eur J Radiol 1999; 31:110–124.

6. Rigauts H. A one year experience with the multislice helical CT. J Belge Radiol 1999; 82:273–276.
7. Rydberg J, Buckwalter KA, Caldemeyer KS, Phillips MD, Conces DJ, et al. Multisection CT: scanning techniques and clinical applications. Radiographics 2000; 20:1787–1806.
8. Rubin GE, Shiau MC, Schmidt AJ, et al. Computed tomographic angiography: historical perspective and new state-of-the-art using multi detector-row helical computed tomography. J Comput Assist Tomogr 1999; 23(suppl 1):83–90.
9. Rubin GD, Shiau MC, Leung AN, et al. Aorta and iliac arteries: single versus multiple detector-row helical CT angiography. Radiology 2000; 21:670–676.
10. Kachelrieß M, Ulzheimer S, Kalender WA. ECG-correlated image reconstruction from subsecond multi-slice spiral CT scans of the heart. Med Phy 2000; 27: 1881–1902.
11. Remy-Jardin M, Remy J, Bahaie F, et al. Clinical value of thin collimation in the diagnostic workup of pulmonary embolism. Am J Radiol 2000; 175:407–411.
12. Patel S, Kazerooni EA, Gross BH. Optimization of small pulmonary artery visualization for pulmonary embolism detection with multidetector CT (abstr). Radiology 1999; 213:471.
13. Nishi J, Kadota M, Yamashita Y, et al. Detection of small lung nodules: the value of retrospective thin slice reconstruction and cine viewing with a multidetector helical CT system (abstr). Radiology 2000; 217:384.
14. Fleischmann D, Rubin GD, Paik DS, et al. Stair-step artifacts with single versus multiple detector-row helical CT. Radiology 2000; 216:185–196.
15. Boiselle PM, Rosen MP, Raptopoulos V. Comparison of CT pulmonary angiography image quality on single and multidetector CT scanners (abstr). 2001 American Roentgen Ray Society Meeting, Seattle, WA, May 2001.
16. Koyama M, Johkoh T, Tomiyama N, et al. Coronal multiplanar reconstruction images from whole lung thin-section CT by multidetector-row CT: differential diagnosis of chronic interstitial pneumonia (abstr). Radiology 2000; 217:383.
17. Eibel R, Tuerk T, Huber AM, et al. Multi-slice thoracic CT for detection of pulmonary nodules: a study on coronal and sagittal STS-MIPs and MPRs (abstr). Radiology 2000; 217:384.
18. Mastora I, Remy-Jardin MJ, Masson P, et al. Multidetector CT imaging of diffuse lung disease: clinical impact of simultaneous reconstruction of contiguous thick and HRCT sections (abstr). Radiology 2000; 217:384.
19. Rubin GD. Data explosion: the challenge of multidetector-row CT. Eur J Radiol 2000; 36:74–80.
20. Tack DM, Bailly J, Muller P, et al. Low dose helical multidetector chest CT in routine practice (abstr). Radiology 2000; 217:383.
21. Simon M, Boiselle PM, Choi JR, et al. Paddle-wheel CT display of pulmonary arteries and other lung structures: a new imaging approach. Am J Radiol. 2001; 177:195–198.

5

CT Fluoroscopy: Use for Thoracic Interventional Procedures

Charles S. White
University of Maryland School of Medicine
Baltimore, Maryland

I. INTRODUCTION

Recent improvements in computed tomography (CT) technology have led to the introduction of CT continuous imaging, also known as real-time CT or CT fluoroscopy. Compared to conventional guidance techniques, CT fluoroscopy may facilitate percutaneous needle and pleural drainage procedures. Computed tomographic fluoroscopy has also proved useful for a newer application, guidance of transbronchial biopsy.

II. COMPUTED TOMOGRAPHY FLUOROSCOPY: TECHNICAL SPECIFICATIONS

Computed tomographic fluoroscopy was first introduced for clinical use in Japan in 1993. The first North American scanner installation was in 1994 and the U.S. Food and Drug Administration approved its use in 1996 [1]. Currently, five vendors provide CT fluoroscopic capability. Our clinical experience has been with the Toshiba Xpress/SX Aspire CI System (Toshiba Medical Systems, Tokyo, Japan).

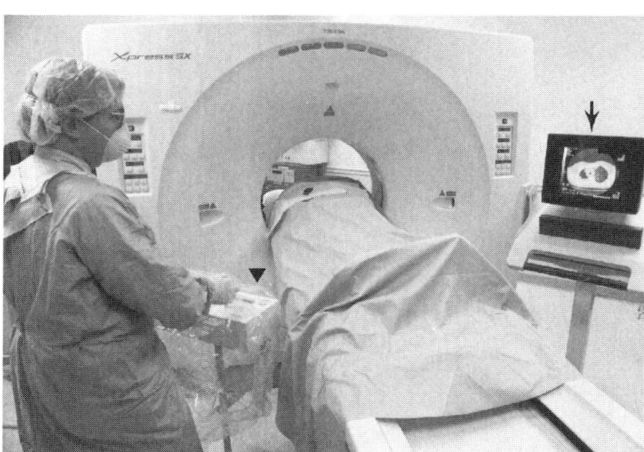

Figure 1 Photograph of the CT fluoroscopy suite that demonstrates the integrated monitor (arrow), control panel (arrowhead), and gantry. Note the sterile cover over the control panel that permits the radiologist to operate the CT fluoroscopy system and manipulate the catheter without compromising sterile technique. (From Ref. 15).

Fluoroscopic CT employs slip-ring technology and can be adapted for use with multislice CT [2,3]. Real-time visualization is accomplished with a fast parallel processor system that permits management of large quantities of data and allows for real-time reconstruction in a 256 × 256 matrix. On our system, after collection and processing of the first 360° of data, each subsequent 60° of data (0.17 sec) are added to the existing data and replace the oldest 60° of data. The first image is displayed 1.17 sec after initiation of CT fluoroscopy. As a result of continuous updating, six images are displayed per second, each reflecting an accumulation of 1 sec of data. The rapid updating of images imparts a real-time effect. A maximum of 100 sec of continuous CT fluoroscopic imaging can be performed and 800 sec of raw data can be stored on the hard drive.

A control panel and monitor are located in the scanning room and can be moved freely to allow the radiologist, wearing a standard fluoroscopic lead apron for protection, to acquire and view CT images optimally without leaving the scanning room (Figs. 1 and 2). The control panel allows selection of the laser light and adjustment of table position, height, and gantry angle. Movement of the table is accomplished with either a joystick on the control panel or a manual sliding mode, which permits the operator to slide the table freely. A button on the control panel or a foot-pedal identical to that used for routine fluoroscopy allows activation of real-time imaging.

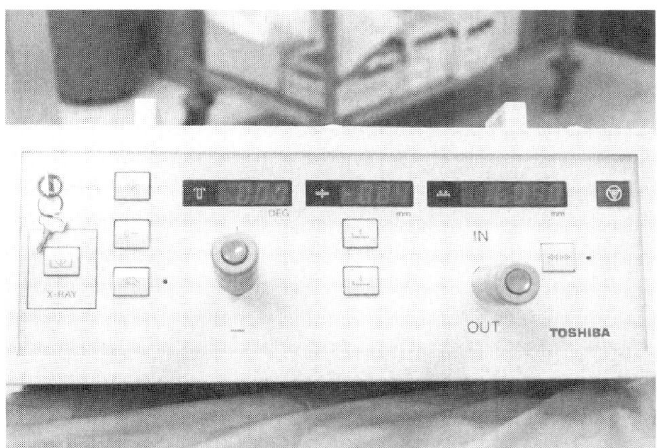

Figure 2 Computed tomographic fluoroscopy control panel. The left joystick adjusts gantry angle and the right joystick controls table movement. Additional functions include power, laserlight, localizer, table height, free-hand sliding mode table position, and emergency weight-off switch.

By placing sterile drapes on the control panel and the foot of the table, the radiologist can view and perform the entire procedure without assistance. Alternatively, an assistant can operate the monitor and table.

Radiation dosimetry is an important consideration when using CT fluoroscopy. Typical radiation dose factors are 80–120 kVp and 30–50 mA/sec. Adjustments are made for the size of the patient and the area being imaged. In the lungs the high contrast between aerated lung and lung abnormalities may permit reduced dose parameters. A dedicated filter allows reduction of dose by 50% compared to that of conventional CT. Absorbed skin dose using a body phantom approximates 20 cGy for an exposure of 50 sec using 120 kVp and 50 mA. Most interventional thoracic procedures require less than 3 min of CT fluoroscopic time [3].

III. PERCUTANEOUS NEEDLE ASPIRATION—CONVENTIONAL IMAGE-GUIDANCE TECHNIQUES

Percutaneous needle aspiration was first reported in the late 1800s. The image-guided approach for sampling lung nodules came into widespread use in the 1960s [2]. Conventional fluoroscopy was the initial technique used for guidance. It is widely available and rapidly performed and allows direct visualization of the nodule during sampling. The use of a C-arm or biplane fluoroscopy permits improved ease of biopsy. Based on several studies, the accuracy of fluoroscopically guided biopsy is 61 to 97% [5].

Conventional fluoroscopy remains the guidance technique of choice in some practices, but it is not suitable for every lesion. Small nodules may be difficult or impossible to identify on orthogonal projections. Using conventional fluoroscopy, the accuracy for biopsy of lesions 2 cm or greater is 80% compared to 60% for lesions less than 1 cm [6]. Even lesions larger than 1 cm may be difficult to visualize and low-density or indistinct nodules often are difficult to identify. Another important limitation of conventional fluoroscopy is that some nodules may be superimposed on normal thoracic structures such as the ribs, hila, or mediastinum. In some instances, biopsy using fluoroscopic guidance may not be advisable if the nodule is adjacent to a major cardiovascular structure such as the aorta [7]. Bullous areas of lung cannot always be recognized on conventional fluoroscopy.

Several investigators have reported the use of ultrasound to assist in thoracic biopsy [8,9,10]. Advantages of ultrasound include real-time imaging, portability, and lack of ionizing radiation. The development of high-resolution, high-frequency probes with dedicated biopsy ports has facilitated use of this technique. However, sonography is limited by attenuation of the beam as it traverses air-filled lung, obscuring nodules that are deep in the lung. Overall, less than 50% of lung masses are accessible to ultrasound guidance [6]. Ultrasound is best reserved for use in biopsy of pulmonary nodules that abut the pleural surface.

Standard CT is the most commonly used guidance technique for lung biopsy. It is safe and accurate. Sensitivity is greater than 90% for malignant lesions but is somewhat lower for benign nodules [11]. For small lung nodules (1.5 cm or less), CT is the optimal technique. Two studies have reported biopsy success rates of 74 and 93%, respectively, for small nodules [12,13]. The advantage of CT in guiding the needle toward the nodule and documenting placement of the needle tip within the nodule is particularly important for small nodules.

The main limitation of standard CT is the lack of real-time visualization. With standard CT, it may take multiple attempts to localize the nodule and direct the needle toward the nodule. After each needle movement, the biopsy team must exit the scanning room while the new needle position is documented. Respiratory motion may alter the relationship of the nodule to ribs and other structures and compensatory adjustment can be difficult in the absence of real-time observation. Finally, sampling of the lesion cannot be observed in real time to assure that the needle tip is within the nodule. The use of CT fluoroscopic guidance overcomes many of the limitations of conventional techniques.

IV. COMPUTED TOMOGRAPHY FLUOROSCOPY OF LUNG NODULES: OPERATOR TECHNIQUE

Two operator approaches may be used to perform CT fluoroscopic biopsy: real-time or interrupted real-time technique. With the real-time technique, the operator directly visualizes the procedure on the CT fluoroscopic monitor while the needle is being advanced and during biopsy of the nodule itself. The particular type of needle chosen is dependent on several factors, including lesion size and location, the sample size desired, and the risk of pneumothorax. If the radiologist wishes to view in real time the needle while it is being advanced or during sampling of the nodule, a modification of technique is required to avoid exposure of the hand holding the needle to the primary radiation beam. A needle holder can be used to overcome this problem. One prototype needle holder is an acrylic resin screw lock device with a handle that projects perpendicular to the needle shaft. The handle on the prototype is somewhat short, placing the operator's hand near the primary radiation beam. A simpler method that increases the distance of the operator's hand from the primary beam is to use a 25-cm metallic sponge forceps to grasp and direct the needle during real-time biopsy [14].

The real-time technique allows coordination of table movement and patient respiration, permitting optimal visualization of the lesion. For instance, a simple maneuver is to slide the table by hand as the patient suspends respiration such that the lesion is brought into view during real-time imaging (couch-top sliding method). Biopsy can then be performed [2]. A related advantage of the real-time technique is the ability to document needle location within the nodule concurrent with aspiration [2]. Movement of the needle into the nodule (puncturing) or ''pushing away'' of the nodule (balloting) by the needle can thus be observed.

The second basic approach to CT fluoroscopic biopsy has been termed the interrupted real-time technique [1]. With the interrupted real-time technique, needle advancement and nodule biopsy are performed without direct visualization but are rapidly confirmed after each needle movement using a short duration of fluoroscopy, often while allowing the patient to remain in the gantry. When the needle tip is clearly identified within the nodule, aspiration is typically done blindly.

Advantages of the interrupted real-time technique compared to the real-time technique described previously include the increased distance of the operator from the primary beam, thus reducing exposure from radiation and obviating the use of a needle holder [15]. The improved tactile sensation provided by direct contact with the biopsy needle during aspiration is also viewed favorably by many operators. A further advantage is that more involved biopsy techniques such as use of a coaxial approach or an automated biopsy device (gun) are facilitated with the interrupted real-time method. A potential disadvantage of the interrupted real-time method is that visualization of complications of the procedure (e.g., pneumothorax) might be delayed. However, this delay is minimal compared to conventional CT. With either the real-time or interrupted real-time technique, tilting of the gantry may prove useful to align the needle and nodule [1].

V. COMPUTED TOMOGRAPHY FLUOROSCOPY TO GUIDE NEEDLE BIOPSY: EARLY CLINICAL RESULTS

To date, the published clinical experience with the use of CT fluoroscopy to guide percutaneous needle biopsy is limited. Katada et al. reported results of 60 CT fluoroscopic procedures in 57 patients, including 36 with CT guided intrathoracic procedures [2]. In their study, the target nodule was punctured on the first attempt in 83% of patients and the average number of passes for all nodules was 1.3.

A diagnostic result was obtained in 32 (97%) of the 33 patients who underwent lung biopsy, including 17 malignant and 15 benign lesions. In a single subcentimeter lesion, the needle tip was visualized in the nodule but there was insufficient tissue for diagnosis. Mean procedure time was 54 min (range 24–139 min) with an average of 74 sec of CT fluoroscopy time for each puncture.

The authors reported 17 (47%) complications among the 36 thoracic procedures, including 16 pneumothoraces and 1 episode of hemoptysis. Five of the pneumothoraces were treated either with aspiration of pleural air or placement of a chest tube. Katada et al. concluded that the real-time capability of the CT fluoroscopy permitted reduction in the number of needle punctures required to perform the biopsy and provided substantial overall advantages over standard CT [2].

The early experience at our institution with CT fluoroscopy to assist in the biopsy of small pulmonary nodules has also been promising [16].

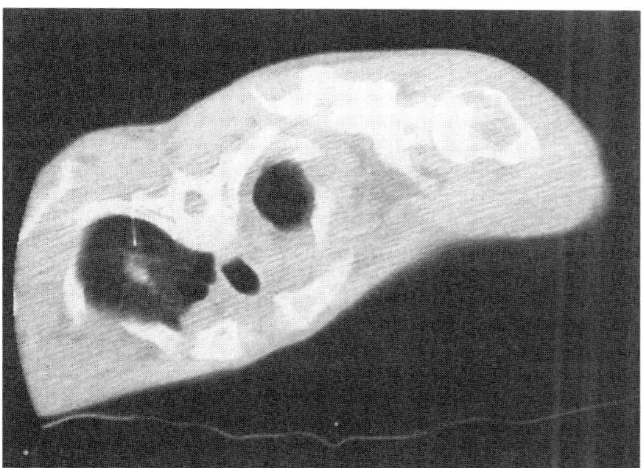

Figure 3 A 56-year-old man with a 1.5-cm left upper lobe nodule. Image from a CT fluoroscopy segment shows the needle traversing an area of bullous disease posterior to the nodule. Adenocarcinoma was diagnosed.

We performed procedures on 17 patients with nodules less than or equal to 1.5 cm. In most cases, we used a coaxial biopsy technique and the interrupted real-time CT fluoroscopy method (Figs. 3 and 4). Similar to standard CT, the needle tip was routinely identified by its characteristic low-density artifact.

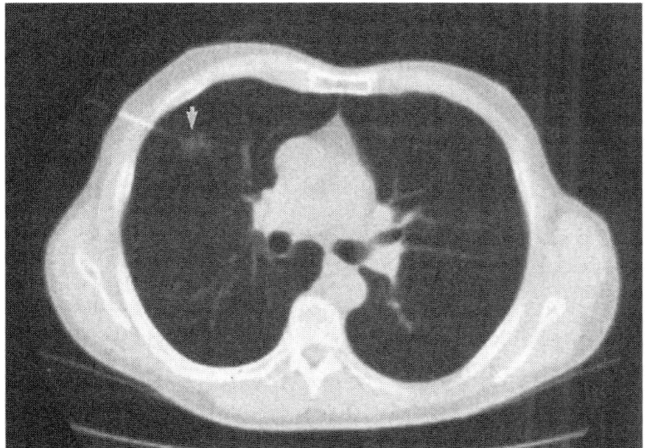

Figure 4 A 65-year-old man with a 1.0-cm right upper lobe nodule. Computed tomography fluoroscopic image shows needle sampling this ill-defined lesion (arrow). A diagnosis of non-small-cell cancer was established.

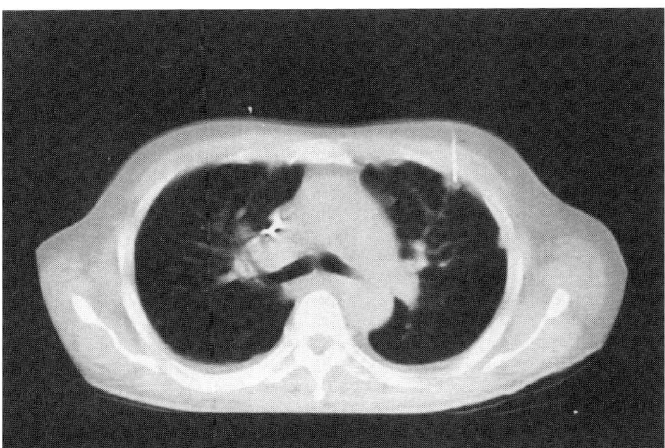

Figure 5 A 67-year-old man with multiple left pleural nodules. Image from a CT fluoroscopic segment demonstrates the needle within a pleural nodule. Biopsy showed sarcoidosis. (From Ref. 14).

We established a diagnosis in 16 (94%) of the 17 lesions, including 11 malignant and 5 benign nodules. A single nondiagnostic biopsy occurred in a patient with small, deep lesion who requested discontinuation of the procedure after a single pass. At surgery, this lesion proved to be a non-small-cell carcinoma. The mean lesion depth in our patients was 7 cm. The mean number of passes was 2.5. The average fluoroscopic time for each puncture was 103 sec. Good image quality was obtained using dose factors of 30 mA and 120 kVp. The mean room time was 91.5 min.

Complications in our series occurred in nine patients (53%), including eight with pneumothorax and one with hemoptysis. Two patients with pneumothoraces required chest tube drainage.

Both our series and that of Katada et al. had similar rates of success and complications [2,16]. It is likely that the increased number of punctures required and higher use of CT fluoroscopic time in our series is due to the smaller size of the nodules. Other factors such as the need for supervision of a resident or fellow may also have contributed.

In addition to use in the lung, we have found CT fluoroscopy guidance valuable to biopsy lesions in the pleura (Fig. 5) and paraspinal region, mediastinum, and chest wall. In these areas, the real-time capability may permit the operator to avoid traversing lung parenchyma.

VI. COMPUTED TOMOGRAPHY FLUOROSCOPY FOR GUIDING PERCUTANEOUS BIOPSY: SUMMARY

Like standard CT, CT fluoroscopy has the advantages of excellent spatial resolution, a wide field of view, optimal imaging of air-filled structures, limited dependence on the operator to obtain images of excellent quality, and the ability to position the biopsy needle in the imaging plane. However, the main limitation of standard CT is the necessity to acquire a series of images after each movement of the biopsy needle, requiring the radiologist to exit the scanning room for each acquisition. Image reconstruction and display take further time. The additional time requirement predisposes to patient movement that may change the needle position in relation to anatomic landmarks. Computed tomographic fluoroscopy obviates leaving the scanning room because images are available in the room and are observed in real time [16].

Potential advantages of the real-time capability of CT fluoroscopy include the ability to visually time the biopsy puncture more easily with the phase of respiration and to allow specific placement of the needle at the edge of the lesion, thereby avoiding the necrotic center of a lesion. If the real-time technique is used, the nodule may be seen to be pushed away (balloted) by the needle, allowing a more rapid puncture technique.

The real-time imaging of CT fluoroscopy permits rapid diagnosis of complications. Hemorrhage is often recognized around the nodule after biopsy and a needle track is often observed upon withdrawal of the needle. A minority of patients develop frank hemoptysis. Pneumothoraces are recognized quickly so that appropriate management can be instituted in a timely fashion (Fig. 6).

An important subjective advantage of CT fluoroscopy is the increased peace of mind that the rapid image display provides for the radiologist. The short time interval between movement of the needle and knowledge of its location and any complications can substantially decrease operator stress related with the procedure.

It is a subjective impression that CT fluoroscopy allows biopsy to be performed more rapidly, particularly for small nodules. However, it is important to recognize that no study has directly compared the duration of procedures done with standard CT and CT fluoroscopy to ascertain if there is a decrease in procedure time with the latter. Likewise, other purported advantages of CT fluoroscopic guidance have not yet been compared directly to those of standard CT.

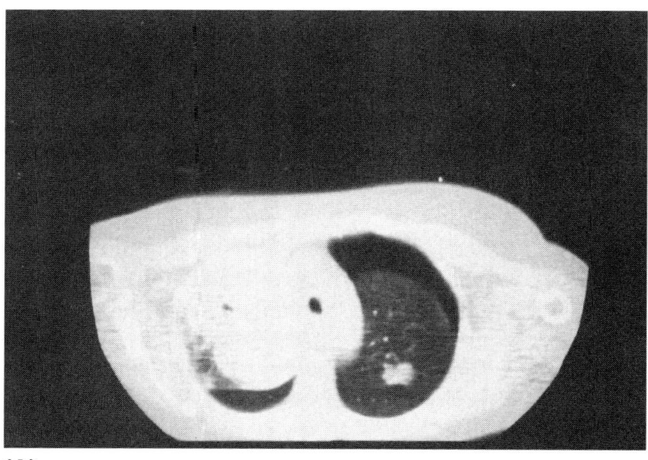

(A)

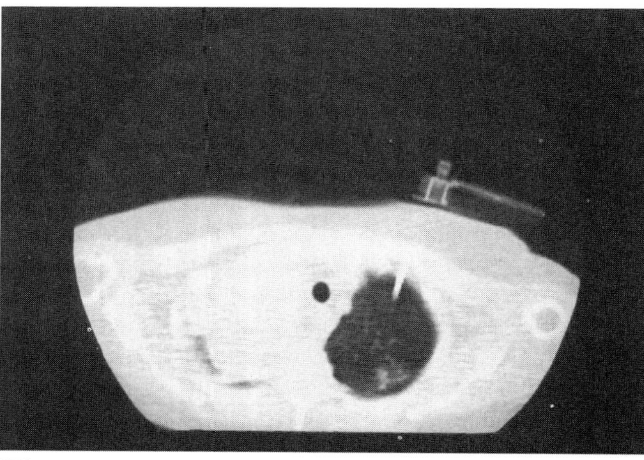

(B)

Figure 6 A 61-year-old man after successful left upper lobe biopsy. (A) Computed tomographic fluoroscopy image obtained moments after the needle was withdrawn shows a moderate anterior pneumothorax. (B) Computed tomography fluoroscopic image after placement of a pleural drainage catheter shows appropriate location of the catheter and minimal residual pneumothorax (From Ref. 14.)

VII. COMPUTED TOMOGRAPHY FLUOROSCOPY: GUIDANCE OF INTRATHORACIC DRAINAGE PROCEDURES

Imaging-guided chest drainage procedures can be used to guide treatment of simple or complicated pleural effusions, pneumothoraces, or mediastinal fluid collections. While pleural collections have been conventionally treated with closed-tube thoracostomy, imaging-guided treatment has been more successful in loculated pleural collections that have septations or substantial fibrinous content. Drainage tubes used in imaging-assisted guidance are generally more easily manipulated, smaller in caliber, and better tolerated [17]. One disadvantage of these tubes is that their smaller size predisposes to obstruction of the tube by debris. Techniques for imaging-guided insertion include fluoroscopy, ultrasound, and CT [18–22].

VIII. CHOICE OF IMAGING MODALITY

Factors involved in the selection of the appropriate imaging modality for drainage of intrathoracic collections include the type of thoracic collection, patient condition, and operator preference.

The size, location, and contents of the collection are important considerations when selecting the appropriate imaging modality for guidance. In general, ultrasound is most useful for drainage of large free-flowing fluid collections [23]. Ultrasound is the technique of choice because it lacks ionizing radiation, is portable, and allows real-time visualization of needle/catheter placement. At times, a free-flowing collection may be less accessible with CT guidance because the fluid collection tends to move to a dependent position in the chest. In contrast, complex fluid collections and air often cannot be distinguished from underlying aerated lung parenchyma by ultrasound and may require CT guidance [24]. The location of the fluid collection may dictate the choice of modality. Structures that are located along the proposed route of catheter insertions such as internal mammary vessels or mediastinal structures may be easier to visualize and avoid with CT guidance. Patients whose condition precludes cessation of respiration present a challenge to the placement of large drainage catheters. The real-time capability of CT fluoroscopy allows visualization of the safest approach to the fluid collection throughout the respiratory cycle, which is important in preprocedure planning [15].

IX. PLEURAL AND MEDIASTINAL FLUID COLLECTIONS

In our practice, pleural drainage is most often requested to treat parapneumonic effusions or empyema [15]. Up to 50% of patients with pneumonia have accompanying pleural fluid [25,26,27]. Most transudates or simple parapneumonic effusions respond to the antibiotic therapy. Drainage catheter placements are usually indicated for exudative effusions, either infectious, inflammatory or neoplastic.

The technical approach for pleural drainage using CT fluoroscopy is similar to that for standard CT. Computed tomographic fluoroscopy is used to plan the site of access to the pleural collection for optimal drainage and patient comfort. The procedure may be performed either in real time by watching the catheter advance into the pleural fluid collection or with an interrupted real-time technique as described for percutaneous needle biopsy. We have generally used the interrupted real-time technique because it minimizes exposure to the operator's hands. Using this technique, the needle is advanced in a stepwise manner with short applications of fluoroscopic CT to document the needle/catheter path [15]. The radiologist stays in the CT suite and initiates CT fluoroscopy via the control panel. The patient remains within the gantry during needle placement.

Either a trocar or modified Seldinger technique may be used to reach the pleural collection. As a rule, large pleural fluid collections that are not adjacent to critical vascular structures may be accessed using a single stick method with a 12–14 French catheter. We typically use hydrogel-coated catheters to easily traverse fascial planes [11].

A modified Seldinger technique is advantageous for more complex collections. In these patients, a Seldinger entry needle is placed into the thoracic collection with CT fluoroscopic guidance. A guidewire is inserted through the needle and coiled. The tract is expanded with serial dilators, after which a pigtail catheter is passed over the guidewire. Dilatation and catheter placement are performed using CT fluoroscopic observation. Documentation of catheter placement with reorientation, as necessary, is achieved with direct CT fluoroscopic observation (Fig. 7). Complex, loculated fluid collections may necessitate multiple drainage catheters or intrapleural fibrinolytic therapy.

Mediastinal fluid collections are uncommon but technically challenging. Potentially drainable mediastinal collections include postoperative abscesses, especially those following esophageal surgery (Fig. 8); infected mediastinal duplication cyst; lymphocele; Boerhaave syndrome; or mediastinal pancreatic pseudocyst [7]. Image-guided mediastinal drainage is technically similar to

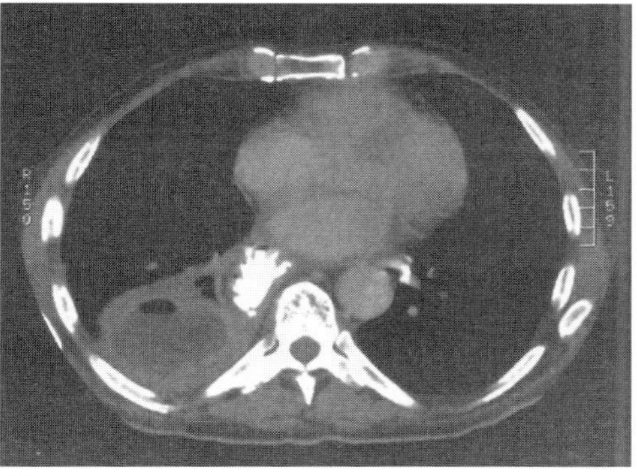

(A)

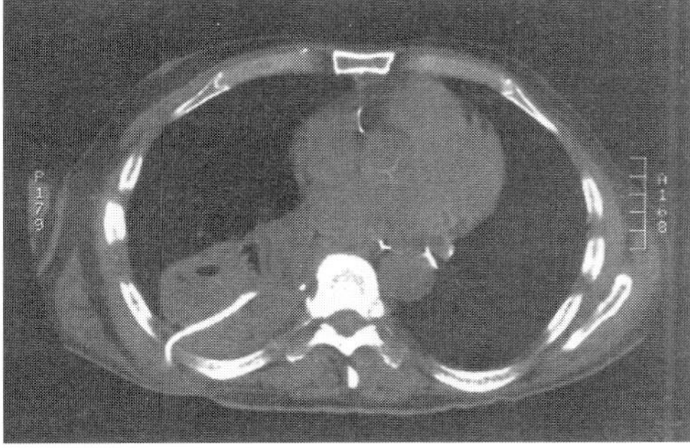

(B)

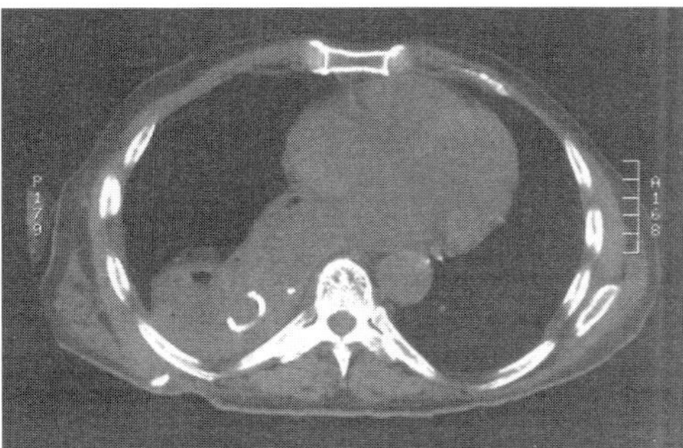

(C)

Figure 7 A 63-year-old man with a loculated pleural collection after esophagectomy with pull-up. (A) Computed tomography scan shows the collection lateral to the contrast filled pull-up. (B and C) Computed tomography fluoroscopic images show placement of pigtail catheter within the fluid collection.

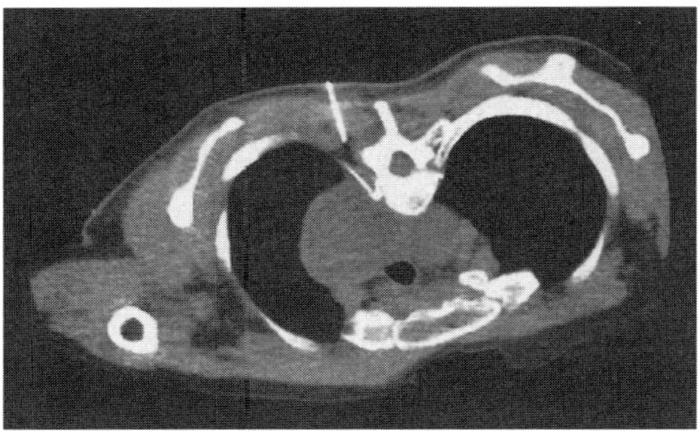

(A)

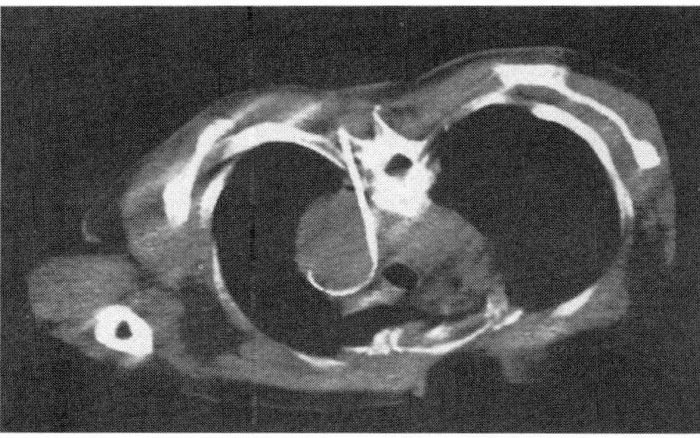

(B)

Figure 8 A 77-year-old man with mediastinal mucocele 2 years after an emergency esophagectomy for perforation. (A) Initial CT fluoroscopy performed for placement of a 19-gauge Seldinger needle into the fluid collection. (B) After guidewire placement and tract dilatation, a pigtail catheter is confirmed to be in the collection.

pleural drainage procedures but particular care is necessary to avoid laceration of the internal mammary and mediastinal vessels, the heart, and other mediastinal structures. For this reason, CT fluoroscopy offers a substantial advantage over other imaging techniques because it permits real-time observation of the needle path [15].

X. PNEUMOTHORAX

Closed-tube thoracostomy placement is useful for a large, symptomatic, or expanding pneumothorax. Radiologists may be required to place a chest tube for treatment of a pneumothorax induced by percutaneous needle biopsy. Small bore drainage tubes are also placed using image guidance for loculated pneumothoraces in patients who have undergone lung volume reduction surgery or lung transplantation or in patients receiving ventilation for the adult respiratory distress syndrome.

The technique for CT-fluoroscopic-guided pneumothorax drainage is similar to that for drainage of pleural fluid collections. Smaller caliber chest tubes (8–10 French) are usually effective but a 12–14 French tube may be required for large pleural tears. Placement of pneumothorax tubes varies based on pneumothorax location and the patient's functional status. Computed tomography fluoroscopy is particularly useful to guide catheter placement in complex, loculated pneumothoraces (Figs. 9 and 10) [15].

In our study of 20 patients who had a variety of pleural and mediastinal collections, we found CT fluoroscopic assistance to be quite valuable, particularly in patients who were not compliant with breathing instructions and those with small or loculated collections [15]. The average procedure time in our case series was 32 min and the average CT fluoroscopic time was 143 sec.

XI. COMPUTED TOMOGRAPHY FLUOROSCOPY: GUIDANCE OF TRANSBRONCHIAL NEEDLE ASPIRATION

Fiber-optic bronchoscopy with transbronchial needle aspiration (TBNA) is useful to sample mediastinal nodes and to diagnose central parenchymal lesions. Enlarged lymph nodes occur in lung cancer and other neoplasms, tuberculosis, and sarcoidosis. Knowledge of nodal status is particularly important to stage lung cancer. Mediastinoscopy, mediastinotomy, and thoracoscopy are valuable surgical techniques for mediastinal staging, but are invasive and require general anesthesia. TBNA with bronchoscopic guidance necessitates only conscious sedation and can be used to sample abnormal lymph nodes that are in proximity to an airway [28,29,30]. Subcarinal and paratracheal lymph nodes are most accessible. One important disadvantage of TBNA compared to surgical techniques is that the target node is not visible through the bronchoscope unless erosion of mucosa has occurred. Typically, the bronchoscopic needle is directed through the airway based on findings identified on the preprocedure CT scan in conjunction with distortions of the airway encountered during the procedure.

Conventional fluoroscopy with a C-arm is often used to guide TBNA in the lung and improve the yield of the procedure. However, in the mediasti-

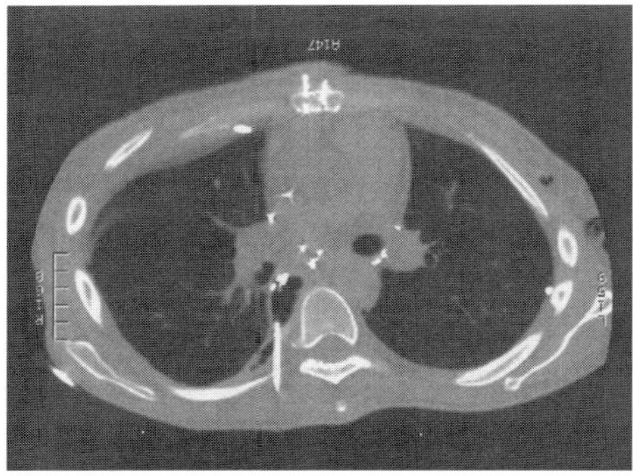

(A)

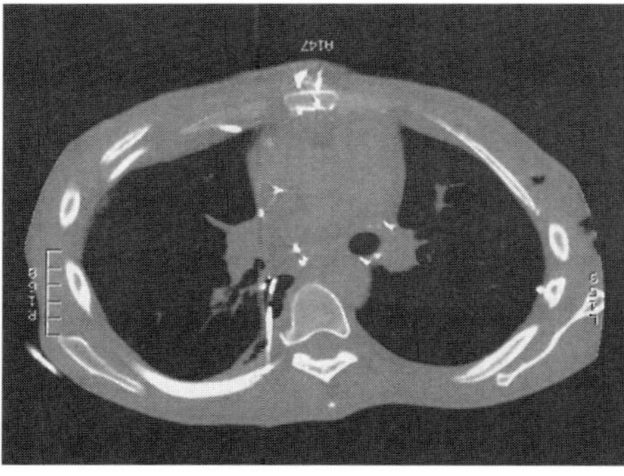

(B)

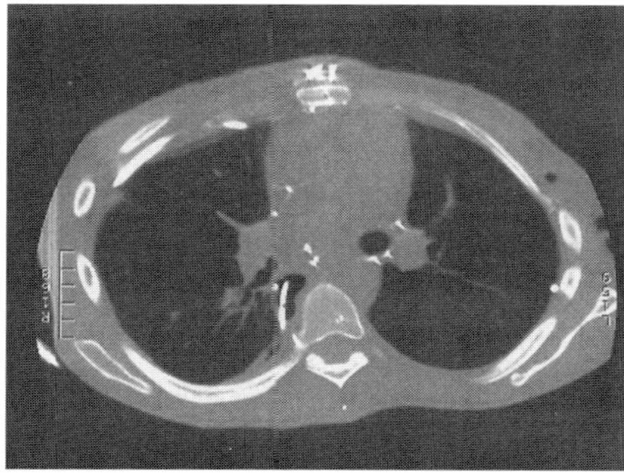

(C)

Figure 9 A 29-year-old man with small residual airspace after undergoing bilateral lung transplantation. (A–C) Images after CT fluoroscopic placement images show the catheter in the right paraspinal airspace. Airspace subsequently resolved.

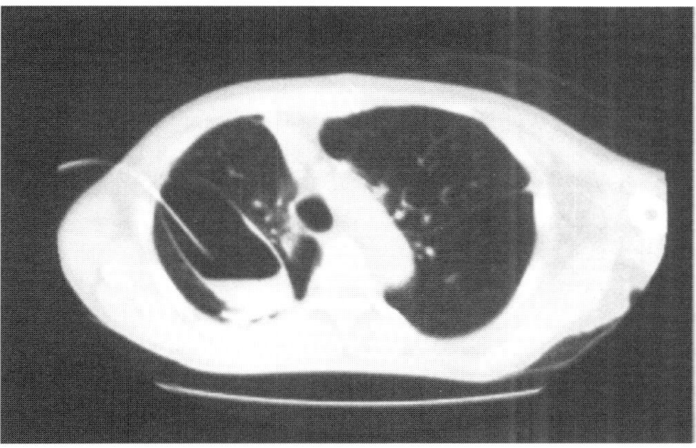

(A)

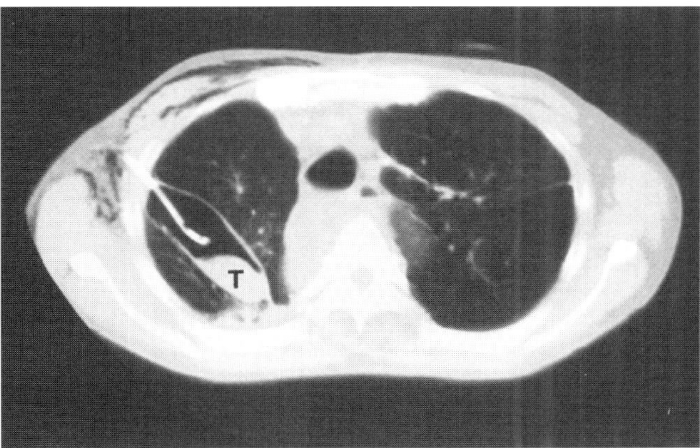

(B)

Figure 10 A 59-year-old man with shortness of breath and a loculated pneumothorax after lung volume reduction surgery. A modified Seldinger technique was used to access the major fissure through a 1-cm pleural window. (A) Computed tomography fluoroscopic image after decompression with an 8 Fr catheter. The patient was symptomatically improved although the pneumothorax is incompletely drained. (B) Computed tomography fluoroscopic image after exchanging the 8 Fr catheter for a 12 Fr catheter with improved decompression. This tube was placed to 20-cm H_20 Pleur-Evac suction. Note thrombus (T), which was present prior to imaging intervention. (From Ref. 15.)

num this technique is limited because of the overlap of structures produced by the two-dimensional fluoroscopic display. In many instances, therefore, the enlarged mediastinal lymph node is not distinguishable using conventional fluoroscopy.

The inability of fluoroscopy to provide adequate visualization of the target lymph node has hindered wider use of TBNA in the mediastinum. Moreover, it has fueled the perception that TBNA is difficult and potentially dangerous and should be performed only by expert bronchoscopists. Most series have indicated that the technique is inferior to that of comparable surgical procedures, with sensitivity ranging from 37 to 90% [29,30]. Thus, many patients who might be candidates for bronchoscopically directed TBNA are referred for surgery. Ultrasound can be used to guide mediastinal TBNA but is limited by the variable image quality and the need for a bronchoscopist with substantial training in ultrasound [31].

Standard CT can also provide image guidance for TBNA [32]. In a study by Rong et al. a successful diagnosis was obtained in 60% of cases of mediastinal adenopathy that underwent TBNA with standard CT guidance. However, similar to its use for percutaneous needle biopsy, standard CT is cumbersome because of the substantial time delay that occurs while the appropriate slice position is identified, the technologist prescribes the sequence and scans the patient, and image reconstruction occurs. During this period, the position of the bronchoscope must remain stationary for several minutes. This time-consuming sequence of events must be repeated for each adjustment of the bronchoscope.

The real-time capability of CT fluoroscopy is valuable in guiding TBNA [33]. Using CT fluoroscopy, each movement of the bronchoscope can be verified quickly on the in-room monitor. The bronchoscopic needle is imaged after it is planted in the airway to assure that it is directed toward the intended biopsy site. Once the needle has been advanced, CT fluoroscopy is used to ascertain that the needle is in the target lesion. Complications such as pneumothorax or hemorrhage are documented quickly.

For lung lesions that are approached nonsurgically, the location of the abnormality determines whether percutaneous needle biopsy or TBNA is chosen. Peripheral lesions, especially those that are subpleural in location are most easily sampled using percutaneous needle biopsy. Central lesions, and particularly those in which a bronchus extends into the lesion, are optimally diagnosed using bronchoscopy with TBNA.

Large central lesions are diagnosed routinely using bronchoscopy with or without fluoroscopic guidance, particularly if a visible endobronchial component is present. Smaller lesions without an endobronchial component are more challenging and require fluoroscopic guidance, ideally with the assistance of a C-arm. However, conventional fluoroscopy is limited in guiding TBNA if the lung nodule is very small. Moreover, it is often difficult to determine the anteroposterior relationship between the needle tip and the nodule even if biplane fluoroscopy is available. Computed tomographic fluoroscopy combines the advantages of the real-time display of conventional fluoroscopy with a three-dimensional display format such that the bronchoscopist can be confident that the needle is in the lesion.

XII. COMPUTED TOMOGRAPHY FLUOROSCOPY TO ASSIST TRANSBRONCHIAL NEEDLE ASPIRATION: CLINICAL EXPERIENCE

We have performed over 35 procedures using CT-fluoroscopic-assisted TBNA, of which the first 27 have been analyzed [34]. The 27 patients were selected to undergo this procedure either because of previous unsuccessful biopsy ($n = 7$) or on the basis of a clinical decision that the lesion might be too small or inaccessible to reach if TBNA was done in a blind fashion. Only one patient had undergone prior percutaneous needle biopsy.

Among the 27 procedures, 15 were performed for mediastinal nodes and 12 for lung nodules or areas of consolidation. The average mediastinal lesion size was 1.7 cm (Fig. 11). Metastatic non-small-cell cancer was diagnosed in 4 patients, and small-cell cancer in 2. Of 9 patients with nondiagnostic TBNA, 2 patients underwent thoracotomy that showed non-small-cell cancer and thus had a falsely negative TBNA. Of the remaining 7 patients, 2 underwent mediastinoscopy that proved negative, 2 had stable adenopathy on a 1-year follow-up, and 3 did not return for further evaluation. Overall, a correct diagnosis was obtained in 10 of 12 (83%) of patients who had clinical or pathological follow-up.

The average size of the lung lesions was 2.2 cm (Figs. 12 and 13). A correct diagnosis was obtained in 8 of the 12 (67%) lung lesions. Diagnoses included non-small-cell cancer in 4 patients with lung nodules and invasive aspergillosis or pseudomonas in 3 immunocompromised patients with ill-defined consolidation. In 1 patient with a nondiagnostic TBNA, a lung nodule resolved spontaneously, suggesting a true negative result. Another patient with a nondiagnostic TBNA proved at surgery to have a metastatic spindle cell sarcoma. In the remaining 3 patients with nondiagnostic TBNA, all of whom

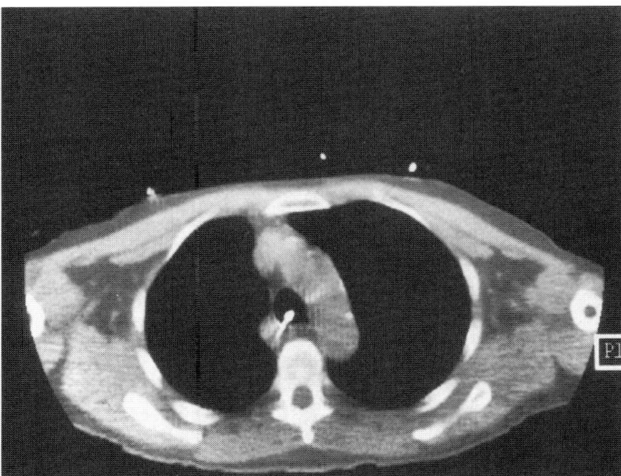

Figure 11 A 72-year-old man with a right paratracheal node. Computed tomography fluoroscopic image shows bronchoscopic needle in the node. Diagnosis was non-small-cell lung cancer.

were immunocompromised, the lesions resolved with broad-spectrum antibiotics, suggesting an infectious etiology.

The mean total room time was just over 1 hr. The mean time from first to last use of the CT scanner is 49 min. The average duration of use of CT fluoroscopy was 228 sec. Using dose factors of 120 kVp and 30–50 mA, the approximate range of skin entrance doses for the procedures was 8–52 cGy.

We identified several factors that may have led to failure to diagnose mediastinal or lung lesions by TBNA. In most cases of mediastinal adenopathy, the target lymph nodes were only slightly enlarged (1–2 cm) and therefore constitute a subset that is known to be difficult to diagnose by TBNA. Several of the patients had undergone previous TBNA using conventional fluoroscopic guidance with indeterminate results, so that obtaining a specific diagnosis was probably more difficult than in a typical population referred for bronchoscopy. In several instances, the needle was convincingly documented in the lesion but no definitive pathologic result was obtained, suggesting sampling error (Fig. 14). In certain patients with mediastinal or lung abnormalities, the bronchoscope could not be manipulated in a manner that would allow the needle to reach the lesion despite imaging guidance.

Two TBNA needle sizes are available (19 and 21 gauge). The 19-gauge aspiration needle was more easily visualized with CT fluoroscopy than the

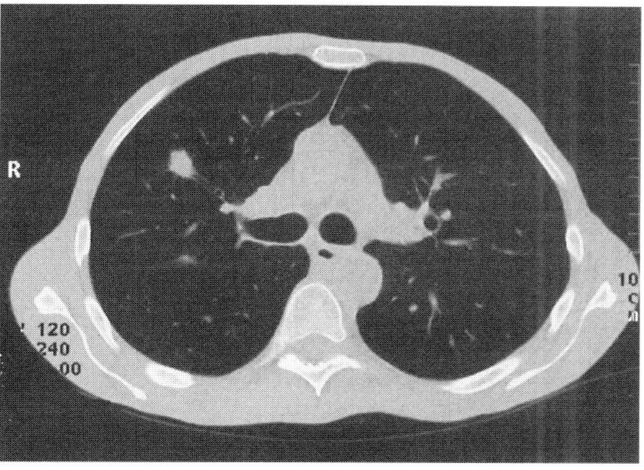

(A)

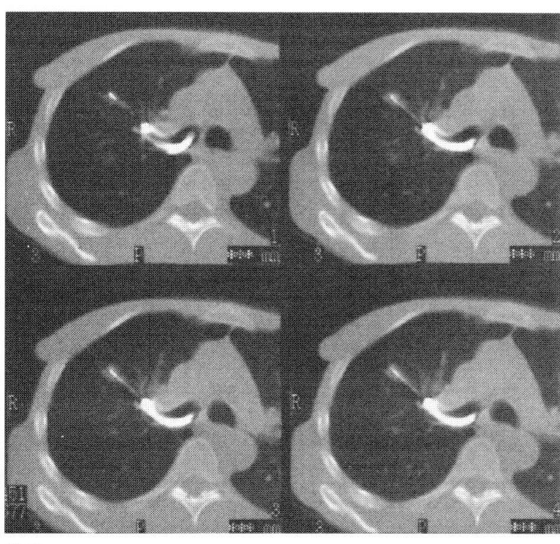

(B)

Figure 12 A 41-year-old man with right upper lobe nodule. (A) Computed tomography scan filmed on lung windows shows a bronchus extending into the lesion. (B) Multiple images from a CT fluoroscopic acquisition show the needle within the nodule. Windowing adjusted for best display. Diagnosis was non-small-cell lung cancer.

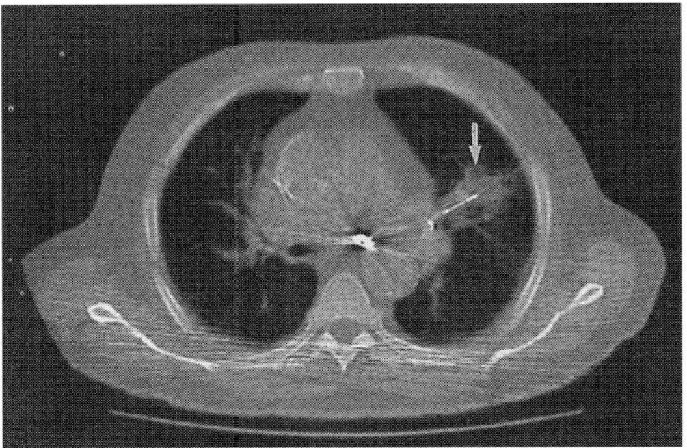

Figure 13 A 74-year-old man with acute leukemia and left upper lobe consolidation. Computed tomography fluoroscopic image shows the needle within the infiltrate (arrow). A diagnosis of aspergillus was made.

21-gauge needle, although both were readily visible. The bronchoscope itself created substantial artifact but this artifact did not interfere with identification of the needle position. The bronchoscopic artifact was not present when subcarinal nodes were aspirated because the needle and bronchoscope were not in the same imaging plane. Malposition of the biopsy needle in the lung was easily observed on CT fluoroscopy (Fig. 15). Often, the needle was identified in the incorrect subsegment and CT fluoroscopy proved valuable to direct

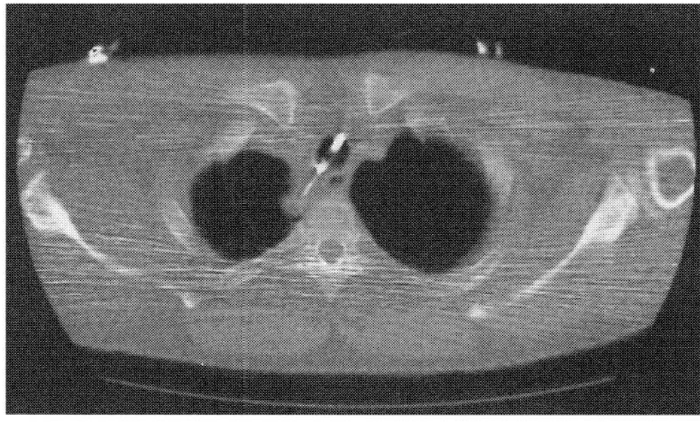

Figure 14 A 49-year-old man with a right apical medial nodule. Computed tomography fluoroscopic image shows needle apparently within lesion. Only benign bronchial cells were aspirated. Lesion subsequently proved to be lung cancer.

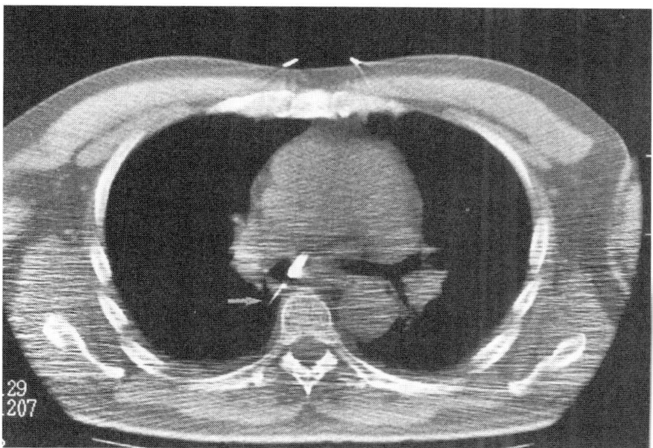

Figure 15 A 66-year-old man with a subcarinal lymph node. Computed tomography fluoroscopic image shows inadvertent needle placement in the lung (arrow). No complication occurred.

repositioning. Complications such as pneumothorax and hemorrhage in the lung could be detected rapidly although neither occurred in our series. Other investigators have reported a favorable experience using CT fluoroscopy to guide TBNA of mediastinal lymph nodes [35].

Our experience indicates that CT fluoroscopy may increase the diagnostic accuracy of inexperienced bronchoscopists by showing the precise location of the bronchoscopic needle in relation to the target lesion. By increasing confidence in needle placement, it may also encourage more experienced bronchoscopists to use a large gauge needle when necessary.

XIII. MISCELLANEOUS APPLICATIONS

The real-time guidance capability of CT fluoroscopy may also be used for other thoracic procedures that are difficult to perform with nonfluoroscopic CT. For example, we have used CT fluoroscopy to evaluate the extent of a sinus tract in a patient with a draining cutaneous wound by observing the distribution of injected contrast in real time (Fig. 16). Computed tomographic fluoroscopy, because of its real-time capability, may be valuable

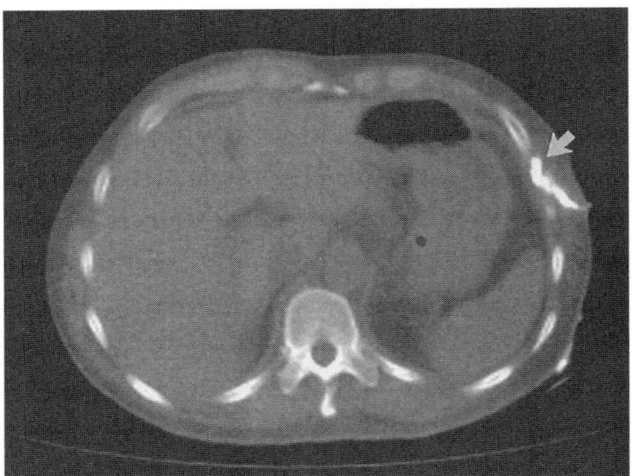

Figure 16 A 41-year-old man with a draining sinus tract. Computed tomography fluoroscopic image acquired immediately after contrast injection shows contrast pooling adjacent to the left lateral ribs (arrow). No fistula was identified.

to assess other dynamic processes such as tracheomalacia and sternal instability.

REFERENCES

1. Daly B, Templeton PA. Real-time CT fluoroscopy: evolution of an interventional tool. Radiology 1999; 211:309–315.
2. Katada K, Kato R, Anno H, Ogura Y, Koga S, Ida Y, Sato M, Nonomura K. Guidance with real-time CT fluoroscopy: early clinical experience. Radiology 1996; 200:851–856.
3. Daly BD, Regits W, White DE. Patient radiation dose during CT fluoroscopy guided percutaneous interventional procedures. Radiology 1999; 213:285.
4. Dahlgren S, Nordenstrom B. Transthoracic Needle Biopsy. Stockholm: Almqvist and Wiksell, 1966:1–32.
5. Weisbrod GL. Transthoracic needle biopsy. World J Surg 1993; 17:705–711.
6. Klein JS, Zarka MA. Transthoracic needle biopsy. Radiol Clin North Am 2000; 38:235–266.
7. Van Sonnenberg E, Casola G, Ho M, Neff CC, Varney RR, Wittich GR, Christensen R, Friedman PJ. Difficult thoracic lesions: CT guided biopsy experience in 150 cases. Radiology 1988; 167:457–461.
8. Hsu WH, Chiang CD, Hsu JY, Kwan PC, Chen CL, Chen CY. Ultrasound-guided

fine-needle aspiration biopsy of lung cancers. J Clin Ultrasound 1996; 24:225–233.
9. Ulrik Knudsen D, Moller Nielsen S, Hariri J, Christensen J, Kristensen S. Ultrasonographically guided fine-needle aspiration biopsy of intrathoracic tumors. Acta Radiologica 1996; 37:327–331.
10. Yang PC, Luh KT, Sheu JC, Kuo SH, Yang SP. Peripheral pulmonary lesions: ultrasonography and ultrasonically guided aspiration biopsy. Radiology 1985; 155:451–456.
11. Westcott JL. Direct percutaneous needle aspiration of localized pulmonary lesions; results in 422 patients. Radiology 1980; 137:31–35.
12. Li H, Boiselle PM, Shepard JO, Trotman-Dickenson B, McLoyd TC. Diagnostic accuracy and safety of CT-guided percutaneous needle aspiration biopsy of the lung; comparison of small and large pulmonary nodules. Am J Radiol 1996; 167: 105–109.
13. Westcott JL, Rao NR, Colley DP. Transthoracic needle biopsy of small pulmonary nodules. Radiology 1997; 202:97–103.
14. White CS, Meyer CA, Templeton PA. CT fluoroscopy for thoracic interventional procedures. Radiol Clin North Am 2000; 38:303–322.
15. Meyer CA, White CS, Wu J, Futterer SF, Templeton PA. Real-time CT fluoroscopy: usefulness in thoracic drainage. Am J Radiol 1998; 171:1097–1101.
16. Templeton PA, Fournier RS, Meyer CA, White CS, Futterer SF. Lung nodules 1.5 cm or smaller in size: CT biopsy success using CT fluoroscopy. Radiology 1997; 205:174.
17. Ulmer JL, Choplin RH, Reed JC. Image-guided catheter drainage of the infected pleural space. J Thorac Imaging 1991; 6:65–73.
18. Klein J, Schultz S. Interventional chest radiology. Curr Probl Diagn Radiol 1992; 21:219–268.
19. Patz EF, Goodman PC, Erasmus JJ. Percutaneous drainage of pleural collections. J Thorac Imaging 1998; 13:83–92.
20. Stavas J, vanSonnenberg E, Casola G, Wittich GR. Percutaneous drainage of infected and noninfected thoracic fluid collections. J Thorac Imaging 1987; 2: 80–87.
21. Tarver RD, Conces DJ. Interventional chest radiology. Radiol Clin North Am 1994; 32:689–709.
22. VanSonnenberg E, Wittich GR, Goodacre BW, Zwischenberger JB. Percutaneous drainage of thoracic collections. J Thorac Imaging 1998; 13:74–82.
23. O'Moore PV, Mueller PR, Simeone JF, Saini S, Butch RJ, Hahn PF, Steiner E, Stark DD, Ferrucci JT Jr. Sonographic guidance in diagnostic and therapeutic interventions in the pleural space. Am J Radiol 1987; 149:1–5.
24. Silverman SG, Mueller PR, Saini S, Hahn PF, Simeone JF, Forman BH, Steiner E, Ferrucci JT. Thoracic empyema: Management with image-guided catheter drainage. Radiology 1988; 169:5–9.
25. Light RW, Girrard WM, Jenkinson SG, George RB. Parapneumonic effusions. Am J Med 1980; 69:507–512.

26. Tartle DA, Potts DE, Sahn SA. The incidence and clinical correlates of parapneumonic effusions in pneumococcal pneumonia. Chest 1978; 74:170–173.
27. Bartlett JG, Finegold SM. Anaerobic infections of the lung and pleural space. Am Rev Respir Dis 1974; 110:56–77.
28. Hashim SW. Baue AE, Geha AS. The role of mediastinoscopy and mediastinotomy in lung cancer. Clin Chest Med 1982; 3:353–359.
29. Utz JP, Patel AM, Edell ES. The role of transcarinal needle aspiration in the staging of bronchoscopic carcinoma. Chest 1993; 104:1012–1016.
30. Wang KP. Transbronchial needle aspiration and percutaneous needle aspiration for staging and diagnosis of lung cancer. Clin Chest Med 1995; 16:535–552.
31. Shannon JJ, Bude RO, Orens JB, Becker FS, Whyte RI, Rubin JM, Quint LE, Martinez FJ. Endoscopic ultrasound-guided needle aspiration of mediastinal adenopathy. Am J Resp Crit Care Med 1996; 153:1424–1430.
32. Rong F, Cui B. CT scan directed transbronchial needle aspiration biopsy for mediastinal nodes. Chest 1998; 114:36–39.
33. White CS, Templeton PA, Hasday JD. CT-assisted transbronchial needle aspiration: usefulness of CT fluoroscopy. Am J Radiol 1997; 169:393–394.
34. White CS, Weiner EA, Patel P, Britt EJ. Transbronchial needle aspiration: guidance with CT fluoroscopy. Chest 2000; 118:1630–1638.
35. Goldberg SN, Raptopoulous V, Boiselle PM, et al.. Improved diagnostic yield for transbronchial mediastinal lymph node biopsy using CT-fluoroscopic guidance. Radiology 2000; 216:764–767.

6
Update of High-Resolution CT of the Lungs

Jannette Collins
University of Wisconsin Medical School
Madison, Wisconsin

I. INTRODUCTION

Superimposition of structures limits the sensitivity, specificity, and diagnostic accuracy with which acute and chronic lung disease can be diagnosed with chest radiography [1]. It can be difficult to determine if a chest radiograph is normal or abnormal. High-resolution computed tomography (HRCT) is not always abnormal in patients with respiratory symptoms but is abnormal in the majority of patients with significant lung disease. Compared with chest radiography, HRCT better defines the morphology and distribution of disease, correlates better with histologic findings, is more accurate in defining chronicity of disease, and is a better guide for biopsy.

Reviewed in this chapter are the basic principles of HRCT, current applications and indications for the use of this technique, and the characteristic HRCT findings associated with a variety of pulmonary disorders. Special emphasis is placed on interpretation of the mosaic attenuation pattern and HRCT features of bronchiolar disease.

II. HIGH-RESOLUTION COMPUTED TOMOGRAPHY TECHNIQUE

Coining of the term ‘‘HRCT’’ is credited to Todo et al. [2], who described the potential use of this technique in the Japanese literature in 1982. The first reports of HRCT in English date to 1985 [3–5], and since that time, HRCT techniques have undergone dramatic development.

Compared with conventional CT, HRCT requires use of the thinnest collimation possible (1–1.5 mm), image reconstruction with a high-spatial frequency (‘‘bone’’) algorithm, increased kVp (120–140) or mA (140–240; mAs 240–400), and use of the largest matrix size available (512 × 512). A range of recommended window settings are available, reflecting differences in personal preference. What is important is that at least one consistent window setting be used. Window mean values ranging from -600 to -700 HU and widow width values ranging from 1000 to 1500 HU are appropriate [6].

With thicker collimation, volume averaging reduces the ability of CT to resolve small structures, such as branches of small airways or vessels, and slight increases or decreases in lung attenuation. Use of a high-spatial frequency algorithm reduces image smoothing and increases spatial resolution, making structures appear sharper. One drawback to this is increased visibility of noise, which can be offset somewhat by increasing the number of photons or scan time (milliamperes-seconds). Because increased scan times can result in increased motion artifacts, it is desirable to limit scan time to 1–2 sec. Increased kilovolts or milliamperes is desirable in large patients in whom noise is a bigger problem, always keeping in mind that increasing scan technique also increases the radiation dose to the patient. This is usually of little clinical concern since with HRCT, radiation is limited to a few thin scan levels. HRCT scanning at 10- 20-mm intervals results in 12 and 6%, respectively, of the radiation dose associated with conventional CT [7].

The ability of HRCT to resolve fine lung structures depends on their orientation relative to the scan plane [8]. Structures measuring 0.1 to 0.2 mm in thickness can be seen if they are largely oriented perpendicular to the scan plane and extend through the thickness of the scan plane, whereas similarly sized structures that are oriented horizontally within the scan plane will not be visible because of volume averaging with the air-filled lung, which occupies most of the thickness of the voxel. Normal interlobular septa, measuring 0.1 to 0.2 mm in thickness will occasionally be seen on HRCT. Bronchi or bronchioles measuring less than 2 to 3 mm in diameter and having a wall thickness of approximately 0.3 mm are usually invisible in the peripheral lung because they have courses that lie roughly in the plane of the scan.

Routine HRCT is obtained during suspended full inspiration with the patient supine. There is no consensus as to whether scans should be obtained at 1-, 2-, or 4-cm intervals, at three preselected levels or at one or two levels through the lower lungs. HRCT provides a sampling of lung anatomy and is therefore most useful in evaluation of diffuse lung disease, especially when performed in lieu of a conventional CT exam. When patients may have limited disease that manifests as small structures scattered throughout the lungs, such as with low profusion silicosis, HRCT may completely miss the disease. In these cases, HRCT should be performed in conjunction with conventional CT. In patients suspected of having interstitial disease that may be limited to the lung bases, such as asbestosis, HRCT should be performed with the patient in both supine and prone positions when supine images show dependent opacities (Fig. 1).

When patients are suspected of having airways disease, such as obliterative bronchiolitis or asthma, scans obtained during expiration should be obtained to detect air trapping. In normal patients, in most lung regions, lung parenchyma increases uniformly in attenuation during expiration, but in the presence of air trapping lung parenchyma remains lucent on expiration and shows little change in volume [9]. Expiratory HRCT can show air trapping in the absence of abnormalities on inspiratory images.

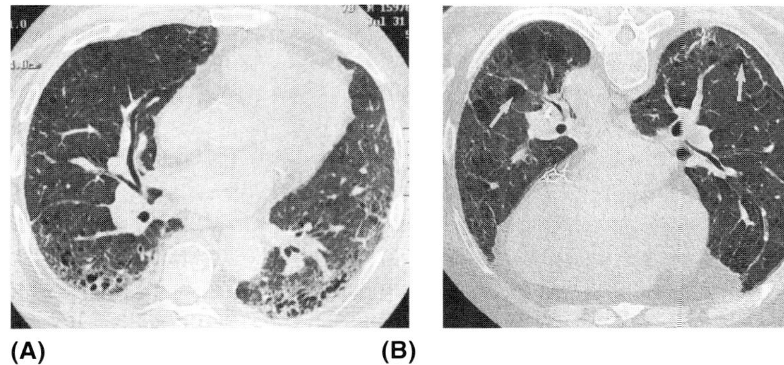

(A) (B)

Figure 1 Supine and prone HRCT. (A) Supine HRCT of a 78-year-old man with congestive heart failure and emphysema shows layers of small "cysts" in the dependent portions of the lungs, suggestive of honeycombing and pulmonary fibrosis. (B) Prone HRCT of the same patient in A 1 day later shows no evidence of honeycombing. There are scattered lucent areas (arrows) representing emphysema and scattered areas of linear atelectasis or scarring. There is decreased ground-glass opacification compared with A as a result of interval diuresis and decrease in pulmonary edema.

Table 1 Indications for the Use of HRCT

1. Unexplained dyspnea in a patient with suspected chronic diffuse infiltrative lung disease
2. Symptomatic patients with known exposures to inorganic dusts such as silica and asbestos, organic antigens, or drugs
3. Immunosuppressed patients with unexplained dyspnea or fever
4. Patients with unexplained hemoptysis
5. Patients with dyspnea or other respiratory symptoms and suspected airways or obstructive lung disease

III. SENSITIVITY AND SPECIFICITY OF HIGH-RESOLUTION COMPUTED TOMOGRAPHY IN THE DIAGNOSIS OF DIFFUSE INFILTRATIVE LUNG DISEASE

Over a hundred different causes of diffuse infiltrative lung diseases have been described, with a yearly incidence of 31.5 and 26.1 per 100,000 men and women respectively [10]. Chest radiographs are relatively inexpensive and easy to obtain and can answer many clinical questions without requiring further diagnostic imaging. However, it is well documented that chest radiographs are limited in both their sensitivity and specificity in patients with diffuse lung disease [11,12].

Up to 50% of patients with proven lung disease on HRCT have normal chest radiographs [13–15]. Both conventional CT and HRCT are more sensitive than chest radiography for detecting both acute and chronic diffuse lung diseases [16–21]. The sensitivity and specificity of HRCT for detecting pulmonary disease are approximately 94 and 96% compared with 80 and 82% for chest radiographs [12,22]. Because of its excellent sensitivity, HRCT can be used to detect lung disease in patients with normal or questionable radiographic abnormalities or who have symptoms or pulmonary function findings suggestive of acute or chronic diffuse lung disease (Table 1), to assess disease activity, and to guide biopsy procedures.

IV. DIAGNOSTIC PATTERNS OF DISEASE ON HIGH-RESOLUTION COMPUTED TOMOGRAPHY

HRCT findings can often be used to limit the differential diagnosis to a few possibilities or, in some cases, can be sufficiently characteristic (in the appro-

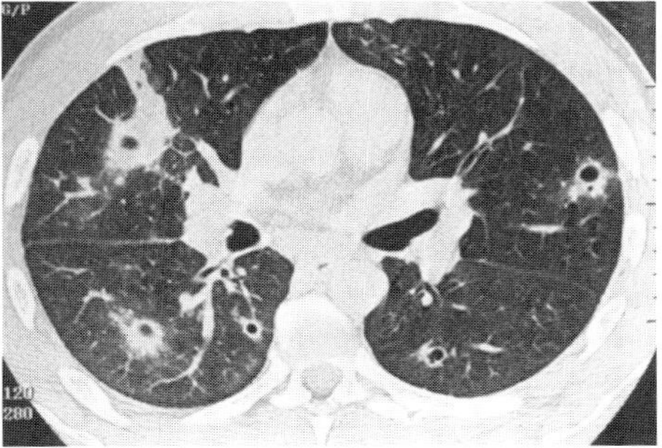

Figure 2 Septic emboli. HRCT of a 32-year-old man with positive blood cultures for *Staphylococcus aureus* shows characteristic cavitating nodules in a predominantly peripheral location.

priate clinical setting) to allow a specific or presumptive diagnosis in the absence of histologic verification (Figs. 2 and 3). Patchy and centrilobular (involving the center of the secondary pulmonary lobule) ground-glass opacities, in a patient with the appropriate exposure history and serologic tests, suggest the diagnosis of acute or subacute hypersensitivity pneumonitis [23] (Fig. 4). Abnormalities are found predominantly in the middle lung zones, and the lung bases are relatively spared.

Sarcoidosis is characterized by nonnecrotizing granulomas distributed

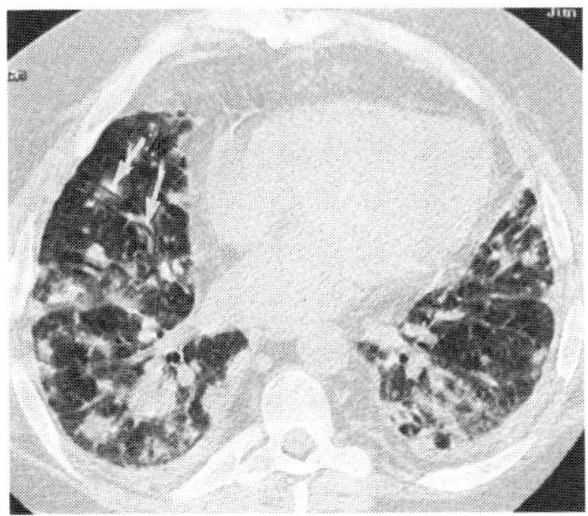

Figure 3 Posttransplant lymphoproliferative disease. HRCT of a 39-year-old man with a history of three renal transplants and on large doses of immunosuppressive drugs shows patchy areas of consolidation in a characteristic bronchovascular distribution. Note air bronchograms (arrows).

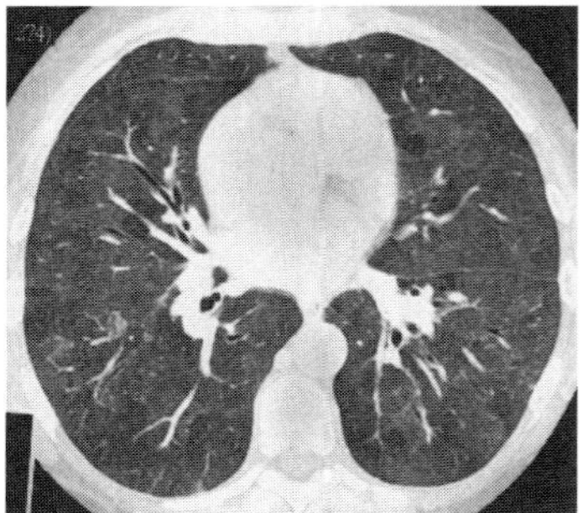

Figure 4 Acute hypersensitivity pneumonitis. HRCT of a 59-year-old woman with fever, chills, dyspnea on exertion, headache, minimal nonproductive cough, fatigue, crackles at the lung bases, and hypoxemia shows multifocal areas of ground-glass opacification in a centrilobular distribution. The patient's symptoms resolved while in the hospital but recurred when she went home, where she was exposed to her pet parakeets. Transbronchial biopsy specimen showed noncaseating granulomas and lymphocytes.

along the lymphatic pathways of the bronchovascular bundles and interlobular septa. The opacities tend to be nodular and predominate in upper and middle lung zones. In later stages, cicatricial changes result in architectural distortion and fibrotic areas of consolidation, with surrounding areas of emphysema, similar to the findings that can be seen in patients with complicated silicosis (Fig. 5). Eliciting an appropriate history of exposure to dusts can be helpful

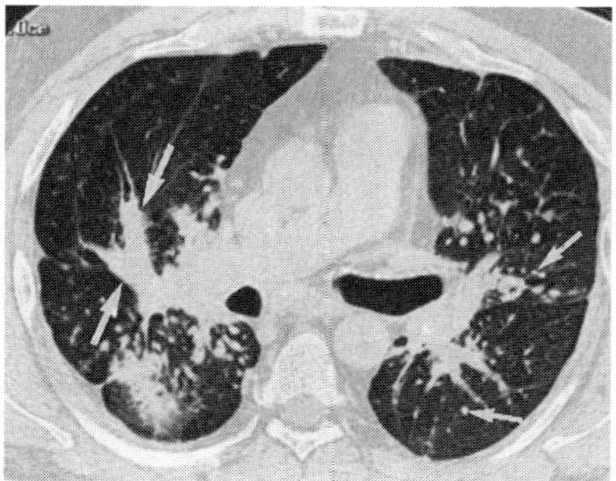

Figure 5 Complicated silicosis. HRCT of a 48-year-old man with a long history as a foundry worker shows numerous small nodules (small arrows) and bilateral conglomerate masses (large arrows) referred to as "progressive massive fibrosis." The same findings can also be seen in sarcoidosis.

in distinguishing the two diseases. In the appropriate clinical setting, classic findings of peribronchovascular (thickening of the axial interstitium surrounding the parahilar bronchi and vessels) and subpleural nodules, especially when associated with central airway abnormalities, should allow a confident diagnosis of sarcoidosis without needing biopsy in most cases [17,24–26].

HRCT of lymphangitic carcinomatosis is characterized by nodular thickening of the interlobular septa without cicatricial distortion of polygonal architecture. Distribution tends to be basilar and peribronchovascular nodularity is often present [27]. A unilateral distribution suggests primary bronchogenic carcinoma as the underlying tumor, as most other tumors result in bilateral lung involvement (Fig. 6).

Smooth subpleural and peribronchovascular thickening associated with increased thickness and number of visible interlobular septal lines without nodularity are characteristics of the interstitial abnormalities seen in pulmonary edema (Fig. 7). The abnormal opacities usually are predominant in the dependent portions of lung. Various degrees of consolidation and ground-glass opacification may be present when there is air-space edema, along with cardiac enlargement, vascular engorgement, and pleural effusions.

Lymphangioleiomyomatosis and pulmonary involvement in tuberous sclerosis are radiologically and pathologically identical. Both are characterized by proliferation of smooth muscle cells along bronchovascular bundles, lymphatics, and pulmonary veins. Numerous small parenchymal cysts are uniformly distributed throughout the lungs and are a characteristic finding on HRCT (Fig. 8) [28,29]. Additional findings that may not be evident on chest

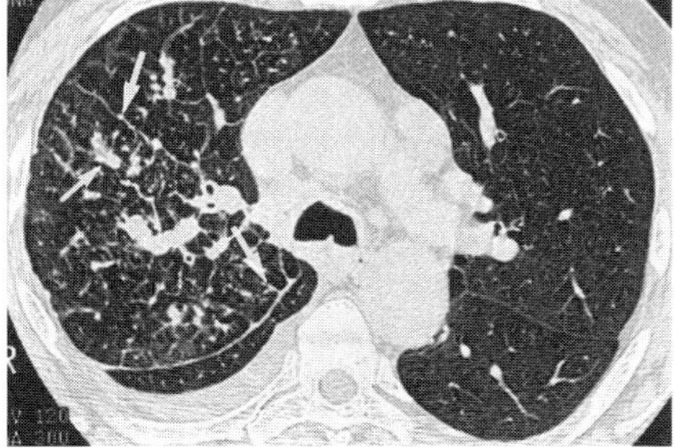

Figure 6 Lymphangitic carcinomatosis. HRCT of a 53-year-old man with large cell bronchogenic carcinoma and symptoms of cough and wheezing shows nodular thickening of the interlobular septa (large arrows) and bronchovascular bundles (small arrow). Unilateral involvement is characteristic of a primary bronchogenic carcinoma.

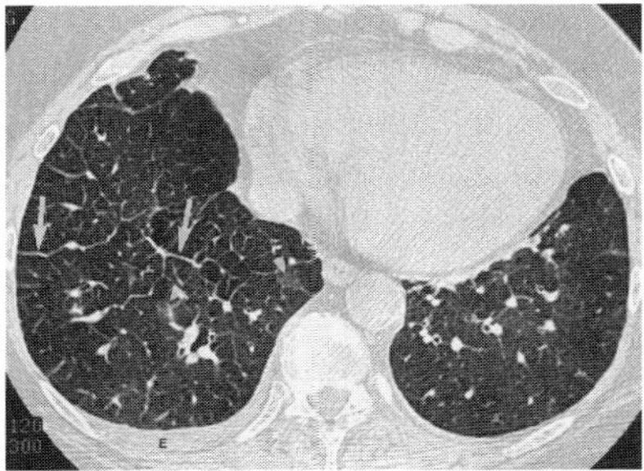

Figure 7 Pulmonary edema. HRCT of a 69-year-old woman shows smooth interlobular septal thickening (Kerley A and B lines, arrows), patchy ground-glass opacification (arrowheads), and a small right pleural effusion (E).

radiographs include pneumothorax, chylous pleural effusion, mediastinal lymphangiomyomatous adenopathy, and renal or hepatic angiomyolipomata.

The parenchymal disease of Langerhan's cell histiocytosis tends to have an upper lung predominance. Even when diffuse, the disease tends to spare the costophrenic angles. Cystic changes and nodules are the predominant HRCT finding (Fig. 9) [30]. Usually, small thin-walled, air-filled cysts or nodules are present. Nodules may progress to cavitated nodules to cysts to confluent cysts. The cysts seen on HRCT in patients with lymphangioleiomyomatosis can have a similar appearance but are generally not associated with nodular changes or an upper lung distribution. The HRCT cystic findings in Langerhan's cell

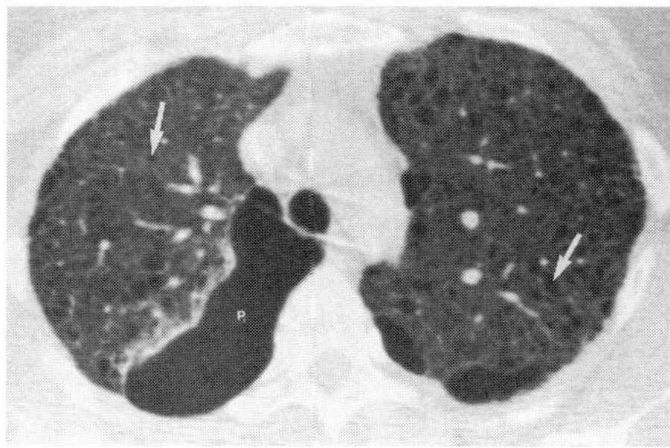

Figure 8 Lymphangioleiomyomatosis. HRCT of a 50-year-old woman with increasing shortness of breath and hemoptysis shows characteristic thin-walled cysts (arrows) with surrounding normal pulmonary architecture. Note pneumothorax on right (P).

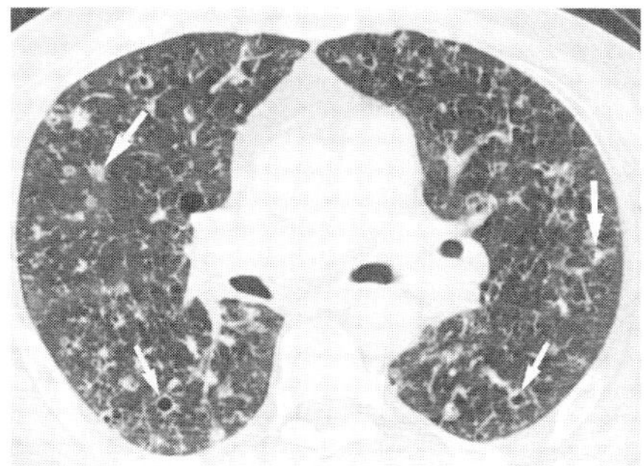

Figure 9 Langerhan's cell histiocytosis. HRCT of an adult male cigarette smoker shows characteristic combination of thin-walled cysts (small arrows) and nodules (large arrows). The upper and middle lungs were predominantly involved.

histiocytosis can also resemble bronchiectasis, but examination of serial sections can differentiate tubular from spherical structures. Cysts in lymphangioleiomyomatosis and Langerhan's cell histiocytosis do not have a peripheral distribution as they do in honeycomb cysts of pulmonary fibrosis.

HRCT findings have been shown to be highly accurate in diagnosing idiopathic pulmonary fibrosis or other causes of usual interstitial pneumonitis (UIP) [31]. UIP is the most common abnormal finding in patients with chronic progressive infiltrating lung disease. It is a histopathological term referring to a pattern of interstitial fibrosis that occurs in patients with various disorders, including idiopathic pulmonary fibrosis, asbestosis, rheumatoid arthritis, mixed connective tissue disease, and scleroderma. The patient's clinical presentation determines the specific diagnosis in these situations. HRCT is often useful in demonstrating the typical features of UIP: patchy reticular, honeycomb, and ground-glass opacities. The abnormalities have a distinctive bibasilar and subpleural distribution. HRCT can be used to assess response to steroid therapy. Patients with UIP who are found to have areas of ground-glass opacity in the absence of significant honeycombing or traction bronchiectasis are more likely to have a response to steroid therapy than are those with only honeycombing or linear or nodular opacities [32]. In the majority of patients who present with clinical features of idiopathic pulmonary fibrosis, the presence of predominately subpleural and bibasilar distribution of fibrosis on HRCT can be sufficiently characteristic to obviate biopsy (Fig. 10) [33,34].

HRCT of emphysema is characterized by bullae or small lucent areas (or both) without the well-defined walls one would expect to see with lung

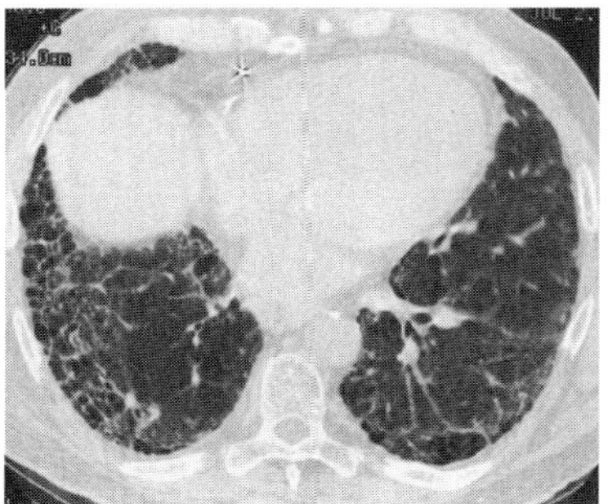

Figure 10 Usual interstitial pneumonitis. HRCT of a 74-year-old man with rheumatoid arthritis shows characteristic rows of small thick-walled cysts in a peripheral, bibasilar distribution.

cysts or honeycombing. HRCT can show changes of centrilobular, panacinar, paracicatricial, and paraseptal emphysema [35]. In some cases, HRCT may show that apparent diffuse infiltrative lung disease on chest radiographs is due to emphysema.

Less than 50% of patients with chronic eosinophilic pneumonia have the classic pattern of peripheral air-space disease involving the middle and upper lung zones on chest radiography [36]. HRCT, unlimited by superimposition of structures, can better display the peripheral distribution of consolidation and ground-glass opacities. The appearance can be identical to bronchiolitis obliterans organizing pneumonia (BOOP). However, in BOOP, bronchial wall thickening and dilatation are frequently found within the areas of consolidation. BOOP can also infrequently be characterized by a central distribution of disease without subpleural involvement.

Bronchiectasis is defined as irreversible dilatation of bronchi. The etiology is usually infectious and bronchiectasis is commonly associated with underlying airway obstruction as occurs with inspissated secretions in patients with cystic fibrosis. The diagnosis of bronchiectasis can be made on HRCT when airways are larger in diameter than the accompanying pulmonary arteries or when small airways are visualized in the periphery of the lungs or along the mediastinal pleural surface. With increasing grades of severity, bronchiectasis can appear smooth-walled (cylindrical), beaded (varicose), or cystic, with clusters of cysts often associated with air-fluid levels. Certain patterns of bronchiectasis are sufficiently characteristic to suggest a specific diagnosis in the appropriate clinical context. For example, central bronchiectasis is a frequent finding in patients with allergic bronchopulmonary aspergillosis. Bronchiectasis associated with ipsilateral hypoplasia of the lung is characteristic of Swyer–James syndrome.

V. PATTERN OF MOSAIC ATTENUATION

A mosaic pattern of attenuation with patchy areas of increased and decreased attenuation is nonspecific and may be seen on HRCT when various infiltrative lung, airway, or vascular diseases are present. When this pattern is caused by regional differences in perfusion due to vascular diseases, it is also known as mosaic perfusion [37] or mosaic oligemia [38]. In cases of infiltrative lung disease, mosaic attenuation results from patchy areas of ground-glass attenuation and interposed normal lung parenchyma. In cases of airway disease, the mosaic pattern results from reflex vasoconstriction secondary to hypoventilation of alveoli distal to airway obstruction and blood flow redistribution to adjacent normal areas of lung. Air trapping in the abnormal lung may also contribute to the reduced attenuation. Infiltrative lung disease and airway disease may be differentiated reliably as the cause of mosaic attenuation on HRCT, whereas vascular disease is often misinterpreted as infiltrative lung disease or airway disease [39].

In infiltrative lung disease, the size of vessels within the areas of ground-glass attenuation is usually similar to that of uninvolved lung, allowing distinction from airway and vascular disease in the majority of cases. In cases of airway and vascular diseases, areas of increased attenuation have relatively large vessels, while areas of decreased attenuation have small vessels [40,41].

Airway diseases that can cause mosaic attenuation can often be recognized by the presence of bronchial dilatation, seen in more than 70% of patients with airway abnormalities [39]. Although air trapping allows early recognition of airway abnormalities, it is not helpful as an isolated finding in the distinction of airway disease from other causes of mosaic attenuation because it can also be seen in patients with infiltrative lung disease and vascular disease [39]. However, when patients are suspected to have small airway disease, isolated air trapping on expiratory HRCT (often with normal inspiratory HRCT) is highly suggestive of asthma or obliterative bronchiolitis (Fig. 11).

In cases of vascular disease, it has been suggested that all areas of the lung, whether they show decreased or increased attenuation, demonstrate the expected increase in attenuation at expiration [40]. However, in a study by Worthy et al. [39], this was not a reliable criterion, as air trapping was also seen in patients with vascular disease. Acute vascular occlusion, resulting in

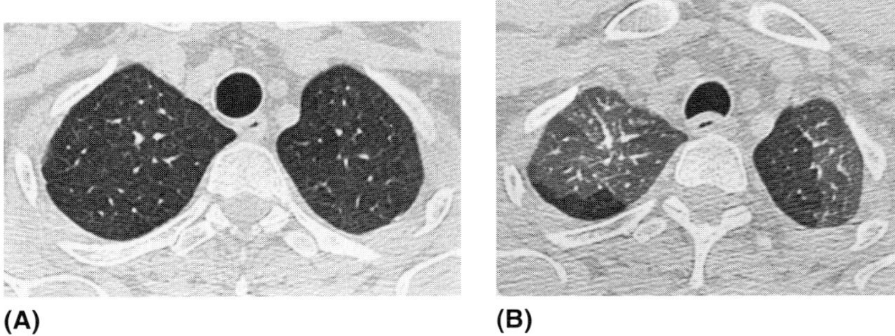

Figure 11 Obliterative bronchiolitis. (A) Inspiratory HRCT of a 40-year-old woman with a heart transplant and decreasing pulmonary function shows no evidence of bronchiolitis. (B) Expiratory HRCT of the same patient in A shows a mosaic pattern of lung attenuation. The lucent areas of lung represent air trapping. Note anterior bowing of posterior membranous trachea on expiration, a normal finding.

a reduced arterial carbon dioxide concentration in the affected lung, can stimulate bronchoconstriction of small airways. Air trapping can then be seen in the affected areas of lung owing to the presence of bronchoconstriction. Bronchial dilatation has also been shown to be a common finding in patients with chronic pulmonary thromboembolism [42]. In the majority of cases of vascular dis-

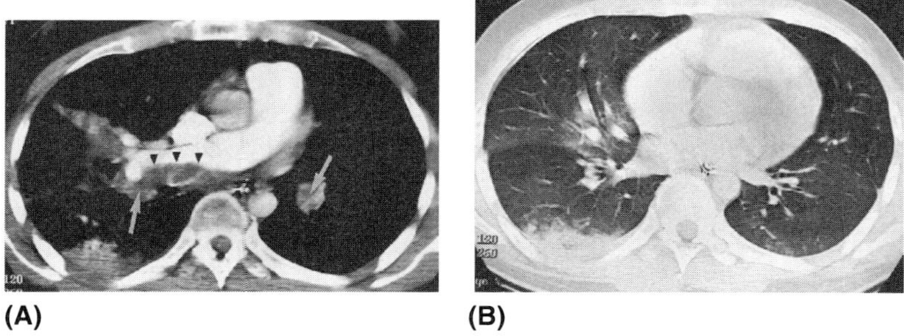

Figure 12 Chronic thromboembolic disease. (A) Helical CT with intravenous contrast material of a 27-year-old man with a history of deep venous thrombosis, shortness of breath, and elevated pulmonary artery pressures shows eccentric clot along the posterior wall of the right pulmonary artery (arrowheads) and clot in the lower lobe branches bilaterally (arrows). (B) HRCT with lung windowing of the same patient in A shows mosaic perfusion.

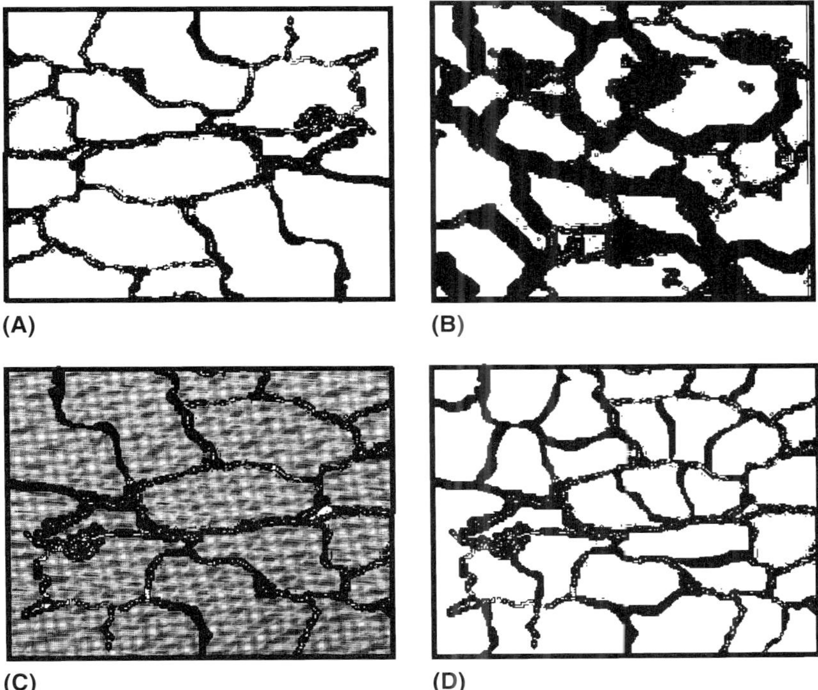

Figure 13 Diagrammatic representations of different causes of ground-glass opacification on HRCT. Each box represents a pixel on a CT scan. Diagrams highlight the nonspecific nature of ground-glass opacification. (A) Pixel contains normal lung parenchyma at full inspiration with normal alveolar walls and alveolar air spaces. Normal amounts of air, blood, and tissue in pixel will yield a certain expected Hounsfield attenuation and will be assigned a gray-scale value. (B) Pixel shows thickening of interstitium of lung, resulting in more ''tissue'' per pixel relative to air, thus increasing the Hounsfield value assigned that pixel. (C) Pixel shows fluid filling alveoli, again increasing Hounsfield value assigned that pixel. (D) Pixel shows normal parenchyma at end of exhalation. Note increased number of alveolar walls per pixel and less air, resulting in increased Hounsfield value assigned that pixel. (From Ref. 43.)

Table 2 Diffuse pattern of GGO on HRCT

Acute rejection of lung transplantation
Adult respiratory distress syndrome
Pulmonary edema
Extrinsic allergic alveolitis
Pulmonary hemorrhage
Infectious pneumonia

ease, mosaic attenuation is caused by chronic pulmonary thromboembolism (Fig. 12), and less commonly by primary pulmonary hypertension or pulmonary capillary hemangiomatosis [39].

Ground-glass opacification (GGO, a hazy increase in lung opacity not associated with obscuration of underlying vessels) as a manifestation of infiltrative lung disease is a nonspecific finding on HRCT with a broad differential diagnosis [43]. GGO can result from partial filling of air spaces, interstitial thickening, partial collapse of alveoli, normal expiration, or increased capillary blood volume (Fig. 13). A pattern approach to the interpretation of GGO on HRCT can help to narrow the differential diagnosis [44]. Some of the patterns to look for include diffuse involvement of the lungs (Table 2, Fig. 14), patchy distribution (Table 3, Fig. 15), focal pattern (Table 4), ''halo'' pattern (Table 5, Fig. 16), peripheral pattern (Table 6), and bronchovascular or centrilobular pattern (Table 7). The ''halo'' sign refers to an area of consolidation sur-

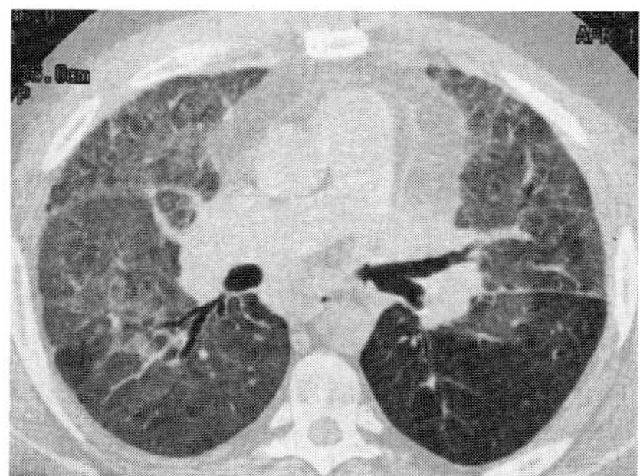

Figure 14 Acute rejection. HRCT of a 38-year-old man after bilateral lung transplantation shows diffuse bilateral ground-glass opacification, correlating histologically with severe acute rejection.

Table 3 Patchy Pattern of GGO on HRCT

Acute rejection of lung transplantation
Adult respiratory distress syndrome
Bronchiolitis obliterans organizing pneumonia
Bronchioloalveolar cell carcinoma
Extrinsic allergic alveolitis
Pulmonary hemorrhage
Infectious pneumonia
Pulmonary alveolar proteinosis

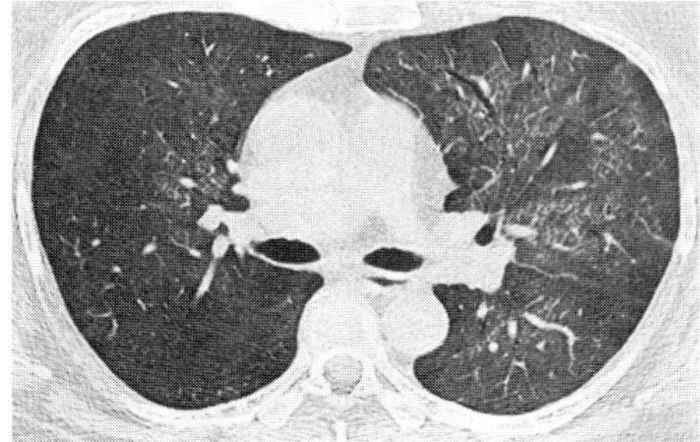

Figure 15 Pneumocystis carinii pneumonia. HRCT of a 56-year-old woman on steroid therapy for autoimmune hepatitis shows characteristic patchy areas of ground-glass opacification.

Table 4 Focal GGO on HRCT

Bronchiolitis obliterans organizing pneumonia
Bronchoalveolar lavage
Bronchioloalveolar cell carcinoma
Pulmonary hemorrhage
Pulmonary infection

Table 5 ''Halo'' Pattern of GGO on HRCT

Invasive pulmonary aspergillosis
Neoplasm, hemorrhagic
Postbiopsy pseudonodule

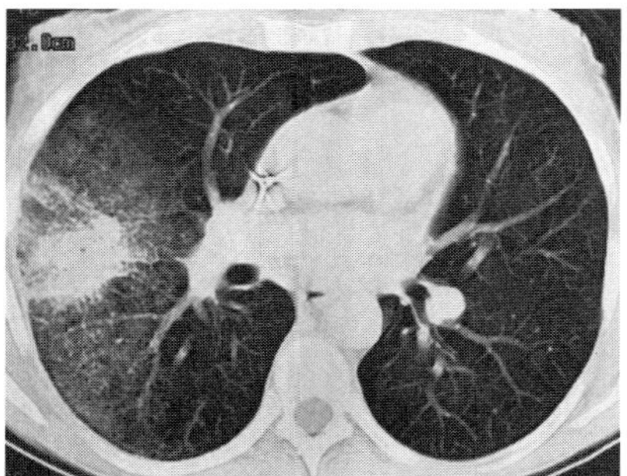

Figure 16 Invasive pulmonary aspergillosis. HRCT of a 50-year-old woman with acute myelogenous leukemia and fever shows focal consolidation in the right upper lobe with surrounding ground-glass opacification (''halo'' sign). In this patient population the halo sign is fairly specific for invasive pulmonary aspergillosis.

Table 6 Peripheral GGO on HRCT

Bronchiolitis obliterans organizing pneumonia
Collagen vascular disease
Desquamative interstitial pneumonitis
Drug toxicity
Eosinophilic pneumonia
Pulmonary fibrosis
Sarcoidosis

Table 7 Bronchovascular or Centrilobular GGO on HRCT

Bronchovascular
Eosinophilic pneumonia
Sarcoidosis
Centrilobular
Extrinsic allergic alveolitis
Respiratory bronchiolitis

rounded by a zone of ground-glass opacification, with this zone often representing hemorrhage.

VI. BRONCHIOLAR PATTERN OF DISEASE ON HIGH-RESOLUTION COMPUTED TOMOGRAPHY

Bronchiolitis and bronchiolectasis are nonspecific inflammatory processes of the small airways caused by many different conditions. Because visibility on HRCT is limited to bronchi more than 2 mm in diameter, normal lobular bronchioles cannot be seen on HRCT. However, diseased bronchioles can be visualized. Direct CT findings of bronchiolar disease include bronchiolar wall thickening, bronchiolar dilatation, and luminal impaction (Fig. 17). Bronchiolar luminal impaction with secretions or fibrotic material manifests as 2- to

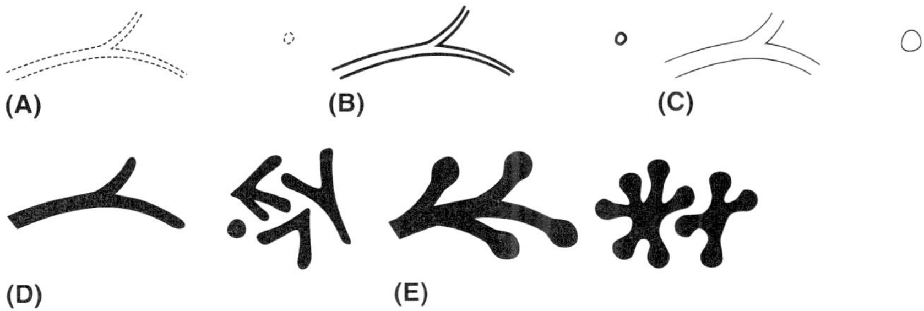

Figure 17 Drawings show normal bronchiole and direct signs of bronchiolar disease. Bronchioles in profile are shown on left and in cross section on right. (A) Normal bronchiole has diameter less than or equal to 1 mm and thin walls and is not usually visible on CT scans. (B) When bronchiolar wall is thickened, CT can show abnormal bronchiole in profile or as ring shadow in cross section in periphery of lung, where bronchioles are usually not seen. (C) Dilated bronchioles become visible on CT when they reach a diameter of 2 mm or greater, the limit of visibility on CT. (D) Impacted bronchioles are shown as centrilobular nodular and linear branching opacities that sometimes form V shapes. (E) Tree-in-bud pattern represents severe bronchiolar impaction with "clubbing" of distal bronchioles and more than one contiguous branching site. Seen in profile, pattern resembles finger-in-glove appearance of impacted bronchi. (From Ref. 43a.)

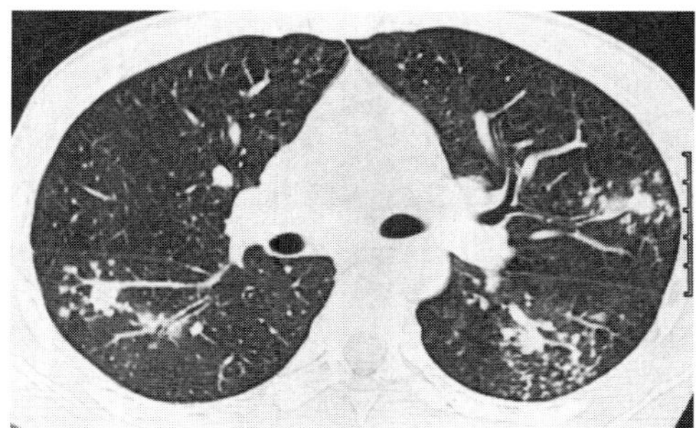

Figure 18 Tuberculosis. HRCT of a 19-year-old man from Bangladesh shows ''tree-in-bud'' pattern of bronchiolar disease in left upper lobe and both lower lobes. This pattern is consistent with active and contagious disease.

4-mm nodular and linear branching centrilobular opacities on HRCT. The ''tree-in-bud'' pattern has been coined to refer to these opacities (Fig. 18), and is analogous to the larger airway ''finger-in-glove'' appearance of bronchial impaction. Indirect signs of bronchiolar disease on HRCT include subsegmental atelectasis and air trapping.

The list of conditions that may exhibit a tree-in-bud pattern on HRCT is extensive, but the etiology is most often an infectious process [45]. Less

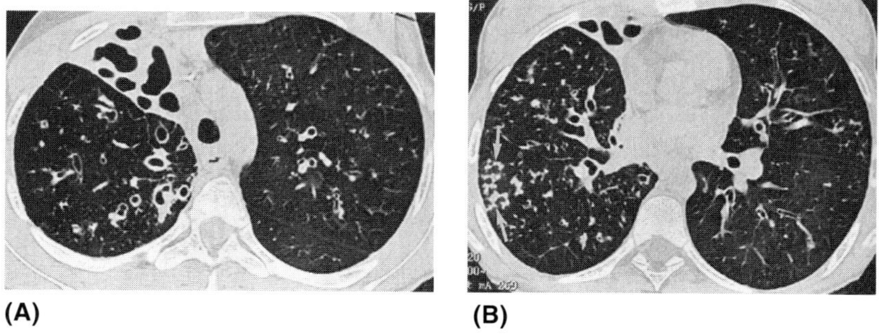

Figure 19 Cystic fibrosis. (A) HRCT of a 15-year-old girl shows dilatation and wall thickening of bronchi and bronchioles. There is destruction and collapse of the right upper lobe. (B) More inferior image of same patient in (A) shows ''tree-in-bud'' pattern of mucoid impaction in the right lower lobe (arrows).

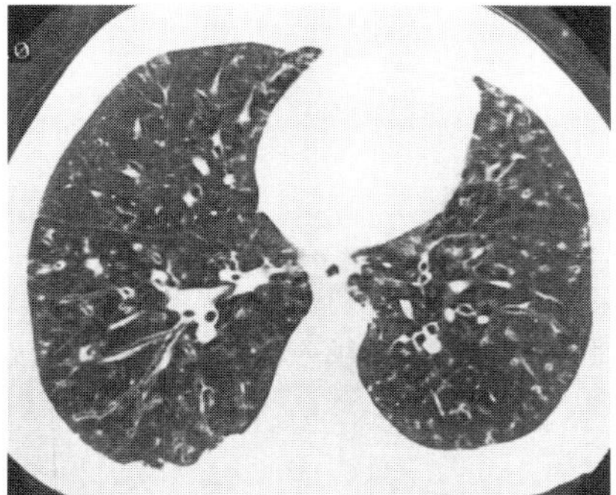

Figure 20 Diffuse panbronchiolitis. HRCT of a 70-year-old Asian male with progressive shortness of breath and chronic sinusitis shows diffuse dilatation and wall-thickening of bronchi and bronchioles and small peripheral nodules in a bronchiolar distribution.

common etiologies include immunologic disorders (allergic bronchopulmonary aspergillosis), congenital disorders (cystic fibrosis; Fig. 19), neoplasms (such as laryngotracheobronchial papillomatosis), aspiration (of gastric contents and oral contrast material), and idiopathic causes (obliterative bronchiolitis, diffuse panbronchiolitis, Fig. 20; and asthma, Fig. 21).

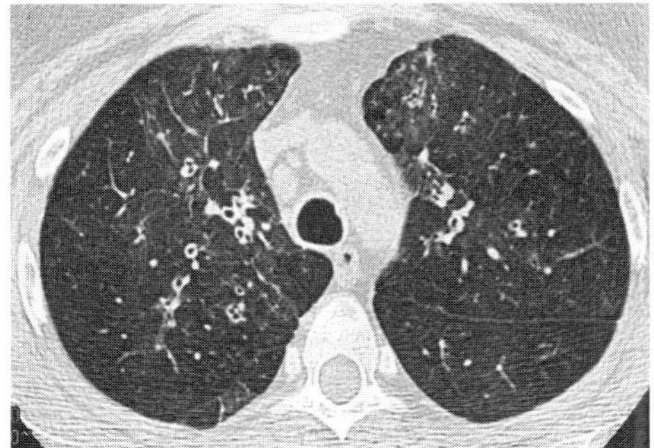

Figure 21 Chronic asthma. HRCT of a 33-year-old woman with chronic refractory asthma and decreasing respiratory function shows dilatation and wall thickening of bronchi and bronchioles. The patient underwent bilateral lung transplantation 6 months later.

REFERENCES

1. Naidich DP. Pulmonary parenchymal high-resolution CT: to be or not to be. Radiology 1989; 171:22–24.
2. Todo G, Itoh H, Nakano Y, et al. High-resolution CT for the evaluation of pulmonary peripheral disorders. Jpn J Clin Radiol 1982; 27:1319–1326.
3. Nakata H, Kimoto T, Nakayama T, Kido M, Miyazaki N, Harada S. Diffuse peripheral lung disease: evaluation by high-resolution computed tomography. Radiology 1985; 157:181–185.
4. Naidich DP, Zerhouni EA, Hutchins GM, Genieser NB, McCauley DI, Siegelmann SS. Computed tomography of the pulmonary parenchyma. Part 1: distal air-space disease. J Thorac Imaging 1985; 1(1):39–53.
5. Zerhouni EA, Naidich DP, Stitik FP, Khouri NF, Siegelman SS. Computed tomography of the pulmonary parenchyma. Part 2: interstitial disease. J Thorac Imaging 1985; 1(1):54–64.
6. Webb WR, Müller NL, Naidich DP. High-Resolution CT of the Lung. 2nd ed. Philadelphia: Lippincott–Raven, 1996:2.
7. Mayo JR, Jackson SA, Müller NL. High-resolution CT of the chest: radiation dose. Am J Radiol 1993; 160:479–481.
8. Webb WR, Müller NL, Naidich DP. High-Resolution CT of the Lung. 2nd ed. Philadelphia: Lippincott–Raven, 1996:13.
9. Webb WR, Stern EJ, Kanth N, Gamsu G. Dynamic pulmonary CT: findings in normal adult men. Radiology 1993; 186:117–124.
10. Coultas DB, Zumwalt RE, Black WC, Sobonys RE. The epidemiology of interstitial lung diseases. Am J Respir Crit Care Med 1994; 150:967–972.
11. Epler GR, McLoud TC, Gaensler EA, Mikus JP, Carrington CB. Normal chest roentgenograms in chronic diffuse infiltrative lung disease. N Engl J Med 1978; 298:801–809.
12. Padley SPG, Hansell DM, Flower CDR, Jennings P. Comparative accuracy of high resolution computed tomography and chest radiography in the diagnosis of chronic diffuse infiltrative lung disease. Clin Radiol 1991; 44:222–226.
13. Gaensler EA, Carrington CB. Open biopsy for chronic diffuse infiltrative lung disease: clinical, roentgenographic, and physiologic correlations in 502 patients. Ann Thorac Surg 1980; 30:411–426.
14. Müller NL. Clinical value of high-resolution CT in chronic diffuse lung disease. Am J Radiol 1991; 157:1163–1170.
15. Thurlbeck WM, Simon G. Radiographic appearance of the chest in emphysema. Am J Radiol 1978; 130:429–440.
16. Lynch DA, Rose CS, Way D, King TE. Hypersensitivity pneumonitis: sensitivity of high-resolution CT in a population-based study. Am J Radiol 1992; 159:469–472.
17. Müller NL, Kullnig P, Miller RR. The CT findings of pulmonary sarcoidosis: analysis of 25 patients. Am J Radiol 1989; 152:1179–1182.

18. Stein MG, Mayo J, Müller N, Aberle DR, Webb WR, Gamsu G. Pulmonary lymphangitic spread of carcinoma: appearance on CT scans. Radiology 1987; 162:371–375.
19. Strickland B, Strickland NH. The value of high definition, narrow section computed tomography in fibrosing alveolitis. Clin Radiol 1988; 39:589–594.
20. Aberle DR, Gamsu G, Ray CS, Feuerstein IM. Asbestos-related pleural and parenchymal fibrosis: detection with high-resolution CT. Radiology 1988; 166: 729–734.
21. Staples CA, Gamsu G, Ray CS, Webb WR. High resolution computed tomography and lung function in asbestos-exposed workers with normal chest radiographs. Am Rev Respir Dis 1989; 139:1502–1508.
22. Padley SPG, Adler B, Müller NL. High-resolution computed tomography of the chest: current indications. J Thorac Imaging 1993; 8:189-199.
23. Rose C, King TE. Controversies in hypersensitivity pneumonitis [editorial]. Am Rev Resp Dis 1992; 145:1–2.
24. Brauner MW, Grenier P, Mompoint D, Lenoir S, de Cremoux H. Pulmonary sarcoidosis: evaluation with high-resolution CT. Radiology 1989; 172:467–471.
25. Bergin CJ, Coblentz CL, Chiles C, Bell DY, Castellino RA. Chronic lung diseases: specific diagnosis using CT. Am J Radiol 1989; 152:1183–1188.
26. Lynch DA, Webb WR, Gamsu G, Stulbarg M, Golden J. Computed tomography in pulmonary sarcoidosis. J Comput Assist Tomogr 1989; 13:405–410.
27. Stein MG, Mayo J, Müller N, Aberle DR, Webb WR, Gamsu G. Pulmonary lymphangitic spread of carcinoma: appearance on CT scans. Radiology 1987; 162:371–375.
28. Lenoir S, Grenier P, Brauner MW, et al. Pulmonary lymphangiomyomatosis and tuberous sclerosis: comparison of radiographic and thin-section CT findings. Radiology 1990; 175:329–334.
29. Müller NL, Chiles C, Kullnig P. Pulmonary lymphangiomyomatosis: correlation of CT with radiographic and functional findings. Radiology 1990; 175:335–339.
30. Brauner MW, Grenier P, Mouelhi MM, Mompoint D, Lenoir S. Pulmonary histiocytosis X: evaluation with high-resolution CT. Radiology 1989; 172:255–258.
31. Primack SL, Hartman TE, Hansell DM, Müller NL. End-stage lung disease: CT findings in 61 patients. Radiology 1993; 189:681–686.
32. Müller NL, Staples CA, Miller RR, Vedal S, Thurlbeck WM, Ostrow DN. Disease activity in idiopathic pulmonary fibrosis: CT and pathologic correlation. Radiology 1987; 165:731–734.
33. Remy-Jardin M, Giraud F, Remy J, Copin MC, Gosselin B, Duhamel A. Importance of ground-glass attenuation in chronic diffuse infiltrative lung disease: pathologic–CT correlation. Radiology 1993; 189:693–698.
34. Wells AU, Hansell DM, Rubens MB, Cullinan P, Black CM, du Bois RM. The predictive value of appearances of thin-section computed tomography in fibrosing alveolitis. Am Rev Respir Dis 1993; 148:1076–1082.
35. Bergin CJ, Müller NL, Miller RR. CT in the qualitative assessment of emphysema. J Thorac Imaging 1986; 1:94–103.

36. Jederlinic PJ, Sicilian L, Gaensler EA. Chronic eosinophilic pneumonia: a report of 19 cases and a review of the literature. Medicine (Baltimore) 1988; 67:154–162.
37. Austin JHM, Müller NL, Friedman PJ, et al. Glossary of terms for CT of the lungs: recommendations of the Nomenclature Committee of the Fleischner Society. Radiology 1996; 200:327–331.
38. Martin KW, Sagel SS, Siegel BA. Mosaic oligemia simulating pulmonary infiltrates on CT. Am J Radiol 1986; 147:670–673.
39. Worthy SA, Müller NL, Hartman TE, Swensen SJ, Padley SPG, Hansell DM. Mosaic attenuation pattern on thin-section CT scans of the lung: differentiation among infiltrative lung, airway, and vascular diseases as a cause. Radiology 1997; 205:465–470.
40. Stern EJ, Swensen SJ, Hartman TE, Frank MS. CT mosaic pattern of lung attenuation: distinguishing different causes. Am J Radiol 1995; 165:813–816.
41. Remy-Jardin M, Remy J, Giraud F, Wattine L, Gosselin B. Computed tomography assessment of ground-glass opacity: semiology and significance. J Thorac Imaging 1993; 8:249–264.
42. Remy-Jardin M, Remy J, Louvegny S, Artaud D, Deschildre F, Duhamel A. Airway changes in chronic pulmonary embolism: CT findings in 33 patients. Radiology 1997; 203:355–360.
43. Collins J, Stern EJ. Ground-glass opacity at CT: the ABCs. Am J Radiol 1997; 169:355–367.
43a. Collins J, Blankenbaker D, Stern EJ. Am J Radiol 1998; 171:365–370.
44. Collins J, Stern EJ. Patterns of ground-glass opacity on computed tomography scanning of the chest. In: Postgraduate Radiology. St. Louis: Abrams and Mosby, 1999; 19:78–91.
45. Aquino SL, Gamsu G, Webb WR, Kee ST. Tree-in-bud pattern: frequency and significance on thin section CT. J Comput Assist Tomogr 1996; 20:594–599.

7

CT Diagnosis of Pulmonary Embolus

Cesario Ciccotosto
Università "G. D'Annunzio"
Chieti, Italy

Lawrence R. Goodman and Lacey Washington
Medical College of Wisconsin and
Froedtert Memorial Lutheran Hospital
Milwaukee, Wisconsin

I. INTRODUCTION

Pulmonary embolus (PE) and deep venous thrombosis (DVT) are two interrelated components of pulmonary thromboembolic disease (PTE). Both are difficult to diagnose clinically and there are many competing tests, some clinical, some laboratory, and some imaging, used for PTE diagnosis. All have strengths and all have drawbacks. As imagers, it is our task to individualize these exams, or combination of exams, to fit the particular patient. A "one approach fits all" strategy is an inefficient use of resources.

Ventilation perfusion (V/Q) scanning has been the keystone imaging modality for the past 40 years. The multi-institutional PIOPED Study [1] demonstrated that a normal ventilation perfusion scan has a 96% negative predictive value and provides sufficient evidence to withhold anticoagulation. Similarly, a high-probability scan coupled with a high-probability clinical suspicion has a 96% positive predictive value for PE. Unfortunately, even using the revised PIOPED criteria for V/Q interpretation, the majority of patients have low or indeterminate probability scans, which are inconclusive for PTE diagnosis and therefore usually require additional imaging [2].

In a patient population with good cardiopulmonary reserve, an inconclusive ventilation perfusion scan and serial negative lower extremity Doppler ultrasounds (LEUS) provide very strong evidence that anticoagulation can be withheld [3]. However, as a single isolated study, a negative lower extremity study does not exclude pulmonary embolism. In fact, approximately one-half of pulmonary embolism patients have negative lower extremity studies.

In a high-risk patient population with inconclusive scintigraphy, pulmonary angiography should follow. This has been the gold standard for many years but is often omitted because it is invasive and because of the perceived risks. A negative pulmonary angiogram indicates that anticoagulation can be safely withheld [4]. Unfortunately, in clinical practice, serial LEUS and pulmonary angiography are not obtained in the majority of eligible patients, and a decision to anticoagulate or not to anticoagulate patients is frequently based on inconclusive scintigraphy and perceived clinical probability, a suboptimal situation [5].

Helical computed tomography (CTA) pulmonary angiography provides a better, but not perfect, alternative to traditional PTE imaging. The current generation of helical and new multislice helical CT scanners provides high-quality axial images of the contrast enhanced pulmonary vessels and lower extremity veins. As in angiography or venography, the clot is displayed directly as a filling defect in the contrast column. Computed tomography is also able to detect other pulmonary and lower extremity diseases that may mimic PTE or DVT.

Computed tomography is not without its drawbacks, however. Many studies have shown that CTA is approximately 90% sensitive [6–10]. Computed tomography will often miss small clots in subsegmental vessels [6]. These very small clots are the same clots, however, that result in inconclusive scintigraphy and a high rate of interobserver disagreement on pulmonary angiography. Respiratory motion also degrades the depiction of the small vessels, resulting in suboptimal scans in 5 to 10% of patients [10]. Despite these limitations, the clinical outcome for patients with negative CTA's who are not anticoagulated is very good. We recently reported a study of 198 CTA negative patients (42% of whom also had LEUS) and 350 scintigraphy negative or low-probability patients (22% of whom had LEUS) who were not anticoagulated. After 3 months of clinical follow-up, the rate of subsequent PE was 1% for negative CT, 0% for normal scintigraphy, and 3.4% for low-probability scintigraphy [11]. For comparison, patients anticoagulated for PE have a 5% incidence of subsequent PE [12]. Computed tomography is also expensive but is cost effective relative to other strategies that require multiple imaging studies in the majority of patients.

A recent addition to the CT armamentarium for PTE is CT venography (CTV). Axial scans through the IVC and lower extremity veins to the knee are obtained 3 minutes after completion of the contrast injection for the pulmonary arterial CT. These studies are easy to perform and appear easy to interpret. Although there are no large studies to date that compare CTV with contrast venography or LEUS, several small studies comparing CTV with lower extremity Doppler show 95% or greater correlation [13–15]. Unlike LEUS, CTV can also evaluate the IVC and iliac veins for DVT. Incorporating the CTV with CTA assures that the pulmonary arteries and lower extremity veins are imaged in every patient. It is very time effective for both patient and referring physician to be able to complete the PTE workup in one 30-min trip to the CT suite.

We believe that scintigraphy, lower extremity Doppler ultrasound, CT of the pulmonary arteries and veins, and pulmonary angiography can be used in a multiarm, cost-effective algorithm that utilizes the strong points of each imaging modality and minimizes the weaknesses of each [6]. The following list outlines our algorithm with its rationale.

1. V/Q scanning: Studies have shown that patients with a normal chest radiograph have a higher likelihood of a definitive scintigraphic answer (normal, very low probability, and high probability). Patients with a normal chest radiograph should start with a V/Q. Inconclusive studies require further imaging directed by the clinical situation.
2. Lower extremity doppler ultrasound: Ultrasound is relatively inexpensive and is highly accurate for symptomatic DVT but is less accurate for asymptomatic (nonocclusive) DVT. Patients with symptoms of DVT should have a lower extremity Doppler ultrasound first. If positive, anticoagulation is indicated. It is up to the individual clinician to decide whether additional imaging for PE is required. A negative scan does not eliminate a PE.
3. Helical CTA and CTV: In patients with abnormal chest radiographs and without signs and symptoms of DVT, CT evaluation of the chest and lower extremities should be performed. Inconclusive studies may require additional imaging.

II. BRONCHOVASCULAR ANATOMY

In interpreting CT pulmonary angiography, it is important to be comfortable with normal bronchovascular anatomy in order to communicate findings accurately and to facilitate comparison of serial studies. For the most part, an embolus is described and located by naming the artery in which it is found. Beyond the central vessels, the artery is called by the name of the adjacent bronchus.

Standard nomenclature for the bronchial segments was established by Jackson and Huber in 1943 [16].

The most important aid to interpreting CT bronchovascular anatomy is the workstation. To interpret CT pulmonary angiography, it is necessary to distinguish pulmonary arteries from veins, and the workstation can greatly simplify this task. First, a workstation with scroll capabilities allows the reader to follow peripheral vessels either to the main pulmonary arteries or to the left atrium. Second, switching between lung and soft-tissue windows shows the relationship of the vessel to a bronchus. Pulmonary arteries parallel the bronchi and pulmonary veins run independently. (The main exceptions to this are the lingular artery and the artery to the posterior subsegment of the left upper lobe. Their origins are somewhat remote from the associated bronchi over short distances [17].) In central parts of the lung, where many vessels and bronchi are in close proximity, it is helpful to note that the upper lobe arteries are usually central to the associated bronchi, and the middle lobe, lower lobe, and lingular arteries are peripheral to the associated bronchi [18].

Beyond these general principles, it is very helpful to know that there is considerable variability in the vascular anatomy at the segmental level and beyond. Most of these variations are minor and can be appreciated at the workstation. Variations usually consist of early bifurcation or the presence of a common trunk or of a multiplicity of vessels in association with a single bronchus. Also, it is common for subsegmental arteries to cross segmental planes. The classic treatise by Boyden [19] on segmental anatomy of the lung was used as a source for the discussion below, along with several articles on cross-sectional anatomy [18,20–22], although the Boyden numbering system was felt to be cumbersome and therefore not used. Boyden's system, however, is included for reference (Table 1) [19].

An example of pulmonary arterial anatomy with labeled vessels is provided for reference (Figs. 1A–1L). The main pulmonary artery originates at the pulmonary valve and extends superiorly and posteriorly where it bifurcates into the right and left pulmonary arteries.

A. Right Pulmonary Arteries

1. Right Upper Lobe

The first branch of the right pulmonary artery is called the truncus anterior; after the takeoff of this vessel, the descending portion of the pulmonary artery is called the interlobar artery, as it lies in the interlobar fissure. The truncus anterior usually begins as a single artery that courses superiorly anterior to

Table 1 Boyden's Numbering System for Segmental Anatomy of the Lung

Boyden Number	Name of Right Lung Segmental Artery	Name of Left Lung Segmental Artery
	Right upper lobe	*Left upper lobe*
A^1	Apical Segment Artery	Apical Artery (to the Apical-posterior segment)
A^2	Anterior Segment Artery	Anterior Segment Artery
A^3	Posterior Segment Artery	Posterior Artery (to the Apical-posterior segment)
A^4	*Right middle lobe*	
	Lateral Segment Artery	Superior Segment Lingular Artery
A^5		
	Medial Segment Artery	Inferior Segment Lingular Artery
A^6	*Right lower lobe*	*Left lower lobe*
A^{7+8}	Superior Segment Artery	Superior Segment Artery
		Anteromedial Basal Segment Artery
A^7		
A^8	Medial Basal Segment Artery	Medial Subsegment Artery
A^9	Anterior Basal Segment Artery	Anterior Subsegment Artery
A^{10}	Lateral Basal Segment Artery	Lateral Basal Segment Artery
	Posterior Basal Segment Artery	Posterior Basal Segment Artery

The numbering system described above applies exactly only if the bronchi and the arteries are precisely parallel, an uncommon scenario. If segments are supplied by arteries that do not directly parallel the bronchi, each artery derives its name from the bronchial segment it supplies. So, for example, a right middle lobe artery may bifurcate into an artery that supplies only a portion of the lateral segment, B^4, and a second artery that supplies the remainder of the lateral segment and the medial segment, B^5. In this case, the first artery is called A^4a, and the second artery is called $A^{5+4}b$. The two major branches of a numbered artery are called a and b, for example, A^3a and A^3b.

the right main bronchus. This most commonly divides into an anterior segmental branch (Fig. 1D) and an upper branch. The upper branch usually divides into apical and posterior segmental branches (Fig. 1C). However, there is commonly a branch from the interlobar pulmonary artery to the posterior segment of the upper lobe and sometimes a branch to the apical segment.

2. Right Middle Lobe

Approximately half of the time, two right middle lobe arteries arise from a common trunk from the right interlobar pulmonary artery, and about half of the time they arise as two separate branches of the interlobar artery (Figs. 1G and 1H). A branch of the medial segmental artery most frequently supplies the anterior aspect of the lateral segment.

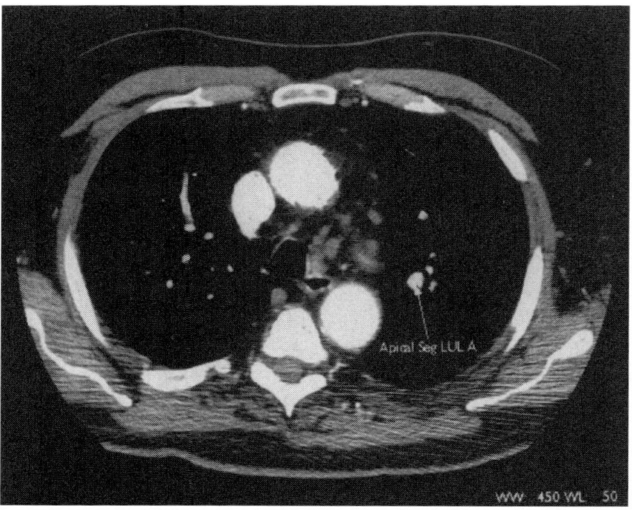

A

Figure 1 Examples are taken from two different patients. (A) Apical segmental artery, LUL. Unlike the common apicoposterior segmental bronchus, this artery frequently has an origin separate from the posterior segmental artery.

3. Right Lower Lobe

Below the origin of the right middle lobe artery or arteries, the interlobar artery becomes the right lower lobe artery. It usually then gives off one or occasionally two posteriorly directed arteries to the superior segment of the right lower lobe (Fig. 1G). This is usually at the same level as, or slightly caudal to, the takeoff of the right middle lobe bronchus. The name of the artery beyond the origin of the superior segmental artery is the pars basalis or basal artery or trunk (Fig. 1H), and this gives off the basal segmental arteries. In slightly more than half of cases, the medial basal segmental artery arises first or arises first as a common trunk with the anterior segmental artery—this representing a very variable artery (Fig. 1J). Finally, the lateral basal and posterior basal arteries arise independently or bifurcate from a common trunk, again with significant variability (Fig. 1K).

B. Left Pulmonary Arteries

Unlike the right upper lobe, the left upper lobe artery arches over the top of the left upper lobe bronchus, which therefore is ''hyparterial.'' Apart from this

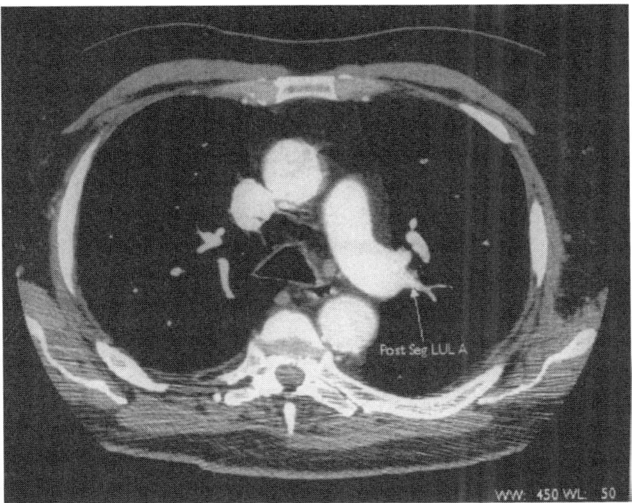

B

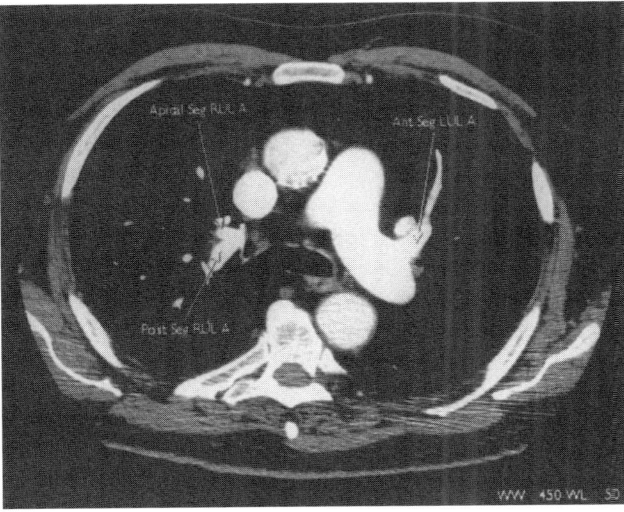

C

Figure 1 (Continued) (B) The posterior segmental artery, LUL. (C) Apical and posterior segmental arteries, RUL, arise from an upper division of the truncus anterior (above the takeoff of the anterior segmental branch), while the anterior segmental artery, LUL, arises independently from the pars anterior.

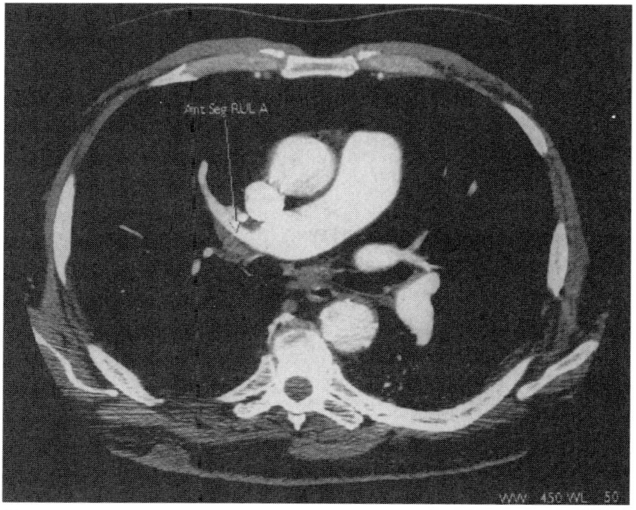

D

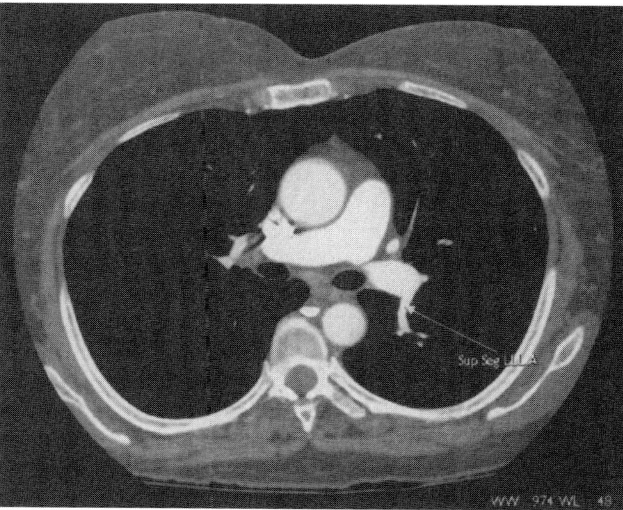

E

Figure 1 (Continued) (D) The anterior segment artery, RUL. (E) The superior segment artery, LLL. This is more commonly single than double and almost always arises above the lingular artery(-ies).

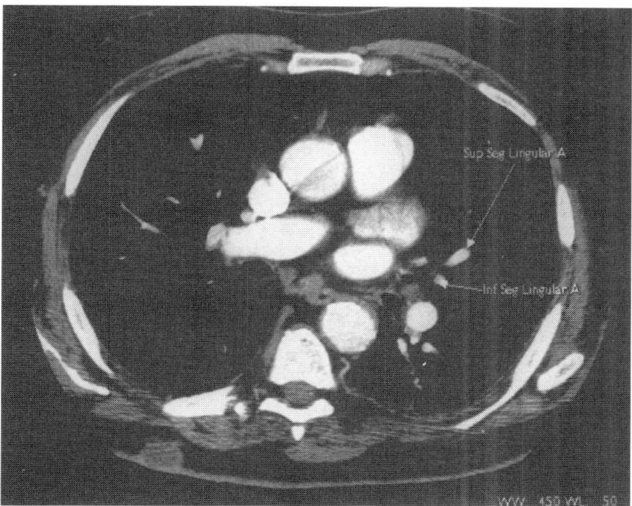

F

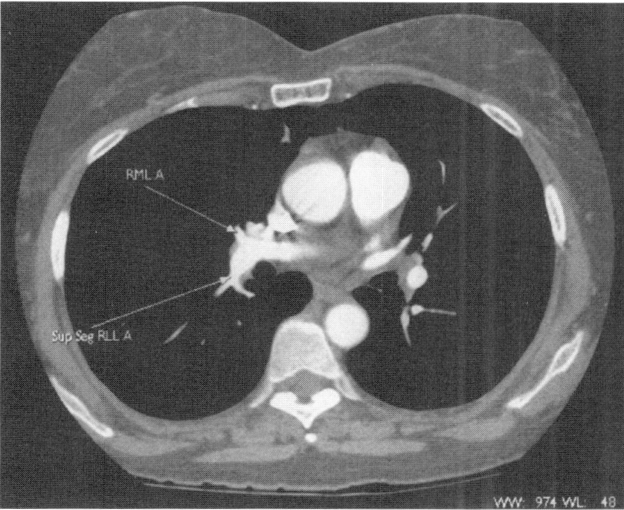

G

Figure 1 (Continued) (F) Segmental branches of the lingular artery. This artery most commonly arises as a single vessel from the interlobar portion of the left pulmonary artery. (G) Right middle lobe artery and the superior segment artery, RLL. The middle lobe artery usually arises immediately above the superior segmental artery but may arise at the same level or below.

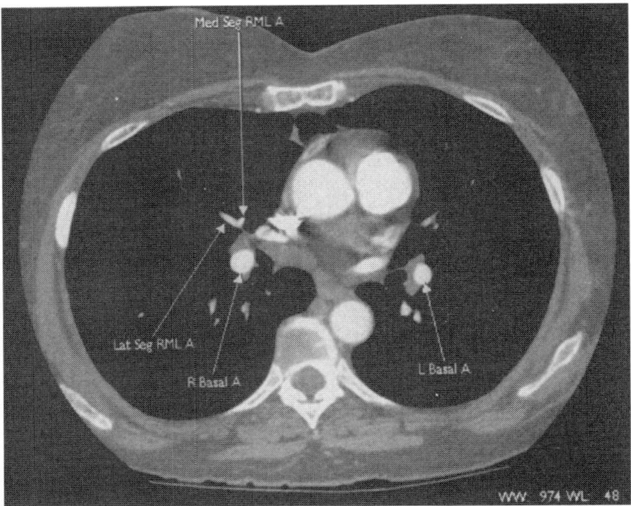

H

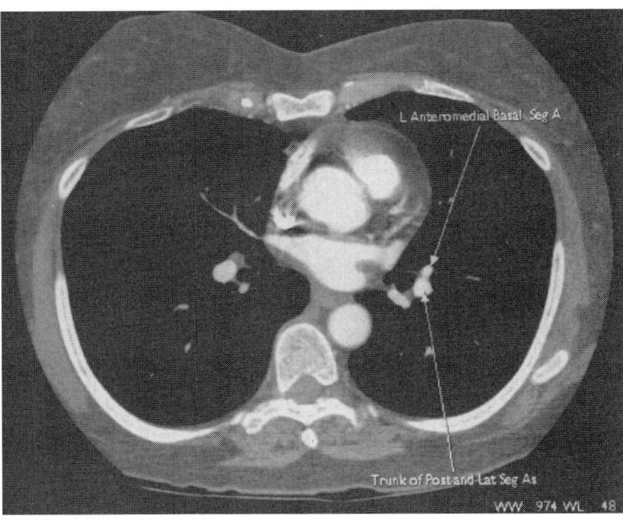

I

Figure 1 (Continued) (H) Medial and lateral segmental arteries, RML. These frequently do not follow the bronchial pattern but cross segmental planes. On each side a basal artery (basal trunk, or pars basalis) supplies the basal segmental vessels. (I) The anteromedial basal segmental artery, LLL. This is usually a common trunk, like the left anteromedial basal segmental bronchus.

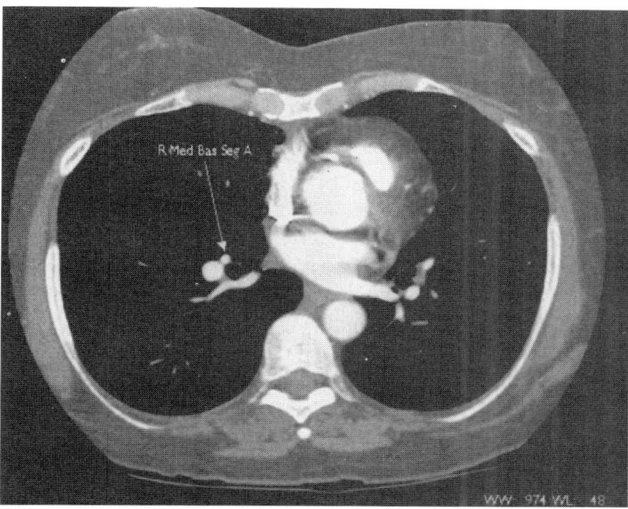

J

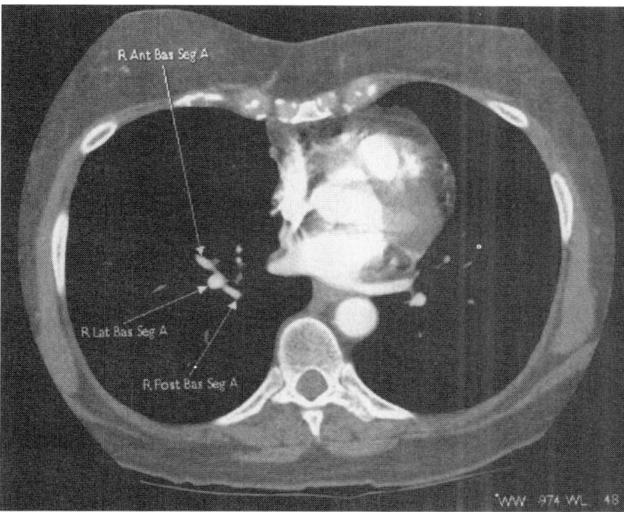

K

Figure 1 (Continued) (J) The medial basal segmental artery, RLL. This is commonly the first branch of the basal artery, sometimes arising in combination with the anterior basal segmental artery or other basal segmental arteries. (K) The anterior, lateral, and posterior segmental arteries, RLL. These are variable in their origins and branching patterns.

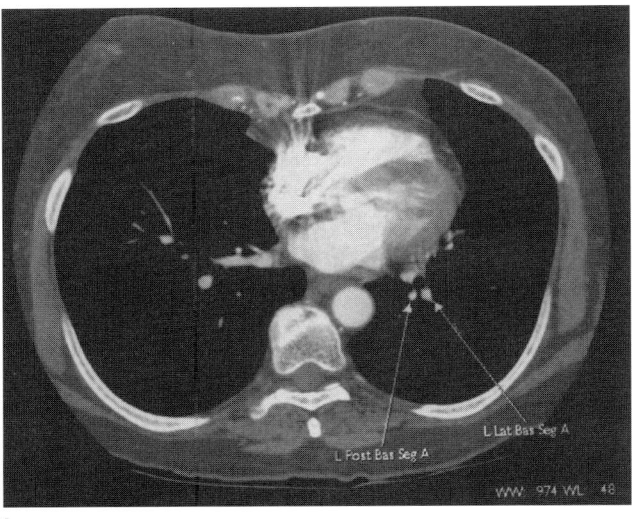

L

Figure 1 (Continued) (L) The lateral and posterior basal segmental arteries, LLL. These may arise, as in this case, from a common trunk or in multiple other configurations.

difference, the arterial branching pattern on the left is quite similar to that on the right. However, there tend to be more separate arteries on the left than the right, with ''scattering of branches along the course of the main artery'' [19].

Left Upper Lobe

Either single or multiple branches arising from the ''pars anterior'' of the left pulmonary artery supply the anterior segment of the left upper lobe (Fig. 1C). Additional branches may arise from this anterior portion and supply portions of the apical and/or lingular segments. Following these branches, apical and posterior arteries usually arise from the superior aspect of the arching left pulmonary artery, and, unlike the apicoposterior segmental bronchus, which usually has a common origin, these two arteries most commonly arise separately (Figs. 1A and 1B).

Interlobar Segment

In contrast to the right side, on the left, the arterial supply to the superior segment of the lower lobe usually arises above the level of the lingular arteries

(Figs. 1E and 1F). Both the superior segmental arteries and the lingular arteries may each arise as a single trunk or as two separate arteries.

Basal Segments

As on the right, the pars basalis or basal trunk gives off arteries to the basal segments on the left. Just as there is usually a single left anteromedial basal segmental bronchus, there is usually a single anteromedial segmental artery (Fig. 1I). However, in about half of cases, the artery to the lateral basal segment arises from a common trunk with this anteromedial branch, separate from a single branch to the posterior basal segment. In the other half of cases, the lateral basal segmental artery arises from a common trunk with the posterior basal segmental branch (Fig. 1L) or in other configurations.

C. Subsegmental Arteries

As stated above, the subsegmental arteries are variable and may cross into adjacent segments. The Boyden system can be used to number subsegmental vessels, but because of the variability and complexity of the subsegmental arterial anatomy, we find it sufficient to identify an embolus as located in a subsegmental vessel arising from a particular segmental artery or located in a particular segment.

D. Venous Anatomy

As Boyden initially indicated, the naming of peripheral venous structures in the lungs is much more difficult than the naming of arteries, as the arteries can be named by the bronchi they correspond to, and thus by the segment they supply, while the veins are located remotely from the bronchi. Centrally, the left upper lobe veins drain into the superior pulmonary vein, and right and left lower lobe veins drain into the right and left inferior pulmonary veins. On the right, upper lobe veins usually form a common superior pulmonary vein that joins with middle lobe veins to form a common superior pulmonary venous confluence. The venous return from the right middle lobe occasionally enters the left atrium separately.

III. TECHNIQUE

The key to effective scanning for pulmonary embolus is careful attention to technique. Since 1992, when Remy-Jardin [23] first reported helical CT for pulmonary embolism, helical scanners have become considerably faster and multidetector scanners have come on the market. This new equipment allows coverage of a larger volume of lung in a shorter period of time while obtaining thinner sections. By the time you read this chapter, further improvements will undoubtedly be in place. Therefore, we deal with the basic concepts of how to optimize technique with the understanding that you can modify the details as appropriate [17,24].

A. Anatomic Volume

Earlier protocols scanned the patient from the inferior pulmonary vein to the aortic arch so that the scan could be completed within a single 24- to 30-sec breath hold. With faster scanning, the area from the lower diaphragm to the aortic arch is easily covered in a single breath hold. Extending the scan to the diaphragm assures that the basilar segmental pulmonary arteries and their proximal subsegmental branches are imaged. After completion of scanning the central area, the apices and the bases are scanned to complete the study of the lung.

B. Scan Direction

Caudal-to-cranial scanning assures that the lung bases, which are most susceptible to image degradation from respiratory motion, are scanned early in the breath hold to minimize respiratory artifact. The direction becomes less important as the scanners become faster and apnea time becomes shorter.

C. Breathing

Minimizing respiratory motion is critical. Most patients can breath hold for the required scan acquisition. Hyperventilation prior to scanning and nasal oxygen may help the marginal patient. In dyspneic patients, slow shallow breathing is usually sufficient to obtain adequate images of the central vessels. In patients on mechanical ventilation, the patient can often be held in apnea during the acquisition or, alternatively, the tidal volume and frequency can be minimized. In sedated intubated patients, a short-acting respiratory paralytic, such as succinylcholine, will assure a brief period of apnea.

D. Scan Parameters

Multiple studies have shown that the thinner the collimation, the better the depiction of the peripheral vessels. Helical images have decreased from 5 to 3 mm in thickness. Multislice scanners allow for 1.25- or 1-mm scans. Similarly, increasing pitch from 1 to 1.7 on helical CT or to 3 or 6 on multislice CT increases speed and decreases patient dose. Diminishing scan rotation time from 1 to .8 or .5 sec increases speed further. Electron-beam CT allows for even more rapid acquisition. With each of these changes, there is a potential decrease in photon statistics and increased noise. This is especially detrimental in large patients, where scan parameters must be altered to increase the amount of radiation and thereby decrease noise.

E. Contrast Material

Intravenous contrast is best administered through an antecubital or central venous catheter. Most centers use nonionic contrast. There is no uniform agreement as to the best injection protocol. Most studies have shown that 100 to 120 cc of full-strength nonionic contrast injected at 3 to 4 cc/sec provides excellent vessel opacification. With the faster scanning protocols, 70 to 90 cc should suffice. (If the lower extremity veins are to be studied also, 100 to 120 cc is probably necessary to provide adequate opacification of the veins.)

There is no universal agreement on the optimal time between onset of contrast injection and scanning. We utilize a preliminary time–density curve to determine the time of peak pulmonary artery enhancement. This utilizes 18 cc of contrast injected over 6 sec while the pulmonary artery is being scanned every 3 sec for 30 sec. The contrast peak is then graphed and 5 sec are arbitrarily added to determine scan delay time (Fig. 2). In the vast majority of patients, the scan delay is 15 to 20 sec. Many centers empirically use a 15- to 25-sec delay without resorting to a time–density curve. In an occasional patient, a specific area is not adequately evaluated on the initial CT because of suboptimal contrast enhancement or respiratory motion. A repeat focal scan through that area can be done using a supplemental 50 cc of contrast and a revised delay based on the prior scan.

F. Venous Studies

At this time, scanning of the IVC and lower extremity veins is a relatively new and a not thoroughly validated technique. Optimal parameters have not been agreed on [13]. A reasonable approach involves scanning from L2 to the knees starting 3 min after completion of the IV contrast injection for the pulmonary arteries. No additional contrast is necessary, although 100 to 120 cc total contrast dose appears to be necessary to obtain adequate enhancement of the veins to 80–100 HU. The ankles are placed together. At our center,

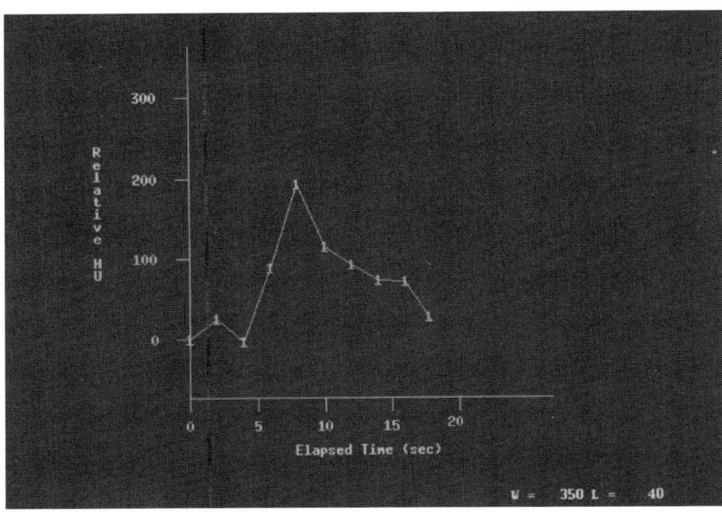

A

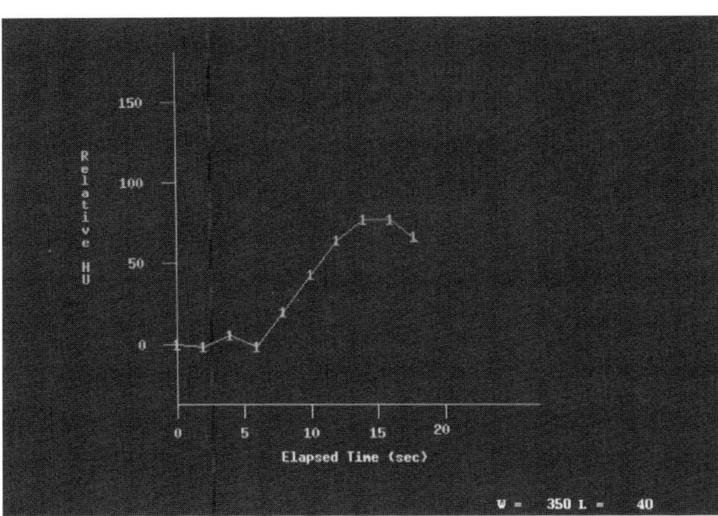

B

Figure 2 Time–density curve. (A) Typical normal time–density curve with peak opacification at approximately 10 sec. Five seconds is then arbitrarily added to determine scan delay. (B) Typical time–density curve in a patient with elevated right heart pressure. The calculated scan delay was 20 sec.

5-mm scans are obtained every 2 cm. Some centers scan continuously, obtaining complete imaging of the veins, but at the cost of increased radiation dose.

G. Filming

The above protocols generate 150 to 250 images, an inconvenient number of slices to read or store on film. We routinely read the scans on a workstation and film every third image at lung and mediastinal windows (20 per film) for archiving. If only small clots are found, demonstration images are filmed in a 4:1 or 6:1 format for future reference.

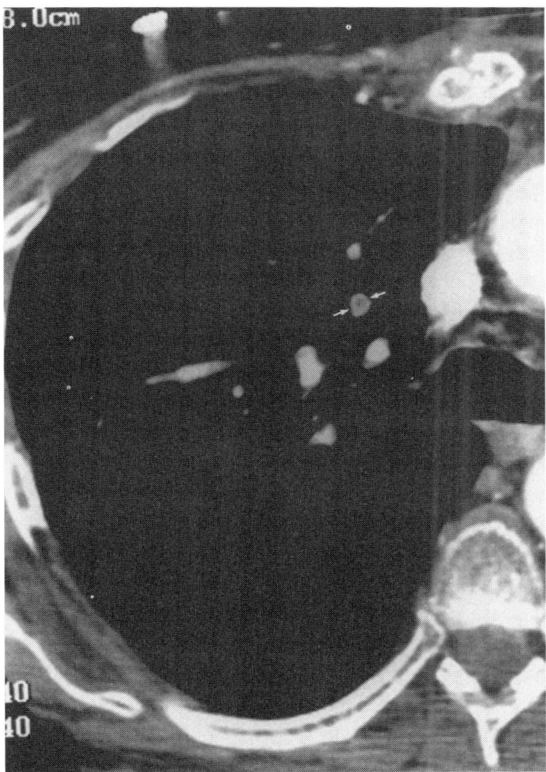

Figure 3 Acute PE. A partial-filling defect is seen in a subsegmental RUL artery, with central low attenuation surrounded by high-attenuation contrast (arrows).

IV. COMPUTED TOMOGRAPHY FINDINGS OF ACUTE PULMONARY EMBOLISM

A diagnosis of pulmonary embolism is made when the embolus is seen as an area of low attenuation in a contrast-enhanced pulmonary artery [24]. Acute pulmonary emboli may be manifested as partial or complete filling defects in vessels, by the "railway track sign," or as mural defects.

A partial filling defect means that clot is seen within a vessel, surrounded by contrast (Fig. 3); a filling defect is complete when the entire artery fails to opacify due to a central filling defect. In the setting of acute embolus, vessels that are completely filled with clot may enlarge (Fig. 4) compared with similar

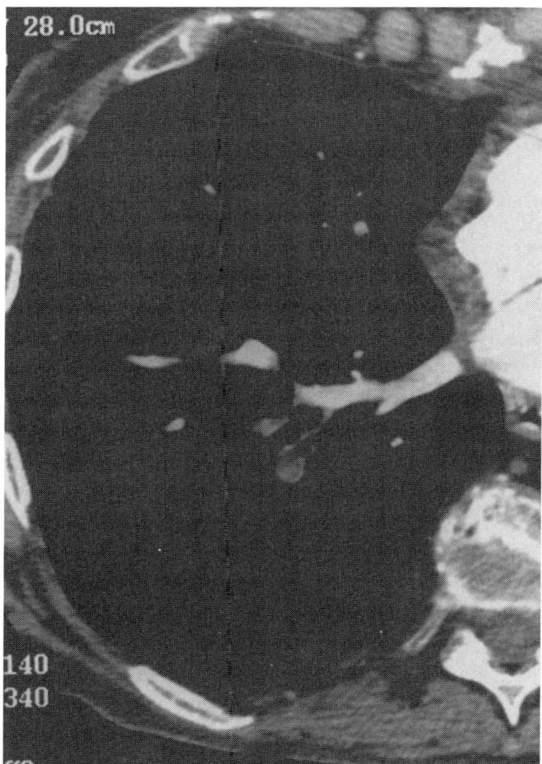

Figure 4 Acute PE. Complete filling defects are seen in the lateral and posterior basal segmental arteries, which appear distended.

vessels of the same generation. This is in contrast to the smaller diameter seen with chronic thromboembolic disease [17]. The ''railway track sign'' is the demonstration of a clot floating within the vessel (Fig. 5), and a mural defect is defined as a clot that appears adherent to the wall of a vessel, with contrast not completely surrounding the clot. In acute thromboembolic disease, mural thrombi usually form acute angles with the vessel walls in vessels that are sufficiently large to examine for this finding (Fig. 6) [17].

There should be a sharp interface between the filling defect of a pulmonary embolism and adjacent contrast, and the filling defect should be seen on more than one image. Looking for these findings should prevent the misdiagnosis of minor mixing inhomogeneity or other artifacts as emboli. The failure to visualize a vessel should not lead to a diagnosis of pulmonary embolism.

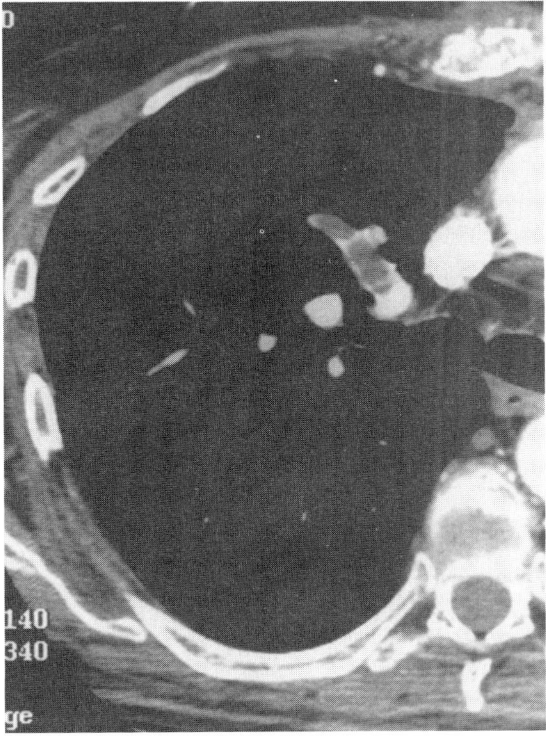

Figure 5 Acute PE. ''Railway track sign'' of clot floating in the anterior segmental RUL artery.

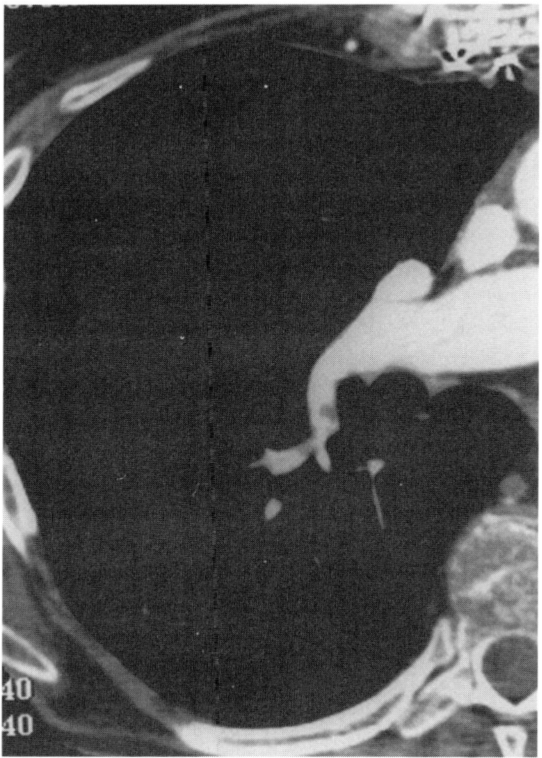

Figure 6 Acute PE. Mural thrombus forming acute angles with the vessel wall in the superior segmental RLL artery.

V. POSTPROCESSING TECHNIQUES

Postprocessing techniques (multiplanar reformation, maximum intensity projection, and virtual angioscopy) are not used routinely in the diagnosis of PE. When transverse sections provide a confident analysis of all the pulmonary arteries, 2D and 3D reformations provide no additional information. Sometimes an in-plane or oblique arterial branch or an area of linear perivascular soft tissue may generate an area of low density that may be confused with PE in the axial plane. This artifact is due to partial volume effect between lung parenchyma or perivascular lymphatic tissue and the contrast enhanced pulmonary artery. The vessels that most often run in the axial plane are the right middle lobe and lingular arteries, the anterior segmental arteries of the upper lobes, and the superior segmental arteries of the lower lobes [25,26]. In these cases, the vessels are displayed better by multiplanar reformations (MPRs) that use data obtained from a contiguous helical data set (Figs. 7 and 8). The images may be reformatted in any anatomical plane (coronal, sagittal, oblique, or curvilinear view). Virtual endoscopy provides a direct view of the intraluminal clot. Its clinical utility has yet to be determined.

Another potential application of MPRs is the evaluation of chronic thromboembolic disease. The creation of MPRs through the longitudinal axis of obliquely oriented vessels can overcome some of the difficulties encountered with axial images in the identification of focal arterial stenoses and webs or in separating eccentric, adherent thrombus from adjacent lymphatic tissue [27].

VI. PITFALLS IN DIAGNOSES

There are many pitfalls in the interpretation of PE, even for the experienced reader [15,22]. The three most important strategies for avoiding pitfalls were discussed above: meticulous technique, understanding of normal anatomy and common variants, and interpretation on a workstation. The remaining major impediments to reading include technical problems that thwart diagnosis and anatomical or disease entities that mimic PE.

A. Technical Problems

Respiratory Motion

Vessel motion will often cause the pulmonary arteries to appear less dense. If the vessels on adjacent images appear normal, and the lung windows reveal respiratory motion in the slice in question, it is almost certainly a respiratory artifact. As a general strategy, pulmonary embolus should be visible on two or more images for confident diagnosis.

Streak Artifacts

Linear artifacts arising from high-density structures, such as the contrast-enhanced superior vena cava, calcified lymph nodes, or surgical clips, can cause apparent lucencies in a contrast-enhanced pulmonary artery. The artifact source is usually readily apparent and the defect is linear in the axial plane.

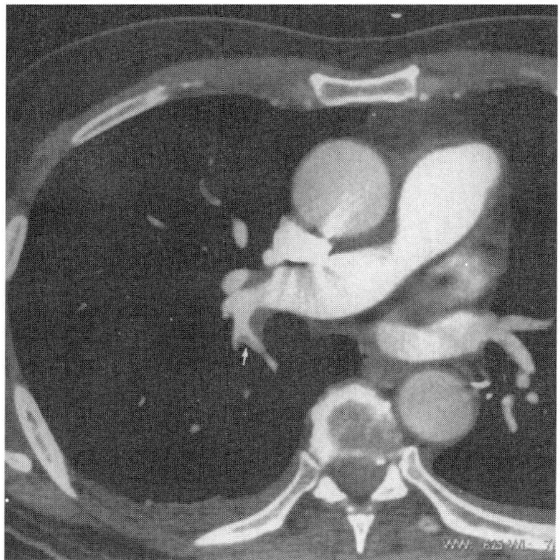

A

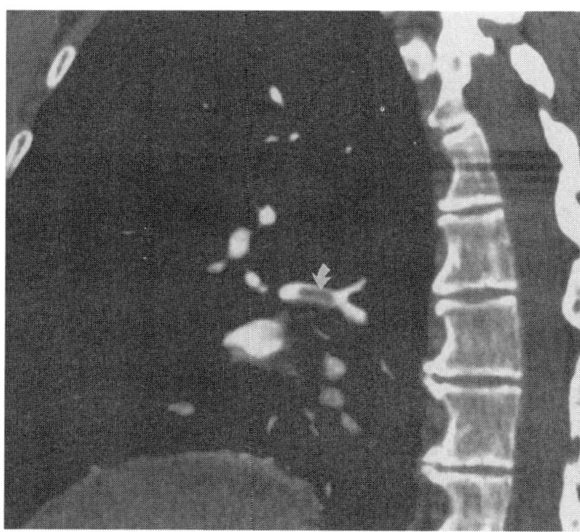

B

Figure 7 Multiplanar reformation. (A) Helical CT angiogram at mediastinal window shows a questionable filling defect at the bifurcation of the superior subsegmental artery of the right lower lobe (arrow). A small embolus is also seen in the anterior subsegmental artery of right upper lobe. There are small bilateral pleural effusions and surgical clips in the left hilum. (B) Sagittal oblique reformation at mediastinal window better depicts intraluminal clot in the superior segmental artery (arrow).

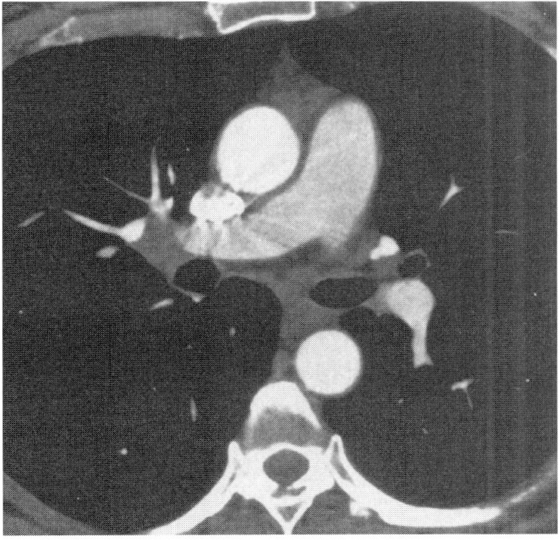

A

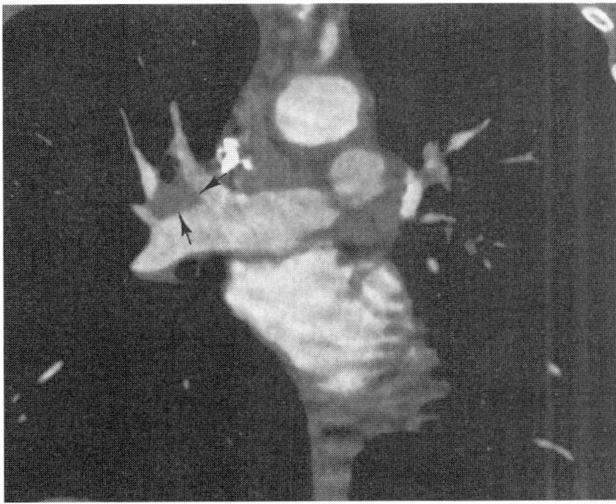

B

Figure 8 Multiplanar reformation. (A) Helical CT angiogram at mediastinal window demonstrates, at the level of right hilum, hypodensity lateral to right pulmonary artery that could correspond to lymphadenopathy or thrombus. (B) Coronal oblique reformation at mediastinal window shows perivascular nature of hypodensity between right superior pulmonary artery and descending pulmonary artery due to lymph nodes (arrows).

Hyperdense Vessels

Small nonocclusive clots may not be visible in densely enhanced larger pulmonary arteries. After routine reading on soft tissue windows, one should reread the images of the proximal arteries at a wider window and higher level. A window width and level of 700/100 HU is applicable to most patients (Fig. 9). Caution should be used in altering window and level because this accentuates artifacts such as inhomogeneous contrast mixing. In general the margins of flow defects are less distinct than the margins of a PE.

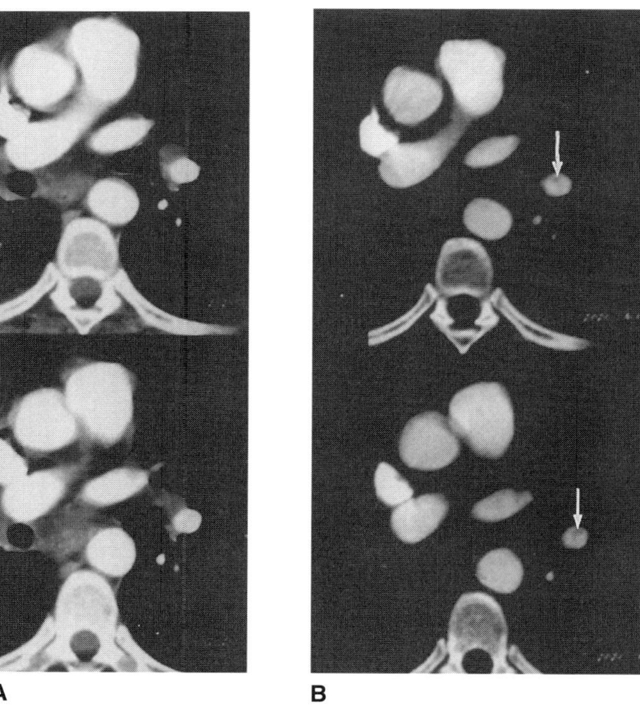

Figure 9 Value cf altering window and level. (A) There is no apparent clot in the left lower lobe pulmonary artery at a window of 450 and a level of 50. (B) At a window of 700, and a level of 100, a small but definite clot is seen on multiple axial images (arrow).

Underenhanced Vessels

If all the vessels are not well enhanced, either the timing of injection was faulty or there was a mechanical problem with the injection, the catheter, or the veins leading to the right heart. Right heart failure may also delay pulmonary artery opacification.

Edge Enhancement

Avoid edge enhancement as used in high-resolution lung algorithms. Edge enhancement causes the margins of the vessels to appear dense. By comparison, the center of the vessel appears more lucent and may be misinterpreted as a PE. A "smooth" or "low spatial frequency" reconstruction algorithm should always be used.

Noisy Images

To avoid excessive noise in large patients, especially at the shoulder and hips, use increased kilovolt peaks and milliampere-seconds thicker slices, and decreased pitch.

B. Anatomical Problems

Vessel Bifurcation

Axial images through the bifurcation of a pulmonary artery often produce the appearance of a central lucency. Workstation paging, above and below, easily identifies these as branch points (Fig. 10).

In-Plane Vessels

Segmental vessels of the middle lobe, the lingula, the superior segments of the lower lobes, and the anterior segments of the upper lobes tend to undulate in and out of the plane or across the plane obliquely, causing pseudofilling defects. Again, cineviewing on a workstation overcomes this problem (Fig. 11). If the contrast column ends in a sharp meniscus, a PE is likely to be present; if it tails off gradually, it is more likely an artifact.

Lymphatic and Connective Tissue

Even in normal patients, there is frequently amorphous lymphatic tissue adjacent to the main, lobar, and proximal segmental vessels. These are often not well-defined "nodes." Lymphatic tissue parallel to the arteries may be volume

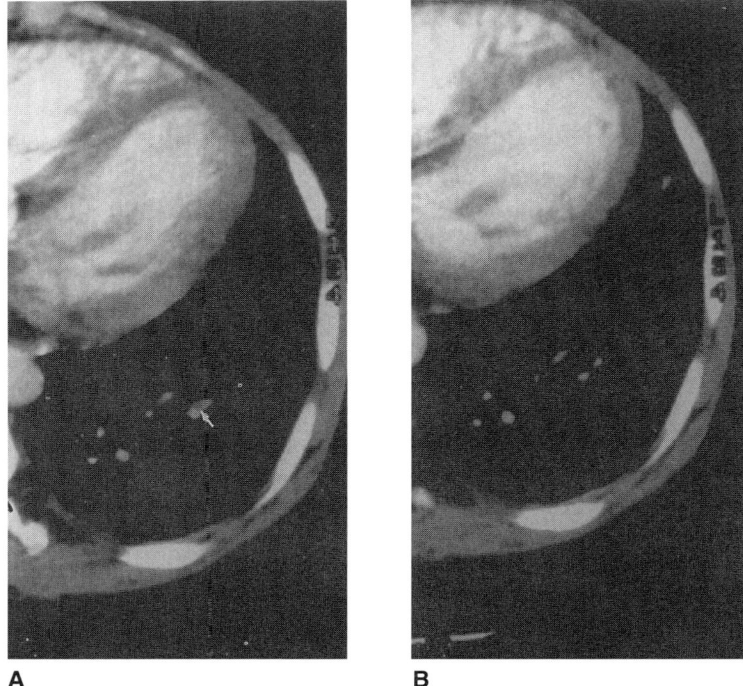

A B

Figure 10 Vessel bifurcation. (A) There appears to be a small lucency in a subsegmental vessel in the left lower lobe (arrow). (B) Shows vessel bifurcation.

averaged ''into'' the adjacent contrast-filled vessel. This is an especially difficult problem at the bifurcation of the right pulmonary artery into the truncus anterior and the interlobar artery and at the origin of the left upper lobe arteries. The lymphatic tissue is usually present over many images and workstation paging usually resolves these issues. It may be especially difficult to distinguish the parallel lymphatic tissue from the wall thickening of chronic pulmonary embolus. Multiplanar reconstructions are especially helpful in solving this problem (Fig. 8).

Mucus Plugs

Mucus-filled small and medium-sized bronchi appear as low-density cylindrical structures, coursing through the lung in exactly the same planes as the

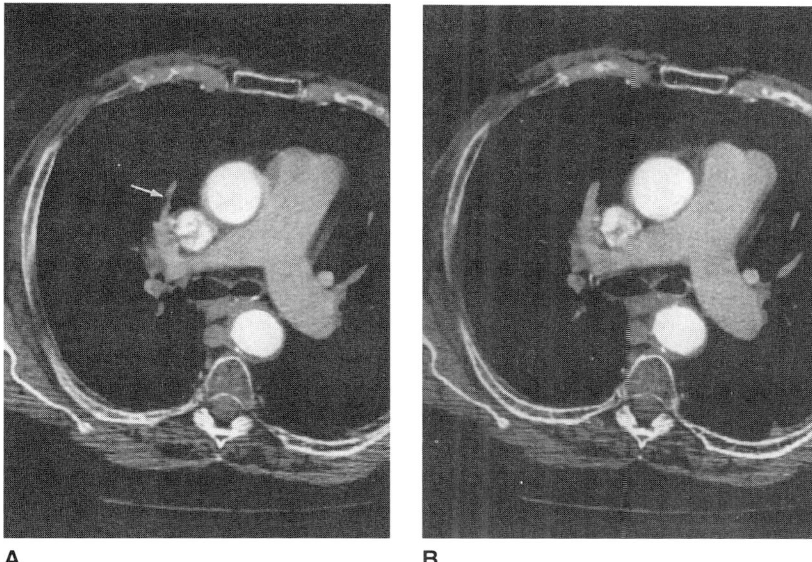

Figure 11 Pseudo-PE due to in-plane vessel. (A) Lucency ''within'' anterior segmental artery of RUL (arrow). (B) At 1.25 mm caudally; the vessel is normal. The scan cephalad to A was no longer in the plane of the vessel (not shown).

pulmonary arteries, and are easily misinterpreted as occluded pulmonary arteries. On mediastinal windows, a contrast-enhanced vessel runs directly adjacent to each of these structures and, on lung windows, no air is visible in the expected location of the bronchus (Fig. 12).

Parenchymal Disease

Atelectasis, pneumonia, emphysema, and so on often distorts pulmonary arteries. In general, with cinepaging, one can follow the distorted vessels into the periphery of the lung. In emphysema, the peripheral vessels are markedly attenuated. The loss of peripheral vessels, without a demonstrable, central filling defect, should not be interpreted as a sign of PE.

Nonenhanced Veins

With faster scanning protocols, it is possible to enhance the pulmonary arteries well before contrast reaches the veins on the initial images. This may simulate a PE.

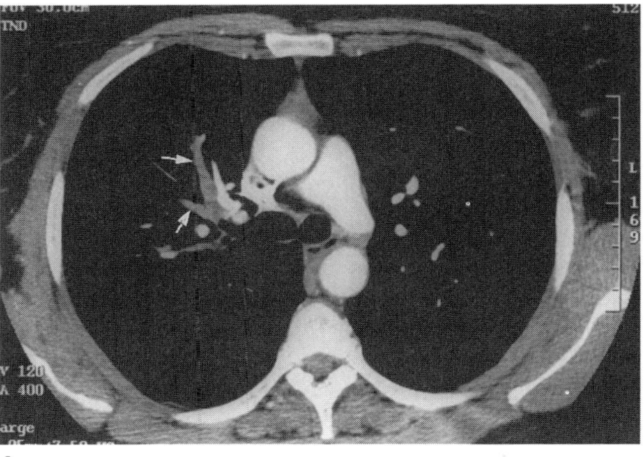

A

B

Figure 12 Mucus plug. (A) There is a branching soft-tissue density supplying the anterior segment of the right upper lobe (arrows). It has the appearance of a clot-filled vessel. However, the contrast-filled pulmonary artery is immediately medial to this area. (B) On the lung windows, there is no air-filled bronchus to the anterior segment of the right upper lobe. One can actually see the cutoff of the air column to the anterior segment of the right upper lobe (arrowhead).

VII. DEEP VENOUS THROMBOSIS OF THE LOWER EXTREMITY

Findings for the diagnosis of acute DVT on CT venography include an intravascular filling defect of low density or total lack of enhancement of a venous region (Fig. 13) [13,28,29]. Ancillary findings of DVT are enlargement of the thrombosed vein, wall enhancement, and perivenous edema (Fig. 14). With acute occlusive thrombosis, the vein enlarges, sometimes to twice the size of the accompanying artery. The vein wall may enhance to a density equal to or higher than muscle density. An additional finding seen in DVT is a focal perivenous soft-tissue infiltration that is probably due to local edema. This finding, not specific for DVT, is most easily detectable in the thigh and popliteal regions where fat surrounds the veins.

For the diagnosis of chronic DVT on CT venography, we have used criteria analogous to criteria used in venography to identify chronic thrombus. In chronic disease, the vein is often smaller than the accompanying artery (Fig. 15), may be calcified, and may not carry contrast-enhanced blood. In addition, extensive collateral veins are an indication that chronic disease is

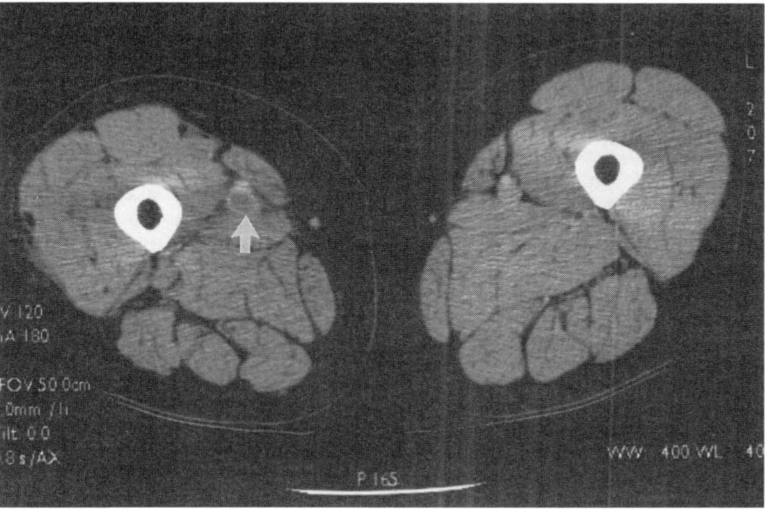

Figure 13 Acute DVT. CT venography image of the midthigh shows a clot in the right superficial femoral vein (arrow). The vein is enlarged. Compare with that of a normal left superficial femoral vein.

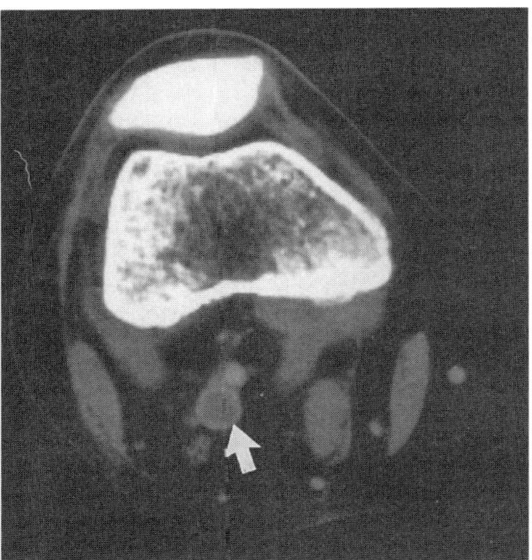

Figure 14 Acute DVT. CT venography image through the knees shows clot in the right popliteal vein. Note expansion of right popliteal vein, the enhanced thick wall (arrow), and the perivenous edema.

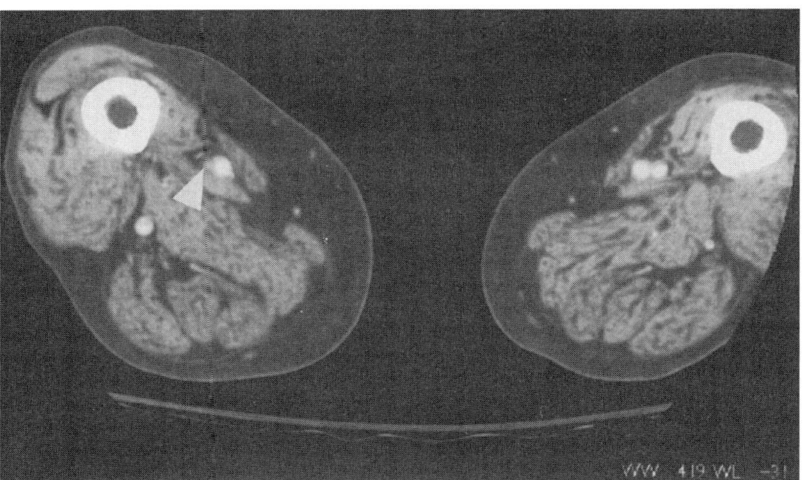

Figure 15 Chronic DVT. CT venography image in patient with chronic DVT. The right superficial femoral vein (arrowhead) is small; compare with that of the normal left superficial femoral vein.

present. Their presence, however, does not rule out acute clot superimposed on chronic clot.

Computed tomography venography can define additional disease (e.g., focal venous aneurysm, abdominal tumor, muscle hematoma, bone fractures, and arterial thrombosis) that has an impact on patient management [27]. Occasionally, incidental findings that will not necessarily affect patient management are revealed, such as a Baker's cyst, or suprapatellar effusions [28,29].

VIII. CHRONIC PULMONARY EMBOLISM

After acute pulmonary embolism (PE), the thrombi usually undergo complete resolution through the process of fibrinolysis, which takes weeks to months [30–32], to reestablish normal pulmonary hemodynamics. With large thrombi, this may take longer. In a study of patients with massive acute PE, despite adequate treatment, some abnormal findings were found at posttherapeutic CTs in 32 patients (52%) after a mean of 11 months [30]. However, for reasons as yet unclear, a small fraction of patients do not experience normal clot lysis. Instead, clots in these patients undergo variable degrees of organization, recanalization, and retraction. The residual strictures, webs, and membranous occlusions cause vascular stenosis. Bilateral chronic pulmonary artery embolism may cause pulmonary artery hypertension (PAH) refractory to medical treatment [31,33].

It is important to recognize chronic pulmonary thromboembolism (CPTE) in order to distinguish it from acute PE, since PAH due to CPTE can potentially be cured by thromboendarterectomy. Diagnostic procedures in these patients may confirm the diagnosis, demonstrate technical operability, and possibly document surgical success. Spiral computed tomography angiography may help us understand changes within the central pulmonary arteries after PE and see morphologic and endoluminal changes due to chronic PE. Results of several studies confirm the value of CT in the diagnosis of CPTE [30,34–38]. Both pulmonary vascular and lung parenchymal abnormalities have been noted.

A. Vascular Abnormalities

Pulmonary angiography is the most widely used technique to diagnose CPTE and to define the location and proximal extent of disease. Pulmonary angiograms usually reveal intimal irregularities, webs, abrupt narrowing, poststenotic dilatation, and tortuous vessels [39]. Residual mural thromboemboli that thicken the wall but do not deform the endovascular contour may be missed at catheter angiography.

Computed tomography may show direct and indirect signs of CPTE. The direct CT findings are visualization of complete obstruction or adherent thrombotic clot (sometimes calcified) (Fig. 16). Adherent clot causes the vessel wall to appear eccentrically thickened (Fig. 17). There may also be evidence of recanalization within the intraluminal defect and arterial stenosis or webs (Fig. 18) [38]. The indirect CT findings are mural irregularities in central and peripheral pulmonary branches, abrupt narrowing of the vessel diameter and abrupt cutoff of distal lobar or segmental artery branches [38]. Computed tomography scans also depict changes of the systemic arterial circulation. In CPTE, the bronchial circulation is increased because peripheral bronchopulmonary anastomoses help maintain the pulmonary circulation. In one study, dilatation and tortuosity of bronchial arteries were seen in 77% of 39 patients with CPTE, and the authors suggested that the presence of visible bronchial arteries on CT is a significant criterion to suggest CPTE [40].

The morphology and shape of the central pulmonary arteries and the heart may be helpful for the diagnosis of CPTE. Additional diagnostic findings include enlargement of the central pulmonary arteries, which are frequently greater in diameter than the aorta. The CT scan is an important tool for detec-

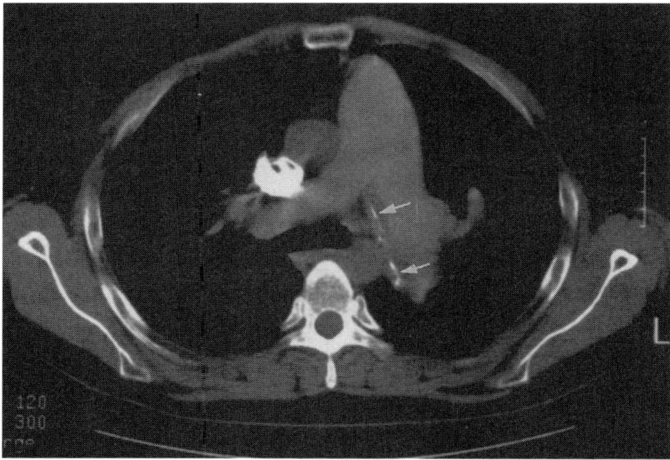

Figure 16 Chronic PE. Suboptimal contrast-enhanced CT in 35-year-old man with chronic pulmonary thromboembolism. There is a mural thrombus with linear calcification (arrows) in the left main pulmonary artery.

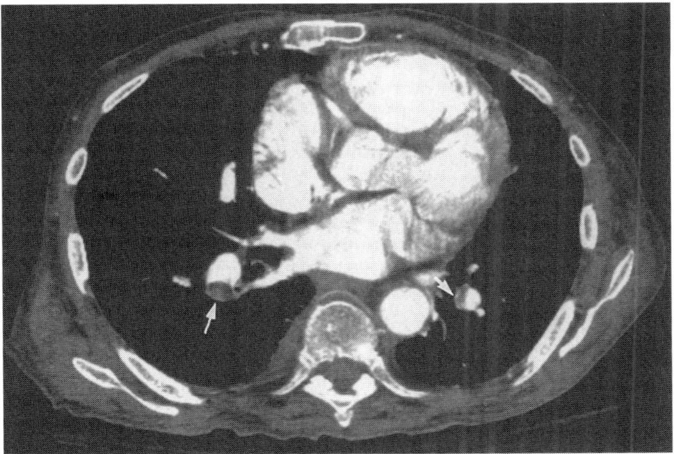

Figure 17 Chronic PE. Computed tomography scan of 60-year-old man with chronic pulmonary thromboembolism. Mediastinal window through midzone reveals marginated mural thrombus in the inferior lobar pulmonary artery, bilaterally (arrows).

tion of PAH: A main pulmonary artery diameter ≧ 29 mm and an increased ratio between the diameter of segmental arteries and corresponding bronchi have high specificity (100%) for predicting the presence of PAH [41]. Patients with CPTE develop right ventricular hypertrophy in response to significant elevation of pulmonary vascular resistance. Over time, right ventricular function deteriorates, even in the absence of recurrent PE, presumably because of the development of hypertensive vascular lesions in the nonobstructed pulmonary artery bed. The right heart dilates [42].

B. Parenchymal Abnormalities

A mosaic pattern of attenuation, with localized areas of decreased and increased attenuation, is a nonspecific finding of CPTE that may be seen on high-resolution CT (HRCT) in various infiltrative lung, airway, or vascular diseases. In CPTE, there are often patchy areas of decreased attenuation and vascularity that correspond to areas of chronically decreased perfusion. They are sharply marginated from adjacent areas with increased or normal attenuation and vessel size that correspond to areas of normal or hyperperfusion (Fig. 19A) [43–45]. Expiratory images may help distinguish the mosaic perfusion of CPTE from that caused by small airways disease. In a study of parenchymal

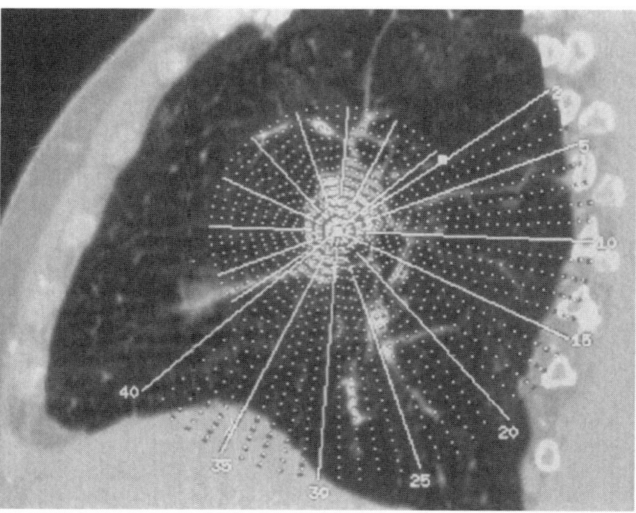

A

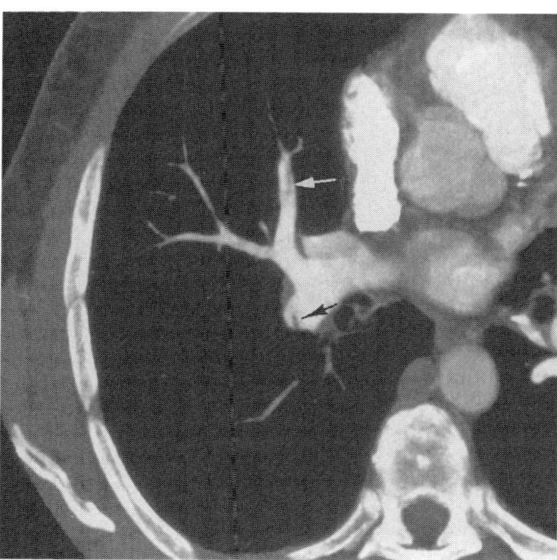

B

Figure 18 Chronic PE: paddlewheel reformation. (A) From a sagittal reformation, 10-mm slice thickness rotational MIP are obtained centered about the right hilum at 4.6° increments [26]. (B) Axial oblique MIP image depicts a linear web in the medial segmental artery of right middle lobe (white arrow) and right lower pulmonary artery (black arrow) due to CPTE.

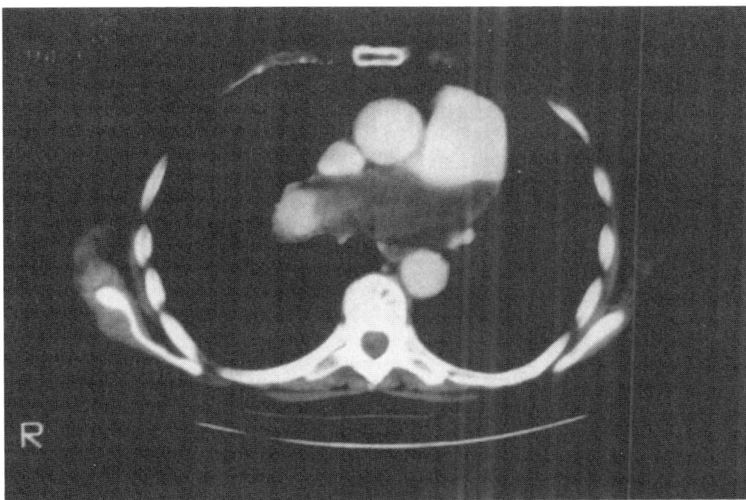

A

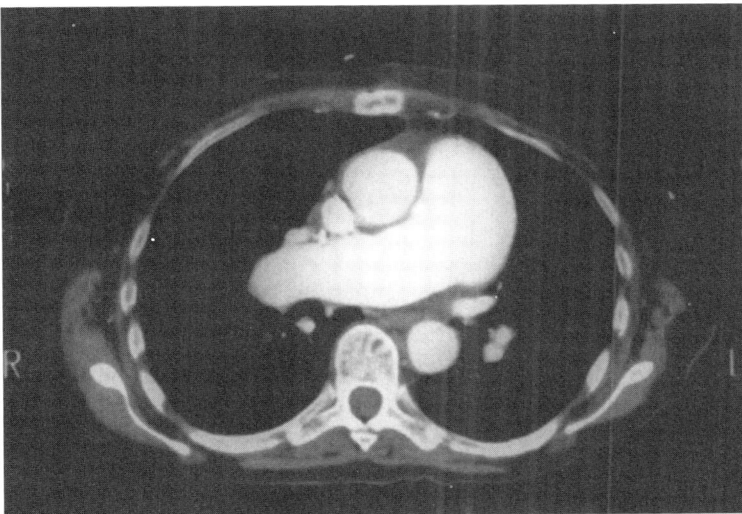

B

Figure 19 Chronic PE. (A) Large chronic PE in main PA and RPA. (B) After thromboendarterectomy, there is residual mild wall thickening of the dorsal wall of the right PA.

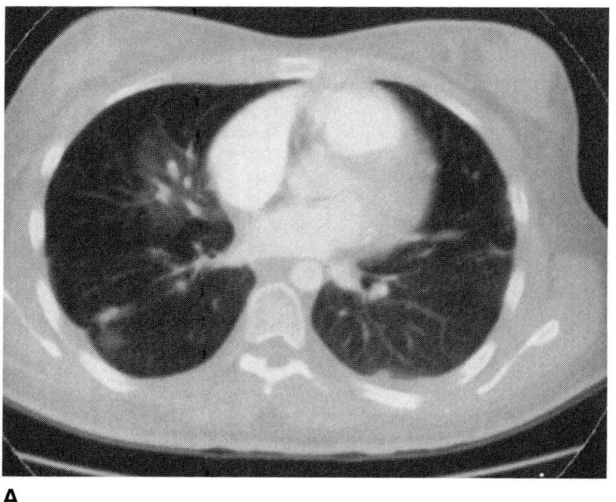

A

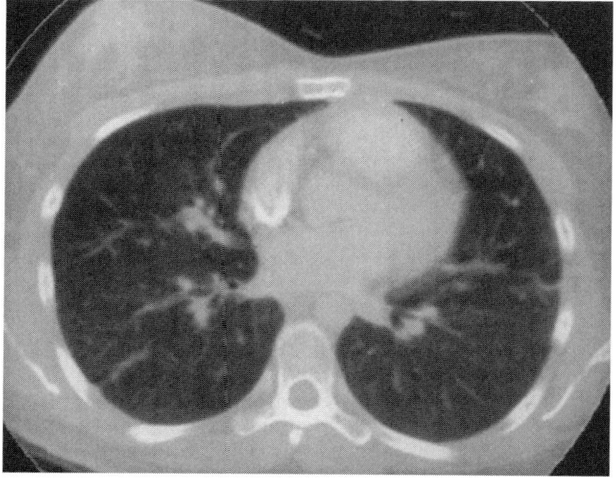

B

Figure 20 Mosaic perfusion of CPTE. (A) Marked variation in attenuation of lung parenchyma and disparity in sizes of segmental vessels at the level of the lower lobes. (B) Marked improvement in mosaic pattern compared to preoperative CT.

abnormalities in 75 patients with CPTE, 58 patients (77.3%) showed mosaic perfusion with normal or dilated pulmonary arteries in areas of relatively increased attenuation [38]. Residual scars from prior pulmonary infarction and cylindrical bronchiectasis are common [46,47].

IX. POSTEMBOLECTOMY FINDINGS

Pulmonary hypertension related to chronic thromboembolic disease may be treated in selected patients with thromboendarterectomy. In this procedure, as described by Jamieson, an endarterectomy of the entire pulmonary vascular bed is performed from the central through subsegmental arteries, while the patient is under circulatory arrest [48]. However, despite the fact that surgical description involves removal of very distal clot from peripheral arteries, according to Bergin et al., preoperative CT angiographic features of patients with good response to surgery include the presence of central pulmonary emboli and limited evidence of small vessel disease [49]. For this reason, CT, which better evaluates the central vessels, can be expected to show dramatic changes after successful surgery.

There is very little literature on the postoperative CT findings after pulmonary thromboendarterectomy. Increased enhancement of pulmonary vessels and improved lung perfusion have been described on MR imaging in a patient who underwent thromboendarterectomy [50]. In our limited experience, as expected, CT demonstrates that the narrowed vessel lumen returns toward normal with enhancement of vessels that previously contained emboli (Fig. 19). The ''thick wall'' of the vessels often return to normal or near normal, and the mosaic perfusion of the parenchyma regresses considerably, but incompletely (Fig. 20). Computed tomography may therefore be an additional tool in evaluating surgical success, to be used with clinical parameters and well-described echocardiographic findings such as right ventricular remodeling and reversal of tricuspid regurgitation.

REFERENCES

1. PIOPED Investigators. Value of the ventilation/perfusion scan in acute pulmonary embolism: results of the Prospective Investigation of Pulmonary Embolism Diagnosis (PIOPED). J Am Med Assoc 1990; 263:2753–2759.
2. Goodman L, Lipchik RJ. Diagnosis of acute pulmonary embolism: time for a new approach. Radiology 1996; 199:25–27.

3. Hull R, Raskob G, Panjuu A, Gill G. A new noninvasive management strategy for patients with suspected pulmonary embolism. Arch Intern Med 1989; 149: 2459–2555.
4. Novelline R, Baltarowich O, Athanasoulis C, Waltman A, Greenfield A. The clinical course of patients with suspected pulmonary embolism and a negative pulmonary arteriogram. Radiology 1978; 126:561–567.
5. Khorasani R, Gudas T, Hikpoor N, Polak J. Treatment of patients with suspected pulmonary embolism and intermediate-probability lung scans: is diagnostic imaging underused? Am J Radiol 1997; 169:1355–1357.
6. Goodman L, Curtin J, Mewissen M, Foley W, Lipchik R, Crain M, et al. Detection of pulmonary embolism in patients with unresolved clinical and scintigraphic diagnosis: Helical CT versus angiography. Am J Radiol 1995; 164:1369–1374.
7. Mayo J, Remy-Jardin M, Müller N, Remy J, Worsley D, Hossein-Foucher C, et al. Pulmonary embolism; prospective comparison of spiral helical CT with ventilation–perfusion scintigraphy. Radiology 1997; 205:447–452.
8. Blachere H, Latrabe V, Montaudon M, Valli N, Couffinhal T, Raherisson C, et al. Pulmonary embolism revealed on helical CT angiography: comparison with ventilation–perfusion radionuclide lung scanning. Am J Radiol 2000; 174:1041–1047.
9. Garg K, Sieler H, Welsh C, Johnston R, Russ P. Clinical validity of helical CT being interpreted as negative for pulmonary embolism: implications for patient treatment. Am J Radiol 1999; 172:1627–1631.
10. Remy-Jardin M, Remy J, Baghaie F, Fribourg M, Artaud D, Duhamel A. Clinical value of thin collimation in the diagnostic workup of pulmonary embolism. Am J Radiol 2000; 175:407–411.
11. Goodman L, Lipchik R, Kuzo R, Liu Y, McAuliffe T, O'Brien D. Subsequent pulmonary embolism: risk after a negative helical CT pulmonary angiogram—prospective comparison with scintigraphy (see comments). Radiology 2000; 215(2):535–542.
12. Hirsh J. Low-molecular-weight heparin: a review of the results of recent studies of the treatment of venous thromboembolism and unstable angina. Circulation 1998; 98:1575–1582.
13. Loud P, Katz D, Klippenstein D, Shah R, Grossman Z. Combined CT venography and pulmonary angiography in suspected thromboembolic disease: diagnostic accuracy for deep venous evaluation. Am J Radiol 2000; 174:61–65.
14. Loud PA, Katz DS, Bruce DA, Klippenstein DL, Grossman ZD. Deep venous thrombosis with suspected pulmonary embolism: detection with combined CT venography and pulmonary angiography. Radiology 2001; 219(2):498–502.
15. Coche EE, Hamoir XL, Hammer FD, et al. Using dual-detector helical CT angiography to detect deep venous thrombosis in patients with suspicion of pulmonary embolism: diagnostic value and additional findings. AJR 2001; 1035–1038.
16. Jackson C, Huber J. Correlated applied anatomy of the bronchial tree and lungs with a system of nomenclature. Dis Chest 1943; 9:319–326.

17. Kuzo R, Goodman L. HCT evaluation of pulmonary embolism: technique and interpretation. Am J Radiol 1997; 169(4):959–965.
18. Jardin M, Remy J. Segmental bronchovascular anatomy of the lower lobes: CT analysis. Am J Radiol 1985; 147:457–468.
19. Boyden E. Segmental Anatomy of the Lungs. New York: McGraw–Hill, 1955.
20. Lee K, Bae W, Lee B, Kim I, Choi E, Lee B. Bronchovascular anatomy of the upper lobes: evaluation with thin-section CT. Radiology 1991; 181:765–772.
21. Lee K, Im J, Kim Y, Jung S, Lee B, Han M, et al. CT anatomy of the lingular segmental bronchi. J Comput Assist Tomogr 1991; 15(1):86–91.
22. Naidich D, Zinn W, Ettenger N, McCauley D, Garay S. Basilar segmental bronchi: thin-section CT evaluation. Radiology 1988; 169:11–16.
23. Remy-Jardin M, Remy J, Wattinne L, Giraud F. Central pulmonary thromboembolism: diagnosis with spiral volumetric CT with the single-breath-hold technique—comparison with pulmonary angiography. Radiology 1992; 185:381–387.
24. Remy-Jardin M, Remy J, Artaud D, Deschildre F, Fribourg M, Beregi J. Spiral CT of pulmonary embolism: technical considerations and interpretive pitfalls. J Thorac Imaging 1997; 12:103–117.
25. Remy-Jardin M, Remy J, Cauvain O, Petyt L, Wannebroucq J, Beregi J-P. Diagnosis of central pulmonary embolism with helical CT: role of two-dimensional multiplanar reformations. Am J Radiol 1995; 165:1131–1138.
26. Simon M, Boiselle PM, Choi JR, Rosen MP, Reynolds K, Raptopoulos V. Paddle-wheel CT display of pulmonary arteries and other lung structures: a new imaging approach. AJR 2001; 177:195–198.
27. Remy-Jardin M, Remy J. Spiral CT angiography of the pulmonary circulation. Radiology 1999; 212:615–636.
28. Katz D, Loud P, Klippenstein D, Shah R, Grossman Z. Extra-thoracic findings on the venous phase of combined computed tomography venography and pulmonary angiography. Clin Radiol 2000; 55:177–181.
29. Baldt M, Zontsich T, Kainberger F, Fleischmann G, Mostbeck G. Spiral CT evaluation of deep venous thrombosis. Semin US Comput Tomogr Mag Reson 1997; 18:369–375.
30. Remy-Jardin M, Louvegny S, Remy J, Artaud D, Deschildre F, Bauchart J-J, et al. Acute central thromboembolic disease: posttherapeutic follow-up with spiral CT angiography. Radiology 1997; 203:173–180.
31. Benotti J, Dalen J. The natural history of pulmonary embolism. Clin Chest Med 1969; 5:403–410.
32. Banas J, Brooks H, Evans G, Paraskas J, Dexter L. Resolution rate of acute pulmonary embolism in man. N Engl J Med 1969; 280:1194–1199.
33. Moser K, Auger W, Fedullo P. Chronic major-vessel thromboembolic pulmonary hypertension. Circulation 1990; 81:1735–1743.
34. Bergin C, Sirlin C, Hauschildt J, Huynh T, Auger W, Fedullo P, et al. Chronic pulmonary thromboembolism: diagnosis with helical CT and MR imaging with angiographic and surgical correlation. Radiology 1997; 204:695–702.
35. Falaschi F, Palla A, Formichi B, Sbragia P, Petruzzelli S, Giuntini C, et al. CT

evaluation of chronic thromboembolic pulmonary hypertension. J Comput Assist Tomogr 1992; 6:897–903.
36. Tardivon A, Musset D, Maitre S, Renot F, Dartevelle P, Simonneau G, et al. Role of CT in chronic pulmonary embolism: comparison with pulmonary angiography. J Comput Assist Tomogr 1993.
37. Roberts H, Kauczor H-U, Schweden F, Thelen M. Spiral CT of pulmonary hypertension and chronic thromboembolism. J Thorac Imaging 1997; 12:118–127.
38. Schwickert H, Schweden F, Schild H, Piepenburg R, Düber C, Kauczor H-U, et al. Pulmonary arteries and lung parenchyma in chronic pulmonary embolism: preoperative and postoperative CT findings. Radiology 1994; 191:351–357.
39. Auger W, Fedullo P, Moser K, Buchbinder M, Peterson K. Chronic major-vessel thromboembolic pulmonary artery obstruction: appearance at angiography. Radiology 1992; 182:393–398.
40. Kauczor H-U, Schwickert H, Mayer E, Schweden F, Schild H, Thelen M. Spiral CT of bronchial arteries in chronic thromboembolism. J Comput Assist Tomogr 1994; 18:855–861.
41. Tan R, Kuzo R, Goodman L, Siegel R, Haasler G, Presberg K. Utility of CT scan evaluation for predicting pulmonary hypertension in patients with parenchymal lung disease. Chest 1998; 113:1250–1256.
42. Moser K, Bloor C. Pulmonary vascular lesions occurring in patients with chronic major vessel thromboembolic pulmonary hypertension. Chest 1993; 103:685–692.
43. Worthy S, Müller N, Hartman T, Swensen S, Padley S, Hansell D. Mosaic attenuation pattern on thin-section CT scans of the lung: differentiation among infiltrative of the lung, airway, and vascular diseases as a cause. Radiology 1997; 205: 465–470.
44. Sherrick A, Swensen S, Hartman T. Mosaic pattern of lung attenuation on CT scans: frequency among patients with pulmonary artery hypertension of different causes. Am J Radiol 1997; 169:79–82.
45. King M, Bergin C, Yeung D, Belezzouli E, Olson L, Ashburn W, et al. Chronic pulmonary thromboembolism: detection of regional hypoperfusion with CT. Radiology 1994; 191:359–363.
46. Bergin C, Rios G, King M, Belezzuoli E, Luna J, Auger W. Accuracy of high-resolution CT in identifying chronic pulmonary thromboembolic disease. Am J Radiol 1996; 166:1371–1377.
47. Remy-Jardin M, Remy J, Louvegny S, Artaud D, Deschildre F, Duhamel A. Airway changes in chronic pulmonary embolism: CT findings in 33 patients. Radiology 1997; 203:355–360.
48. Jamieson S. Pulmonary thromboendarterectomy. Heart 1998; 79(2):118–120.
49. Bergin C, Sirlin C, Deutsch R, Fedullo P, Hauschildt J, Huynh T, et al. Predictors of patient response to pulmonary thromboendarterectomy. Am J Radiol 2000; 174(2):509–515.
50. Kreitner K-F, Mayer E, Voigtlaender T, Thelen M, Oelert H. Three-dimensional contrast-enhanced magnetic resonance angiography in a patient with chronic thromboembolic pulmonary hypertension before and after thromboendarterectomy. Circulation 1999; 99(8):1101.

8
Spiral CT Angiography of the Thoracic Aorta

Timothy John Carroll, Curtis E. Green, and Jeffrey S. Klein
University of Vermont College of Medicine
Burlington, Vermont

I. INTRODUCTION

In recent years, advances in computed tomography (CT) imaging have led to an increasing role for CT angiography in the evaluation of a variety of aortic abnormalities. In this chapter, we review the role of spiral CT angiography in the assessment of congenital and acquired aortic abnormalities and compare this technique to other imaging modalities, including conventional aortography, magnetic resonance imaging, and transesophageal echocardiography.

II. CONGENITAL ANOMALIES OF THE AORTA

A. Embryology

It is not necessary to thoroughly understand the embryological development of the aorta to diagnose the various arch anomalies, but it is useful to have a basic idea about how they arise as it makes the imaging findings easier to understand. In the classic theoretical embryological double arch proposed by Edwards (Fig. 1), there are right and left aortic arches that connect the ascending and descending portions of the aorta [1]. Each gives rise to a carotid and a subclavian artery. In normal development, the left arch persists and the part of the right arch distal to the origin of the right subclavian artery becomes

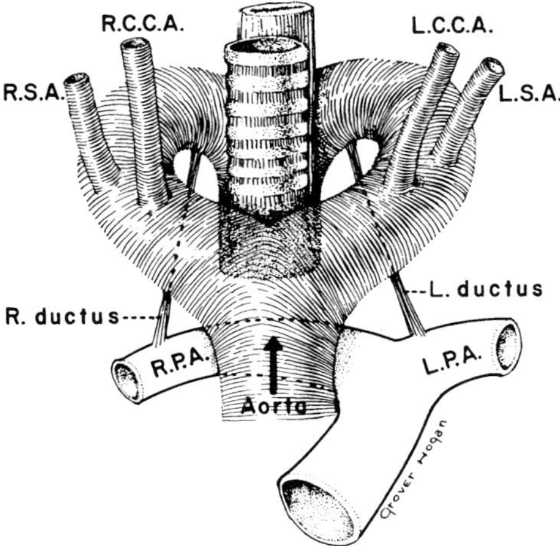

Figure 1 Hypothetical double aortic arch system of Edwards.

atretic. This results in three great vessels arising from the arch: a right brachiocephalic artery composed of the proximal remnant of the right arch and the right carotid and subclavian arteries; a left common carotid artery, and a left subclavian artery. The remnant of the ductus arteriosus, the ligamentum arteriosum, connects the bottom of the transverse arch to the proximal left pulmonary artery. Essentially all of the developmental anomalies of the aortic arch branches can be explained by variations in which part of the embryological double arch becomes atretic.

B. Diagnosis of Congenital Aortic Anomalies and Vascular Rings

A vascular ring results from encircling of the trachea by a combination of the aorta and its branches and the ligamentum arteriosum. If the ring is tight enough, tracheal compression and respiratory compromise may result. It is important to remember that the mere presence of an arch anomaly does not mean that there is a vascular ring. The diagnosis of ring should be made on the basis of symptoms and anatomy, not anatomy alone. When presented with a patient with stridor, the evaluation should begin with a frontal and lateral chest radiographs and a barium esophagram. If these confirm the presence of airway compromise and suggest a vascular cause, further evaluation with cross-sectional imaging can be pursued. In this day and age, there is little, if any, indication for angiographic evaluation of vascular anomalies.

Magnetic resonance imaging (MRI) using spin-echo (black blood) techniques is an elegant method of delineating the mediastinal vascular anatomy in infants, children, and adults with suspected congenital aortic anomalies, particularly vascular rings and aortic coarctation [2]. The lack of need for intravenous contrast and the ability to obtain two- and three-dimensional reformatted images to optimize display of aortic and branch anomalies make MRI the modality of choice in infants and children.

Rapid scanning with contrast-enhanced spiral CT, particularly the recent advent of multidetector-row scanners capable of very rapid scanning with thin collimation and minimal respiratory motion artifact, provides information analogous to MRI [3]. The scanning parameters and contrast administration used for CT aortography in infants and children are tailored to the individual examination, but follow the basic principles of CT aortography as outlined in Table 1. The technique utilized to evaluate suspected congenital aortic anomalies with spiral CT is the same as for the evaluation of acquired aortic disease

Table 1 Helical CT Scanning Protocol for Thoracic Aortic Disease

Procedural element	Protocol
Anatomic cephalocaudal extent of scan	Apices → bases
Scan milliamp, kilovolt peak settings	220 mAs, 120 kVp
Duration of helical exposure	20–30 sec
Pitch	2.0:1 (single-detector CT) 6.0:1 (MDCT) Table speed = 15 mm/rot.
Collimation	5 mm (infants = 3 mm) (single-detector CT) 2.5 mm (MDCT)
Display field of view	Widest rib → widest rib from AP scout
Patient instructions during scanning	Single breath hold after three maximal breaths
Precontrast scans	None
Contrast type/concentration/volume	Nonionic 300 mg% and 1 cc/kg (infants and children), 150 cc (adults)
Contrast injection rate	1–3 cc/sec
Scan delay from start of injection to scan	40 sec
Reconstruction algorithm	Standard
Reconstruction intervals	Contiguous for filming 3 mm for 3D reconstructions (infants = 2 mm) (single detector CT) 1.25 mm (MDCT)

in the adult population with the following exceptions: in neonates and children a lower exposure technique is utilized to limit radiation dosage, thinner collimation (3 mm) is utilized as less cephalocaudal coverage is needed, and the volume and rate of contrast administration is based on patient weight (2 mL of 300 mg% nonionic/kg injected at 2 mL/sec). Scans are reconstructed at overlapping (i.e., 2 mm) intervals for soft-copy interpretation and two- and three-dimensional reconstruction on a workstation.

C. Double Aortic Arch

Persistence of both aortic arches is an uncommon anomaly that frequently results in tracheal compression. Most patients present early in life although double arch may present as an incidental finding in an asymptomatic patient or as a ''mediastinal mass.'' In the majority of patients the right-sided arch is dominant, being larger, higher, and more anterior than the left-sided arch (Fig. 2). Each arch gives rise to a carotid and a subclavian artery. In some patients the left arch is atretic. In this case double arch cannot readily be distinguished from right arch with aberrant left subclavian artery and a left ligamentum. Surgical repair consists of division of the nondominant arch and ligamentum.

D. Right Aortic Arch

Persistence of the right aortic arch with atresia of the left occurs in approximately 1/2200 persons without congenital heart disease. The incidence in certain congenital anomalies such as Tetralogy of Fallot and persistent truncus arteriosus can be as high as 50%. Most persons with right aortic arch are completely asymptomatic and come to medical attention because the right arch is misdiagnosed on chest radiographs as a mediastinal mass. There are two common types of right arch: those with mirror-image branching of the great vessels (Type I) and those with aberrant origin of the left subclavian artery (Type II).

In the Type I right arch, the first vessel arising from the arch is a left brachiocephalic artery, followed in order by the right common carotid artery and the right subclavian artery. This anomaly results from atresia of the embryonic double arch distal to the left subclavian artery. These rarely cause symptoms of any kind, but are almost always associated with congenital heart disease.

In the Type II arch, the order of origination of the great vessels is left common carotid, right common carotid, right subclavian artery, and left sub-

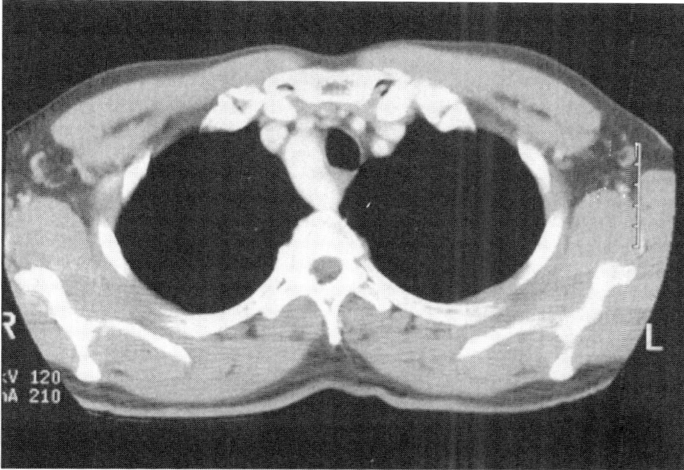

A

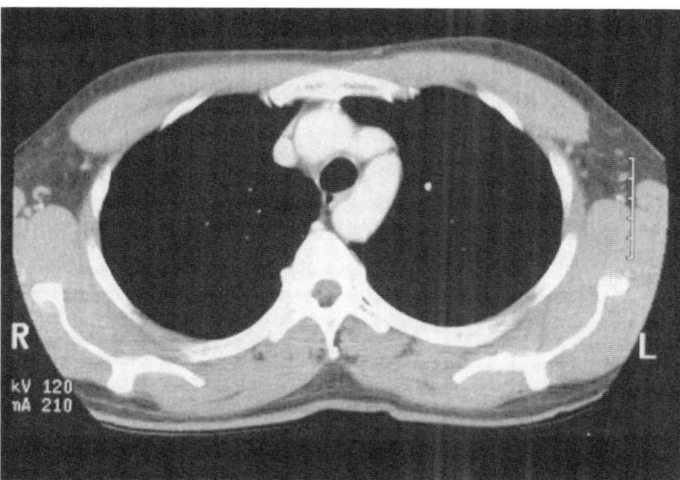

B

Figure 2 Double aortic arch. (A) Contrast-enhanced spiral CT through upper chest shows a high right aortic arch. (B) Scan at a more inferior location shows left component of double aortic arch.

clavian artery. In this case the left subclavian artery arises from the proximal portion of the descending aorta, just below the origin of the ductus arteriosus. Because the ligamentum is almost always left-sided, there is the potential for a vascular ring, although it is uncommon for it to be clinically significant.

With both types of right arch, the arch (by definition) passes to the right side of the trachea. In most cases the descending aorta is also on the right, not crossing over to the diaphragmatic hiatus until just above the diaphragm. Occasionally the arch will cross behind the esophagus at the level of the transverse arch, resulting in the so-called retroesophageal right arch. These patients usually have an aberrant left subclavian artery and may be more likely to complain of dysphagia than those in whom the aorta descends on the right.

The CT appearance of the Type I arch is the exact mirror image of the typical left arch. With Type II right arch the first branch of the aorta, the left common carotid, tends to be smaller than the typical brachiocephalic artery. The aberrant left subclavian artery, arises from the aorta just below the arch and courses posterior to the esophagus before ascending to resume its normal course (Fig. 3).

E. Left Aortic Arch with Aberrant Right Subclavian Artery

Aberrant origin of the right subclavian artery occurs when the embryological right arch becomes atretic between the origins of the right common carotid artery and the right subclavian artery and is said to occur in between 1/200 and 1/250 persons. The incidence is increased in Tetralogy of Fallot and coarctation of the aorta. The situation is a mirror image of the Type II right aortic arch, with the right subclavian artery arising from the proximal descending aorta. The right ductus almost always disappears and this anomaly is therefore rarely associated with a vascular ring. The origin of the aberrant vessel may be quite dilated, in which case it is referred to as the diverticulum of Kommerell. Occasionally the diverticulum of Kommerell enlarges to the point where it compresses on the esophagus (Fig. 3). Traditionally these have been blamed for dysphagia (dysphagia lusoria), but not all clinicians and investigators accept a causal association. An aberrant right subclavian artery may present as a right supraclavicular mass on the frontal chest radiograph and may be more prone to aneurysm formation than the normally arising right subclavian artery.

F. Coarctation and Pseudocoarctation of the Aorta

Coarctation of the aorta is a rare lesion in adults and is not likely to be discovered incidentally during chest CT for other indications. Magnetic resonance

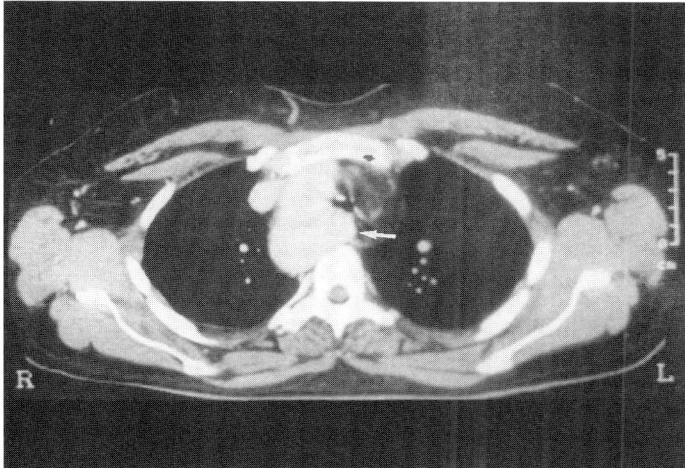

A

B

Figure 3 Right aortic arch with aberrant left subclavian artery. (A) Contrast-enhanced CT through upper chest in a patient with dysphagia shows a right aortic arch with an aberrant left subclavian artery (arrow) coursing toward the left in a retroesophageal location. (B) Scan through the apices shows the normal position of the left subclavian artery (arrow).

imaging is the preferred method for evaluation of coarctation. The coarctation is almost always just distal to the origin of the left subclavian artery although lower thoracic and abdominal coarctations occur. The area of narrowing may be quite discrete and easily missed on axial images, but should be apparent on reconstructed sagittal images. Dilatation of the descending aorta and left subclavian artery may be the only clues to the presence of coarctation on the axial images. Dilatation of the ascending aorta is not uncommon and may result from systemic hypertension or a stenotic aortic valve, the latter related to the high incidence of bicuspid aortic valve in patients with aortic coarctation.

Pseudocoarctation of the aorta is caused by kinking or folding of the proximal portion of the descending aorta and frequently results in a mass on the frontal chest radiograph. The diagnosis can be suspected from the lateral chest radiograph where the actual kink is sometimes visible. Because CT is the primary modality for evaluation of mediastinal masses, one is more likely to encounter a patient with pseudocoarctation than with coarctation. Pseudocoarctation is thought by some to be a form fruste of coarctation, in part because it also has a high association with bicuspid aortic valve and an increased incidence in Turner's and Noonan's syndromes. By definition there is absent or a trivial pressure gradient across the pseudocoarctation and surgical repair is rarely necessary. On axial CT images one sees a very dilated proximal descending aorta that usually extends higher than normal. The left subclavian artery may arise from either above or below the kink. Sagittal reconstructions nicely demonstrate the folded aorta and great vessel origins.

G. Cervical Aortic Arch

Cervical arch is a rare anomaly, most commonly seen on the right side with the arch extending into the high right paratracheal region, displacing the trachea. It is usually asymptomatic in adults although children may present with either a vascular ring or tracheal compression. Clinically it may present as a pulsating neck mass. The diagnosis is straightforward on axial or reconstructed images as the cervical portion of the aorta can be readily demonstrated to be continuous with the ascending aorta and separate from the great vessels.

III. ACUTE AORTIC DISEASES

This group of diseases comprises three conditions that typically present with acute chest pain: aortic dissection and two recently detailed entities that have similar clinical and radiologic features, aortic intramural hematoma and penetrating atherosclerotic ulcer of the aorta (Fig. 4). The widespread availability and use of cross-sectional techniques, including transesophageal echocardiography (TEE), spiral CT, and MR angiography, have allowed greater recognition of aortic dissection and its variants. This section focuses on the pathologic and imaging findings in these acute aortic diseases, with an emphasis on the characteristic CT features of each entity.

A. Aortic Dissection

Aortic dissection is the most common and lethal of the acute aortic disorders, with a reported incidence of 0.2–0.8% [4]. Risk factors for the development of aortic dissection include hypertension, cystic medial necrosis due to connective tissue disease (i.e., Marfan's and Ehlers-Danlos syndrome), congenital lesions such as bicuspid aortic valve and aortic coarctation, pregnancy, trauma, and arteritis. Patients who develop intramural hematomas, a variant of aortic dissection described below, may in a minority of cases develop communications with the aortic lumen thereby progressing to true dissection. Thoracic aortic aneurysms are more prone to dissection, as aortic wall tension is directly related to luminal diameter (Laplace's law). There is a male predominance for the diagnosis in most reported series. Symptoms on presentation include chest pain radiating to the back, syncope, and shortness of breath. Acute aortic dissection is defined as dissection detected within 2 weeks of the onset of symptoms, while chronic dissection is older than two weeks [5]. Since the clinical presentation may mimic myocardial infarction, pulmonary embolism, and other conditions, the diagnosis is often elusive.

The main pathologic feature of aortic dissection is an intimal tear within a weakened vessel wall that allows aortic blood to form a false channel that runs parallel to the true aortic lumen within the outer two-thirds of the aortic media (Fig. 4C). There are two classification systems for aortic dissection that are based on the origin of the intimal tear and the extent of aortic involvement: the Debakey classification and the Stanford classification. In the Debakey system, a Type I dissection arises from a tear in the ascending aorta at the sinotubular junction and involves both ascending and descending aorta, while a Type II dissection affects only the ascending aorta. When the intimal tear arises just distal to the ligamentum arteriosum and extends distally to involve the descending aorta, it is classified as a Type III dissection. Debakey Type III dissections can be further subclassified as Type IIIa when the dissection is limited to the descending aorta and IIIb when there is extension into the abdominal aorta and iliac arteries [6]. The Stanford classification divides aortic dissection into two categories: Type A dissection with involvement of the

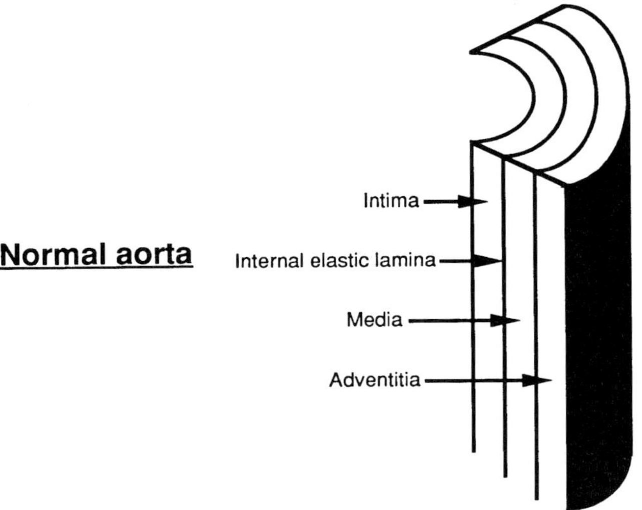

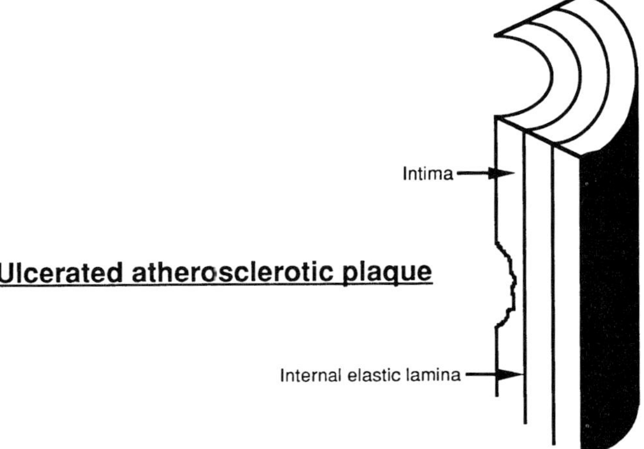

Figure 4 (A–E) Diagram of aortic dissection and its variants.

Aortic dissection

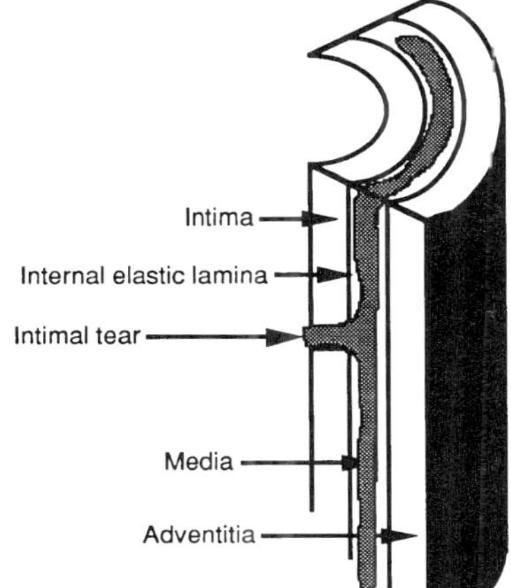

C

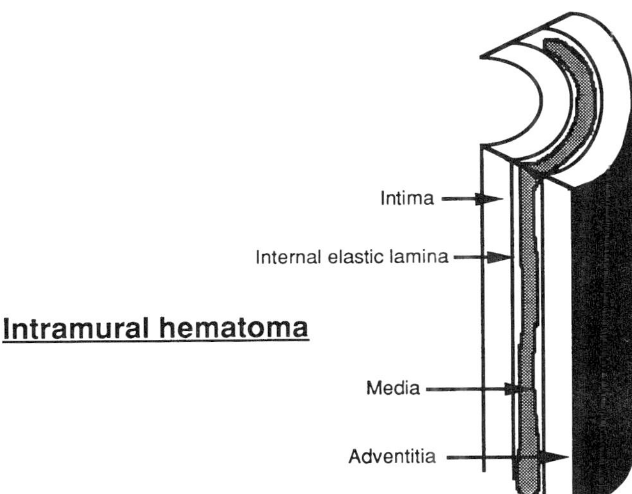

D

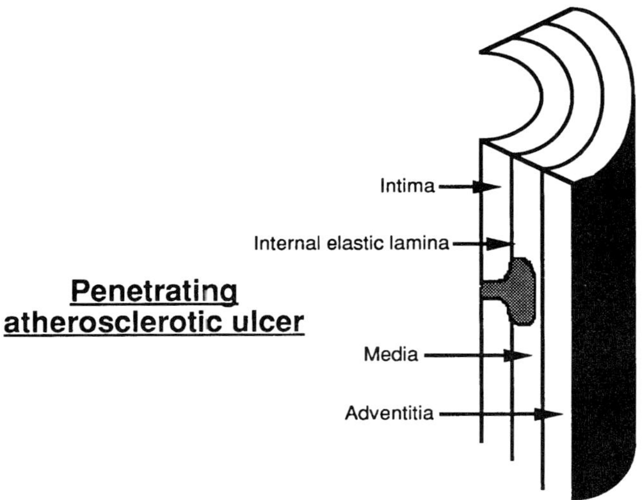

Figure 4 Continued

ascending aorta with (Fig. 5) or without extension distally into the arch or descending aorta, and Type B dissection limited to the descending aorta. Approximately two-thirds of aorta dissections are Type A and one-third is Type B. The Stanford classification system has become the more widely utilized system, as there has been significant data published on the therapeutic and prognostic implications of Type A versus Type B aortic dissection.

The chest radiograph is of limited value in the evaluation of suspected aortic dissection. Some patients with aortic dissection show mediastinal widening, aortic dilatation, and indistinctness of the aortic knob on frontal chest radiographs. Medial displacement of intimal calcifications greater than 1.0 cm from the lateral aortic margin has been described as an insensitive but fairly specific finding of aortic dissection in the appropriate clinical context, but this finding is not of value in the aortic knob where the arch is foreshortened and the calcification is unlikely to lie in the same coronal plane as that portion of the distal aortic arch that forms the lateral margin of the aortic knob.

Emergent cross-sectional imaging will almost invariably be necessary when acute aortic dissection is suspected. In institutions where transesophageal echocardiography is available on an emergent basis, this exam, although invasive and quite operator dependent, can be performed at the bedside and

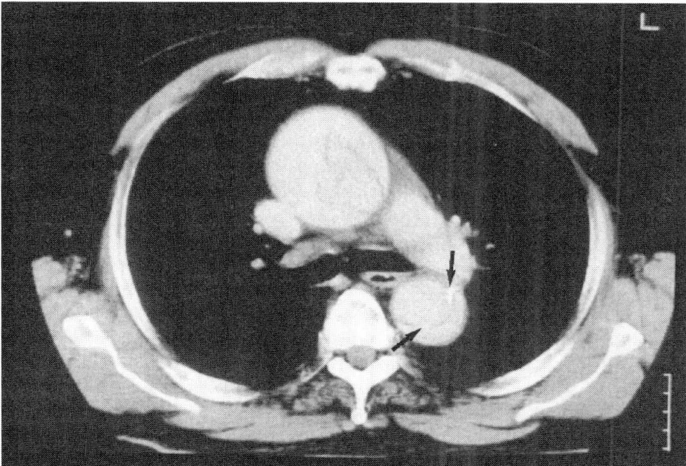

A

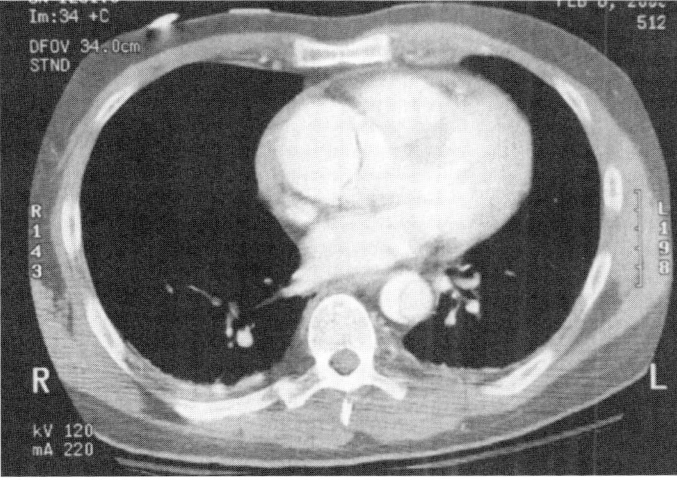

B

Figure 5 Stanford type A aortic dissection. (A) Enhanced scan at the tracheal carina shows an intimal flap within a dilated ascending aorta extending into the descending aorta with flow in both true and false lumina. Note displacement of intimal calcifications in the descending aorta (arrows). (B) Scan at the level of the aortic root shows the intimal flap at the sinotubular junction in the ascending aorta. The false lumen is anterolaterally situated in the ascending aorta and posterolateral in the descending aorta. (C) Scan through the proximal arch vessels shows the intimal flap extending into the proximal brachiocephalic and left subclavian arteries.

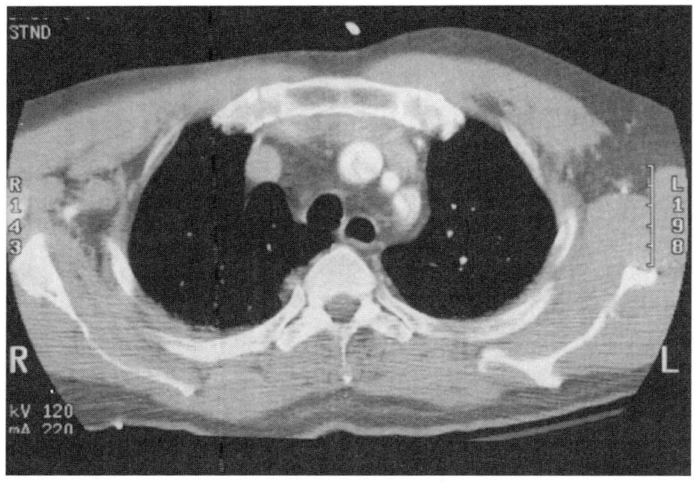

C

Figure 5 Continued

provides rapid assessment of the aorta, including the presence or absence of an intimal flap, the status of the aortic valve, the presence of pericardial fluid, and the functional status of the myocardium. Limitations include availability; the inability to assess the status of the great vessels; and occasional difficulty in visualizing the entirety of the ascending aorta, arch, and descending aorta. Prior to the advent of spiral CT in the early 1990s, magnetic resonance appeared to be the modality of choice, with a reported sensitivity and specificity of 98% [7]. In addition to its high accuracy for diagnosis, additional advantages of traditional (spin-echo and gradient-echo) MR include lack of need for iodinated contrast and the simultaneous evaluation of the aorta and great vessels, heart, and pericardial space in multiple planes. More recently the development of contrast- (i.e., gadolinium)- enhanced MR angiography has provided exquisite detail of the aorta and arch vessels with significantly reduced acquisition times, allowing complete aortic evaluation in a single-breath-hold acquisition. Recent studies have confirmed the excellent accuracy of MR for imaging aortic dissection but the more widespread availability of spiral CT and the greater ease of monitoring unstable patients in the CT suite has made this technique the more widely utilized imaging procedure for evaluation of suspected acute aortic disease, including dissection. Magnetic resonance is of particular value in monitoring the success of nonoperative management of dissection and in the postoperative follow-up of surgically managed patients.

Conventional contrast angiography, while often utilized in the past for detecting the presence and extent of disease in aortic dissection, has been largely supplanted by the cross-sectional modalities described above. Angiography has been shown to be less sensitive than spiral CT, MR, and TEE for the diagnosis of dissection. However, if percutaneous techniques at managing aortic dissection, including percutaneous fenestration of the aorta and stent-graft obliteration of the lumen, become more widely employed, there may be increasing utilization of catheter angiography for both diagnostic and therapeutic purposes.

Spiral computed tomography has become a mainstay in the imaging diagnosis of suspected acute aortic dissection due to its widespread availability and high image acquisition speed; proximity to the emergency room at most institutions; uniform high-quality axial and multiplanar-reconstructed images; and ability to simultaneously assess the entire aorta and arch vessels, pericardial space, and the remainder of the thorax. In a 1996 study by Sommer and colleagues, spiral CT had a 100% sensitivity and specificity in the detection of aortic dissection [8]. The technique used for the evaluation of acute aortic dissection is shown in Table 2. Initial unenhanced scans are performed to detect medially displaced intimal calcifications or to visualize an intimal flap in patients with severe anemia [9], with either finding indicating the presence of a false lumen. In addition, the presence of an aortic intramural hematoma that may mimic aortic dissection clinically is depicted on unenhanced scans as a crescentic region of intramural high attenuation that can be mistaken for a thickened aortic wall if only contrast-enhanced scans are obtained. In patients with significant renal insufficiency, either of these findings on unenhanced CT may be sufficient for appropriate diagnosis and triage without the risk of inducing contrast-mediated renal failure.

The contrast-enhanced CT scans obtained in patients with suspected dissection should begin above the aortic arch to include the proximal arch vessels and extend to the level of the common iliac arteries inferiorly. Since a large number of axial images are obtained with the use of thin collimation and overlapping reconstruction, particularly with the newer multidetector-row CT scanners, the study is most easily interpreted on a workstation where cineviewing is possible and multiplanar reformatted images, particularly oblique sagittal reconstructions, can be created. The CT diagnosis of aortic dissection is made by detection of an intimal flap separating the true from false lumen (Fig. 5). In type A dissections, the false lumen is typically seen along the right anterolateral wall of the ascending aorta and spirals as it extends distally to lie along the left posterolateral wall of the descending aorta. While it is often helpful in Type A dissections to determine the presence of involvement of the arch vessels, this does not usually alter the surgical approach to the patient.

Table 2 Helical CT Scanning Protocol for Suspected Aortic Dissection

Procedural element	Protocol
Anatomic cepahlocaudal extent of scan	Apices to iliac bifurcation
Scan mAs, and kVp	220 mAs, 120 kVp
Duration of helical exposure	30–45 sec
Pitch	2.0:1 (single detector CT) 6.0:1 (MDCT) Table speed = 15 mm/rot.
Collimation	5 mm (single-detector CT) 2.5 mm (MDCT)
Display field of view	Widest rib → widest rib from AP scout
Patient instructions during scanning	Breath-hold after three maximal breaths
Precontrast scans	Apices to bases using 7-mm collimation, pitch 1.5:1, reconstructed at 10.5-mm intervals (single-detector CT) Apices to bases using 5-mm collimation, pitch 6:1, reconstructed at 2.5-mm intervals (MDCT)
Contrast type/concentration/volume	Nonionic 300 mg% 150 cc
Contrast injection rate	3 cc/sec
Scan delay from start of injection to scan	40 sec
Reconstruction algorithm	Standard
Reconstruction spacing	Contiguous for filming 3 mm for 3D reconstructions (single-detector CT) contiguous for filming 1.25-mm intervals for 3D reconstructions (MDCT)

Computed tomography findings associated with dissection include pericardial or pleural effusion and aortic dilatation.

While the primary goal of imaging is to establish the presence of a dissection, the complications of aortic dissection are also readily depicted on spiral CT. These include aortic branch vessel occlusion, specifically involvement of the arch vessels or renal or mesenteric vessels; aneurysm formation; hemopericardium with tamponade; and rupture with mediastinal or pleural hemorrhage (Fig. 6). The presence of aortic regurgitation or the development of myocardial infarction from proximal extension of a dissection are best evaluated on TEE.

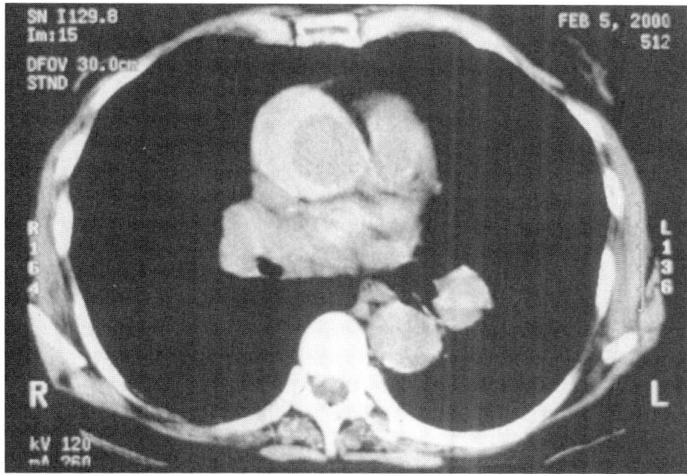

A

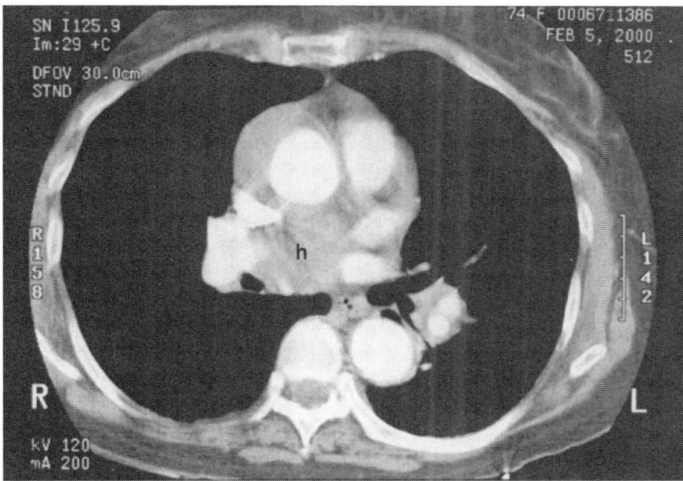

B

Figure 6 Ruptured thrombosed Type A aortic dissection. (A) Unenhanced CT shows crescentic high attenuation material surrounding the ascending aorta. (B) Contrast-enhanced scan at the same level as (a) shows no enhancement of the crescentic density, indicating either a thrombosed false lumen or an intramural hematoma. There is hematoma (h) within the middle mediastinum and surrounding the left lower hilar arteries. Surgery confirmed a thrombosed Type A dissection with mediastinal leakage, which was successfully repaired.

The role of computer-generated two-dimensional (multiplanar or MPR) and three-dimensional (multiplanar volumetric or MPVR) reconstructions in the evaluation of aortic dissection is limited. While single-voxel-thick (two-dimensional) oblique sagittal MPRs and curved planar reformations (CPRs) obtained parallel to the long axis of the thoracic aorta allow for simultaneous display of the entire aorta and arch vessels, the additional diagnostic value provided is minimal. CPRs can help depict the relationship of the intimal flap to great vessel ostia [10]. Volumetric reconstructions (MPVRs) performed with maximum intensity projection (MIP) and shaded surface display rendering techniques have a limited ability to depict intimal flaps and therefore are the least valuable of the reconstruction algorithms in evaluating aortic dissection.

There are several pitfalls in the interpretation of CT aortography for the diagnosis of dissection. These include factors that can produce the false appearance of an intimal flap and insufficient vascular enhancement to allow detection of an intimal flap [11]. The most common cause of a pseudodissection is a curvilinear streak artifact in the ascending aorta related to the pulsatile movement of the aortic wall between end diastole and end systole [12]. These artifacts are typically seen along the left anterior and right posterior aspects of the ascending aorta and are minimized by use of a 180° linear interpolation reconstruction algorithm [13]. Other common causes of streak artifacts in the aorta include dense contrast in the left brachiocephalic vein (from a left arm contrast injection) or superior vena cava and mediastinal clips or in-dwelling tubes or catheters. In addition, any high-attenuation structure that contacts the enhancing aortic lumen can simulate an enhancing false lumen and produce the appearance of an intimal flap. These include an enhanced left brachiocephalic, superior intercostal, or left inferior pulmonary vein and curvilinear atelectasis of the left lower lobe.

The natural history of medically managed acute Type A dissection is associated with a 3-month mortality rate of 90% [5], rendering surgical repair the treatment of choice in Type A dissection in operative candidates. Alternatively, the survival rate for medically managed Type B dissection is 73% at 1 year: This in combination with a high rate of paraplegia and death (up to 65%) in surgically managed Type B dissections warrants medical therapy in this group unless there is the development of aneurysm, rupture, or proximal extension into the arch and ascending aorta. Although the traditional approach to Type A dissection is immediate surgery and Type B medical management, recent data suggest that some Type A dissections, particularly where the diagnosis is delayed several days after onset of symptoms or patients are considered poor surgical candidates, may be managed with semielective surgery or even aggressive medical therapy alone with good outcomes. Patients with Type B dissections complicated by ischemic injury to the kidneys, spinal cord, bowel, or legs; rapid enlargement; rupture; intractable pain; or proximal extension require surgical repair.

B. Intramural Hematoma

Intramural hematoma (IMH) of the aorta is an acute clinical entity that represents a hemorrhage confined to the aortic media in which there is no intimal tear (Fig. 4D). It is thought to arise from rupture of the vasa vasorum within the aortic media and as in aortic dissection tends to affect hypertensive patients, although it can result from trauma or develop as a complication of a penetrating atherosclerotic ulcer. Since only first recognized as a distinct radiographic entity in 1985 [14], it is likely that a significant percentage of cases of IMH have been traditionally misclassified as "atypical" aortic dissections. In support of this concept is the finding that at one institution a retrospective review of 214 patients originally classified as aortic dissection showed 17 (8%) that met the imaging criteria for IMH [15].

Patients with IMH tend to be older at age of presentation than those with aortic dissection, particularly when compared to Type A dissection associated with Marfan's syndrome. As in classic dissection, pain radiating to the back is the most common presenting complaint. Unlike classic dissection, most patients with IMH (70%) have involvement limited to the descending aorta, and branch vessel occlusion is very uncommon. Based on a similar mode of presentation to classic dissection and severity of this disorder, most experts recommend classifying IMH in a manner analogous to that of aortic dissection (i.e., Type A with ascending aortic involvement and Type B limited to the descending aorta).

Transesophageal echocardiography can depict IMH but this diagnosis is often difficult to distinguish sonographically from mural thrombus within a dilated aorta. Computed tomography has a 96% sensitivity for the detection of intramural hematoma [16]. Noncontrast-enhanced CT demonstrates a high-attenuation crescent-shaped thickening of the aortic wall that extends in the cephalocaudal direction without significant compromise of the vascular lumen (i.e., there is a concave interface between the hematoma and the aortic lumen) (Fig. 7A). There may be medial displacement of intimal calcifications and the aorta is often dilated or aneurysmal. Following intravenous contrast administration, there is lack of enhancement of the hematoma, no intimal flap is identified, and the hematoma appears hypodense relative to the enhancing aortic lumen (Fig. 7B). It may be difficult to distinguish IMH from atherosclerotic

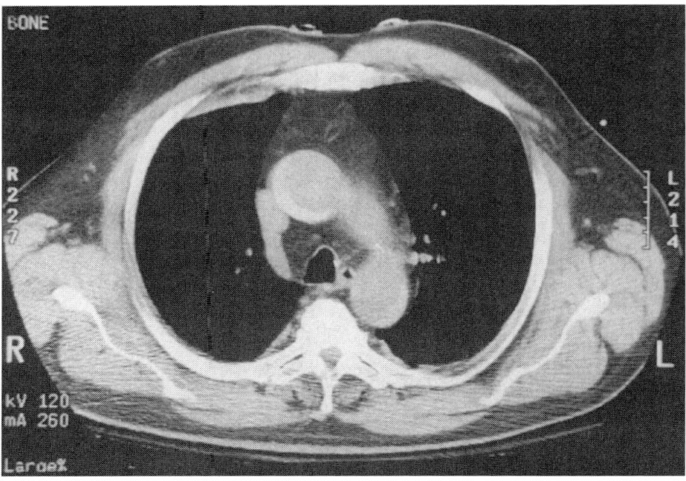

A

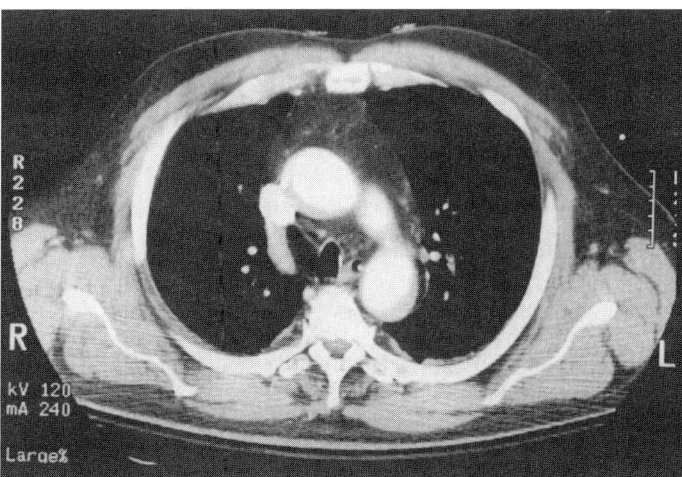

B

Figure 7 Intramural hematoma (Type A) of the aorta. (A) Unenhanced CT just below the aortic arch shows crescentic high attenuation material within the ascending and descending aorta. (B) Following contrast administration, there is no enhancement of the crescentic material.

thickening of the aorta or thrombus within an aortic aneurysm. The presence of a high-attenuation smooth crescentic intramural density on precontrast scans that does not enhance and the absence of an intimal flap usually allows for accurate diagnosis. While the distinction from an acutely thrombosed aortic dissection is more difficult, an IMH, unlike a dissection, does not typically spiral around the circumference of the aorta, as it extends longitudinally. MRI, particularly with the use of dynamic cine-gradient-echo (GRE) sequences, is particularly accurate for assessing IMH and is used as the primary method of diagnosis in some institutions [17,18]. Aortography is insensitive to the detection of intramural hematoma unassociated with penetrating atherosclerotic ulcer as the thickened aortic wall is difficult to appreciate and distinguish from atherosclerotic disease.

The prognosis for patients with IMH depends on the type or extent of hematoma formation, the age of the patient, and the presence of comorbid conditions. Most centers with experience managing IMH recommend an operative approach to Type A IMH, since there is a high rate of rupture with resultant pericardial tamponade or mediastinal hemorrhage or the development of intimal disruption with dissection in these patients [15,17,19]. Most patients with Type B IMH have good short-term outcome with aggressive medical control of hypertension. However, close clinical and cross-sectional imaging follow-up within the first 10–14 days of presentation is recommended to detect progressive aortic involvement or dilatation (Fig. 8) or progression to typical dissection, conditions that might warrant a more aggressive approach.

C. Penetrating Atherosclerotic Ulcer

Penetrating atherosclerotic ulcer (PAU) is an ulcer that develops within an atherosclerotically diseased portion of the thoracic or rarely the abdominal aorta, penetrating the internal elastic lamina and into the aortic media and associated with a localized intramural hematoma (Fig. 4E) [20]. This most often develops in elderly hypertensive patients with severe atherosclerotic disease and most commonly affects the descending thoracic aorta (90%) [15]. While ulcerated atherosclerotic plaques limited to the aortic intima may be detected as incidental findings on contrast-enhanced thoracic CT, most patients with PAU present with chest and back pain indistinguishable from type B aortic dissection. In most cases the ulcerating lesion is limited in extent by the locally advanced atherosclerotic disease present within the adjacent portion of the aorta, although extension along the length of the aorta or through the media and adventitia with pseudoaneurysm formation can occur. As with IMH, the diagnosis of PAU among patients presenting with acute aortic syn-

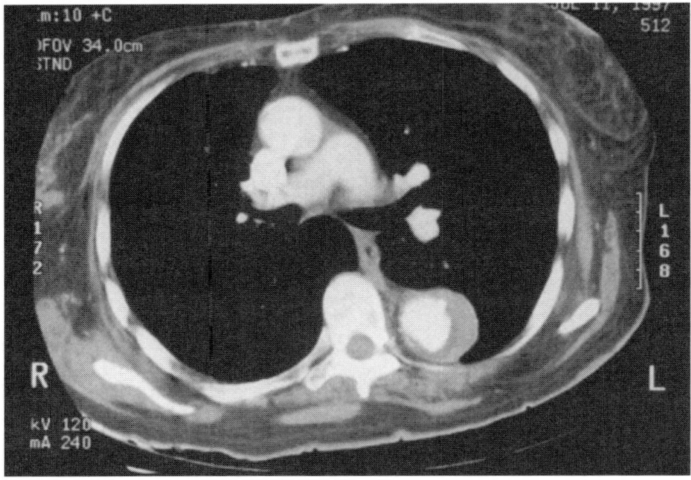

A

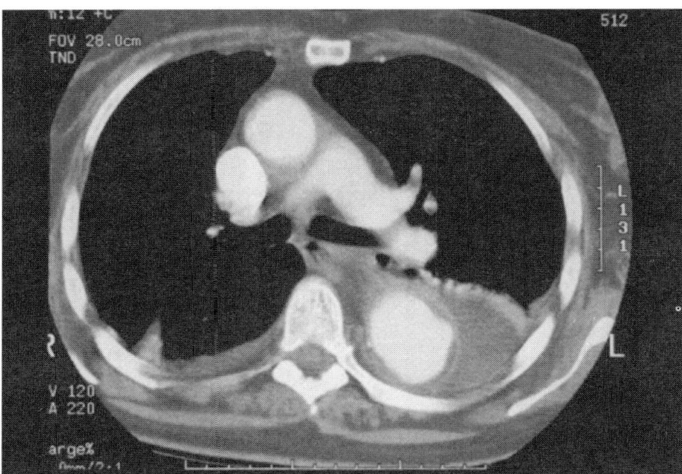

B

Figure 8 Intramural hematoma (IMH) with rapid development of aneurysmal dilatation. (A) Contrast-enhanced scan shows a mildly dilated descending aorta with a mural crescent of high-attenuation material representing an IMH. (B) Repeat CT obtained 48 hr later due to persistent pain shows aneurysmal dilatation of the descending aorta with development of a left pleural effusion. (C) Oblique sagittal maximum intensity projection (MIP) image obtained from the scan in (B) shows fusiform aneurysmal dilatation of the middescending aorta. Left thoracotomy performed emergently showed impending rupture of an aneurysmal descending aorta with a subadventitial hematoma.

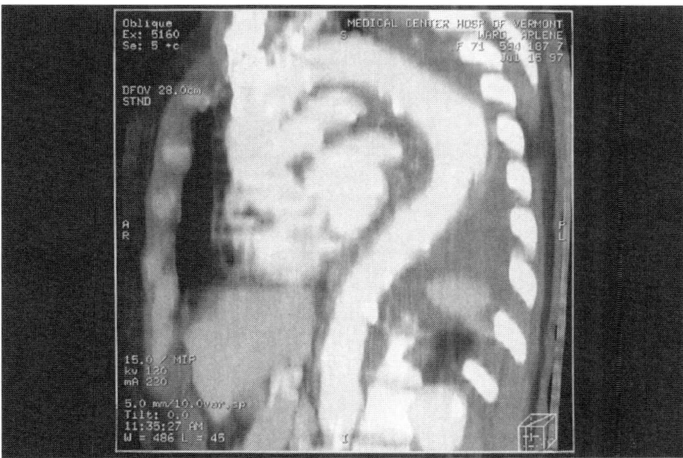

C

dromes was likely underrecognized in the era prior to cross-sectional imaging with CT: In the above-mentioned series from Coady and colleagues at Yale University, 19 (9%) of 214 patients initially diagnosed as aortic dissection were found to have PAU on review of imaging, surgical, and pathologic studies [15].

Contrast-enhanced spiral CT with the use of axial and planar reconstructions is the primary method of diagnosis of PAU. The characteristic finding is a localized ulceration penetrating through the aortic intima within the mid to distal third of the descending aorta (Fig. 9) [21,22]. There may be inward displacement of intimal calcifications, allowing distinction from an ulcerated atherosclerotic plaque limited to the intima (Fig. 4C). Focal thickening of the adjacent aortic wall is seen, representing the associated intramural hematoma. The cephalocaudal extent of the ulceration is most easily appreciated on coronal or sagittal reconstructions. While MR and TEE can depict the ulceration and associated intramural hematoma without the need for intravenous contrast, the lower inherent spatial resolution of these techniques and more widespread access to CT makes contrast-enhanced spiral CT the modality of choice for suspected PAU. Aortography can depict PAU projecting from the aortic lumen if filmed in tangent to the ulcer crater.

Complications of PAU include progression to classic aortic dissection, embolization of material from the ulcer into the distal arterial circulation, extensive intramural hematoma formation, and development of a pseudoaneurysm with subsequent rupture (Fig. 10). Branch vessel occlusion does not

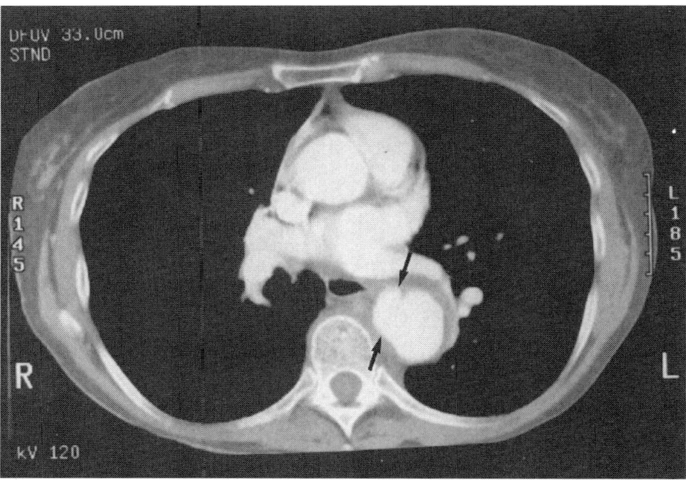

A

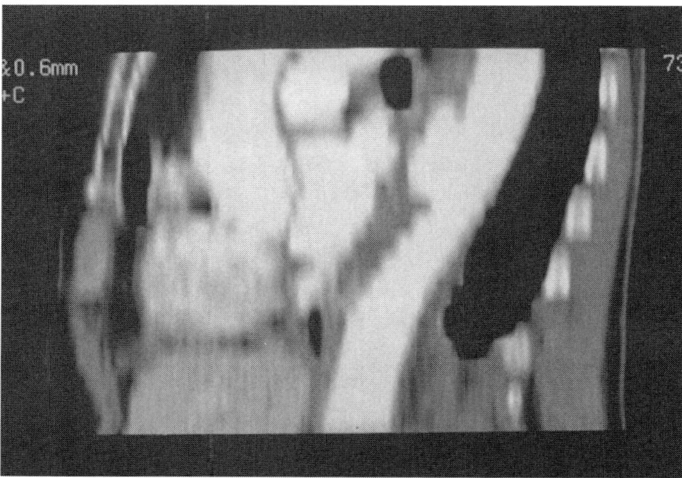

B

Figure 9 Penetrating atherosclerotic ulcer of the aorta. (A) Contrast-enhanced CT shows an ulcer (arrow) projecting anteromedially from the middescending aorta. (B) Oblique sagittal reconstruction shows the ulcer in profile.

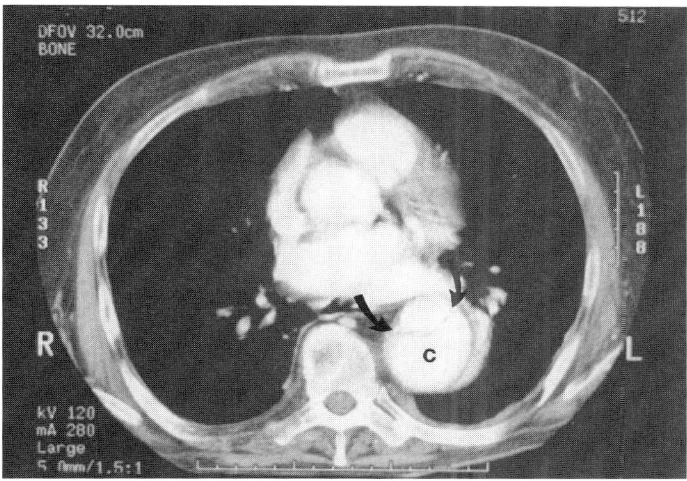

A

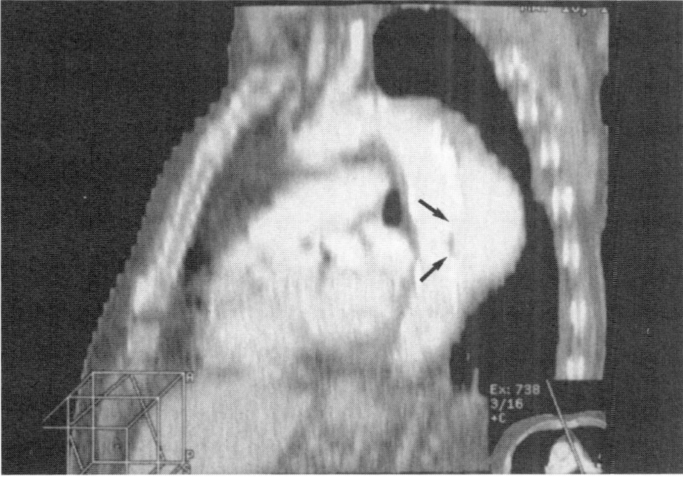

B

Figure 10 Pseudoaneurysm complicating penetrating atherosclerotic ulcer. (A) Contrast-enhanced CT at level of left atrium shows a large collection (c) enhancing simultaneously with the aortic lumen. Note medially-displaced intima with calcifications (curved arrows). (B) Oblique sagittal reconstruction shows a pseudoaneurysm with its neck (straight arrows) seen in profile. The aneurysm and penetrating ulcer were surgically confirmed.

occur in uncomplicated PAU. Although patients with descending PAUs, particularly those with significant contraindications to surgery, can be managed conservatively, several series have shown a tendency for PAUs to progress to aneurysm formation with an incidence of rupture exceeding 40%. This rate of rupture is significantly higher than that seen in classic aortic dissection or IMH [22,23]. Therefore, nonoperated patients should be followed closely with repeat cross-sectional imaging studies obtained within days of initial presentation to detect complications. Patients that require surgical intervention typically undergo replacement of the diseased aortic segment with an interposition graft [24], a procedure that is more extensive than repair of an intimal flap in aortic dissection and is associated with a higher incidence of paraplegia due to spinal cord ischemia [25].

IV. TRAUMATIC AORTIC INJURY

Traumatic injury to the aorta (TAI) accounts for approximately 15% of all deaths due to motor vehicle accidents. While 90% of patients with TAI die before reaching a medical facility, those that survive to reach the hospital have a 30–40% mortality within the first 24 hr [26]. It is in these patients that a rapid and accurate diagnosis of TAI is critical to survival.

The mechanism responsible for TAI in cases of blunt trauma is felt to be a shear injury to the aorta from rapid deceleration. The injury is usually the result of a high-speed motor vehicle accident but can also develop from a vertical fall or a plane crash. Those portions of the aorta that are relatively fixed in position are most prone to injury from shearing effects: in survivors of TAI these include the aortic isthmus (90%); aortic root (5–10%); or, less often, the descending aorta at the diaphragmatic hiatus or at the site of a hyperextension injury in the thoracic spine. The resultant aortic injury can range from a focal intimal tear or intramural hematoma to complete laceration or transection of the aortic wall. Injuries to the ascending aorta are almost invariably fatal, as they result in pericardial tamponade and aortic valve disruption. While injuries to the aortic isthmus can likewise be fatal, containment of a mural aortic injury by the adventitia (pseudoaneurysms) or periadventitial tissues (false aneurysms) can prevent exsanguination and allow a patient to survive long enough to be evaluated.

The initial imaging evaluation of suspected aortic injury remains the portable chest radiograph, usually obtained with the trauma patient in the supine position. Radiographic abnormalities suggesting an aortic injury include widening of the mediastinum, obscuration of the aortic knob, thickening of the right paratracheal stripe, a left apical cap, and rightward deviation of the trachea or in-dwelling nasogastric tube, all findings of a mediastinal hematoma. A normal portable chest radiograph, particularly an erect film, has a high negative predictive value for excluding aortic injury (approximately 98%) [27].

It is well recognized that only a small minority of patients that undergo evaluation for TAI will be found to have such an injury, in large part because the clinical evaluation of the trauma patient is difficult and the chest radiograph is a sensitive but nonspecific indicator of TAI. The initial role of CT in the evaluation of TAI was limited due to relatively slow scan speeds and limited resolution in the uncooperative trauma patient. Both the increased availability of spiral CT scanners in trauma centers, with their inherent rapid acquisition time and high contrast and spatial resolution, along with increased utilization of spiral CT for the evaluation of head, spine, abdominopelvic, and musculoskeletal injuries have led to renewed interest in the use of spiral CT in this setting. The early efforts to determine the role of CT in the evaluation of TAI focused on patients with a low to moderate suspicion for TAI and equivocal chest radiographs who were selected for angiography based on the detection of mediastinal hematoma. This was mostly done in an attempt to reduce the percentage of negative catheter aortograms performed [28,29]. More recently, several large series comparing spiral CT to conventional angiography for the diagnosis of TAI have shown that spiral CT is an accurate and cost-effective technique that provides direct evaluation of the aorta while obviating the need for conventional aortography in most clinical settings [30–32]. Despite the excellent published results of spiral CT for TAI, the technique has not gained universal acceptance even where available due to concerns of false negative examinations, particularly in cases where there is no mediastinal hematoma detected. However, it is almost certain that with the advent of multidetector-row technology, spiral CT will eventually supplant aortography to become the definitive tool for the evaluation of TAI.

Aortography remains the gold standard in the evaluation of traumatic aortic injury. It is a safe and highly accurate examination with a negative predictive value for aortic injury approaching 100%. It has a particular advantage over spiral CT for evaluation of the ascending aorta, a region where the spiral CT detection of injury is limited due to motion and streak artifacts. Angiography is, however, an invasive and relatively costly examination that is not as rapidly available as spiral CT in most trauma centers and does not provide the global evaluation of the major organ systems affected in blunt trauma victims that spiral CT affords.

The technique of CT aortography is similar to that described for the evaluation of other aortic diseases (Table 1). In the blunt trauma patient, the

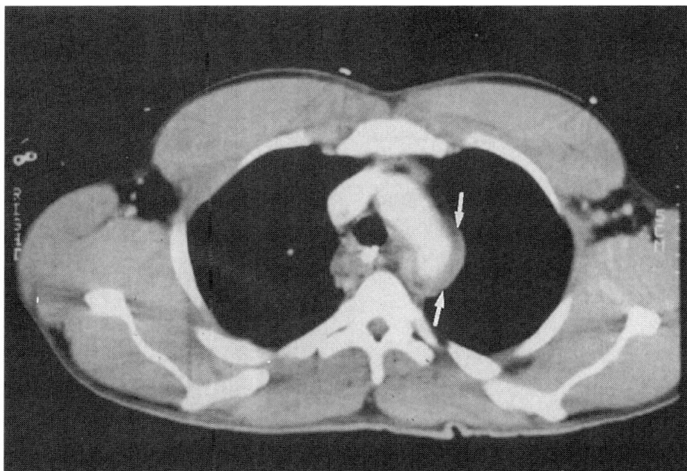

A

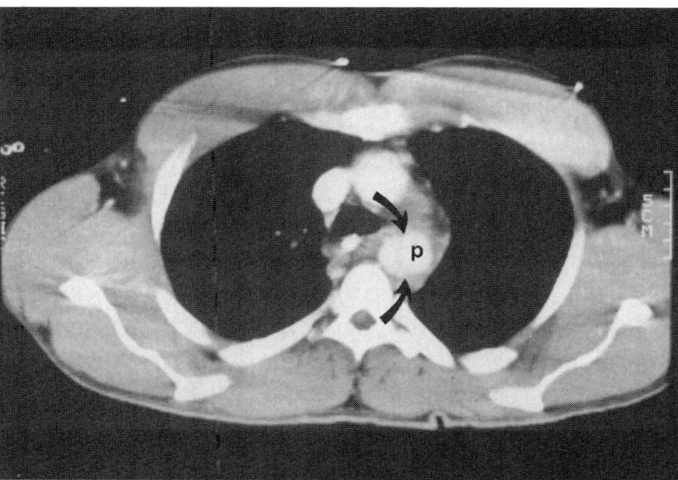

B

Figure 11 Traumatic aortic transection. (A) Contrast-enhanced CT at the level of the aortic arch shows a periaortic (straight arrows) and posterior mediastinal hematoma. Note slight rightward displacement of the trachea and nasogastric tube. (B) Scan immediately below a shows an endoluminal flap (curved arrow) and pseudoaneurysm formation (p).

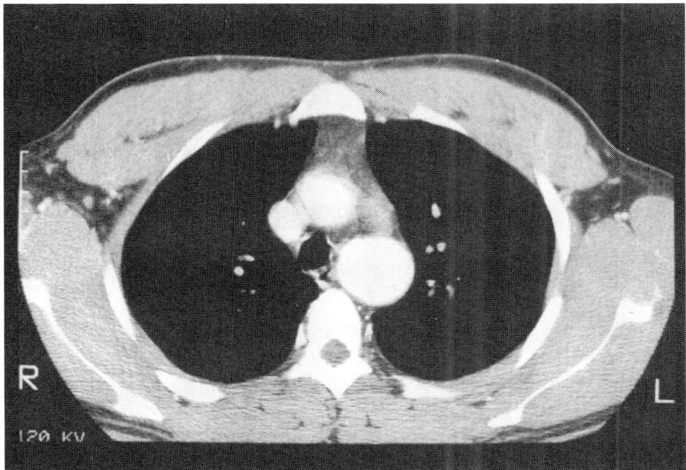

A

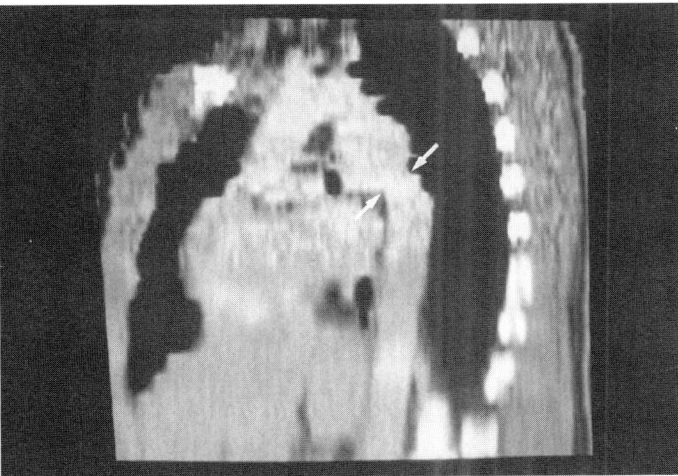

B

Figure 12 Traumatic aortic injury with pseudoaneurysm formation and pseudocoarctation. (A) Contrast-enhanced CT in a patient with a history of a motor vehicle accident 3 years previously shows an aneurysmal proximal descending aorta. (B) Oblique sagittal reconstruction shows the aneurysm of the aortic isthmus with aortic narrowing distal to the aneurysm (arrows). Surgically confirmed aortic transsection with pseudoaneurysm formation.

evaluation of the thoracic aorta and chest is often only part of a more extensive evaluation of the abdomen, pelvis, head, and spine. Since nearly one-third of patients with aortic injury have an abdominal visceral injury or pelvic fracture, most experts recommend performing an abdominal and pelvic CT as a direct extension of the thoracic examination [33].

The spiral CT diagnosis of TAI includes both direct and indirect findings. The detection of a periaortic hematoma, particularly around the aortic isthmus, is an indirect and nonspecific sign of aortic injury but at some centers will lead to an aortogram even in the presence of a normal aorta on CT (Fig. 11). An anterior or posterior mediastinal hematoma usually indicates an injury to the sternum or thoracic spine respectively. The absence of a periaortic hematoma or aortic abnormality on a good-quality spiral CT confidently excludes TAI. Hemopericardium or hemothorax are additional indirect signs of TAI but are most often due to other injuries. Direct findings of TAI include linear intraluminal filling defects that reflect either intimal or mural flaps from aortic laceration or transection, pseudoaneurysm formation, abrupt caliber change (pseudocoarctation) (Fig. 12), and active contrast extravasation.

The distinction between minimal aortic injuries and nontraumatic aortic entities such as a ductus diverticulum, prominent origin of a bronchial artery, and atherosclerosis can be difficult and is often the source of false positive CT aortograms [33]. The subtle aortic abnormality produced by a small intimal flap, mural hematoma, or small pseudoaneurysm may be seen on only two or three contiguous images. Aortography is recommended to delineate such subtle injuries and can usually distinguish between a normal variant or atherosclerotic plaque and a true aortic injury. However, in selected cases transesophageal or intravascular ultrasound may be necessary to better define the aortic abnormality.

V. AORTIC ANEURYSM

An aortic aneurysm is defined as an abnormal permanent dilatation of the aorta. Since the aorta normally dilates with advancing age, the ''normal'' diameter is age dependent, but always less than 4 cm in diameter in the ascending aorta and less than 3 cm in the descending aorta [34]. Approximately 75% of thoracic aortic aneurysms (TAAs) affect the descending aorta, where atherosclerotic disease is most common. In addition, the aortic diameter tapers as it extends distally, with the descending aorta never larger than the ascending aorta. The prevalence of aneurysm increases with age, with an overall incidence of approximately 450 per 100,000 people and a male: female ratio of approximately 3:1 [35]. Concommitant abdominal aortic aneurysms is seen in up to 28% of patients, so the entire thoracoabdominal aorta should be imaged when evaluating TAAs [35].

The etiologies of thoracic aortic aneurysm (TAA) include atherosclerosis, connective tissue diseases such as Marfan's and Ehlers-Danlos syndromes, trauma, aortitis (including syphilis, mycotic aneurysms, and noninfectious inflammatory diseases) (Fig. 13), and aortic dissection. A genetic predisposition to TAA is supported by studies that show a familial aggregation of cases [36].

Thoracic aortic aneurysms are generally divided into true aneurysms and pseudoaneurysms (i.e., false aneurysms) based on their gross and pathological appearance. True aortic aneurysms are usually fusiform in shape and are composed of all three anatomic layers (intima, media, and adventitia). These most commonly arise in the descending thoracic aorta as the result of atherosclerotic disease. Pseudoaneurysms have an absent intimal layer and are contained by the adventitia or periadventitial tissues. They are usually saccular in shape; have a narrow neck where they arise from the aorta; and develop as the result of blunt or penetrating trauma, a penetrating atherosclerotic ulcer, or infection. Pseudoaneurysms may affect any portion of the thoracic aorta (Fig. 14), although traumatic pseudoaneurysms are most often found at the aortic isthmus and those resulting as a complication of PAU are usually seen in the descending aorta.

Plain film findings of aortic aneurysm include a mediastinal mass with peripheral calcification that is contiguous with the aorta, widening of the aortic knob or prominence of the ascending or descending aorta, and mediastinal widening. Aortography can considerably underestimate the size of the aneurysm due to mural thrombus and is rarely obtained in the evaluation of TAA.

Spiral CT aortography and MR have virtually replaced conventional aortography for the detection and characterization of thoracoabdominal aortic aneurysms. Spiral CT allows accurate diagnosis of aortic aneurysm and readily distinguishes this from other mediastinal masses. It demonstrates all features of TAAs, including an accurate assessment of the shape, length, and diameter of the aneurysm; the presence of mural thrombus and calcification; and the relationship of the aneurysm to adjacent intrathoracic structures [37]. Spiral CT is limited by an inability to evaluate the coronary arteries in patients with ascending aortic aneurysms or delineate the intercostal supply to the spinal cord at T8-L1 in those with descending TAAs, information more readily provided by angiography.

While it may be difficult to distinguish mural thrombus in an aortic aneurysm from an intramural hematoma (IMH) or thrombosed aortic dissection, there are several CT findings that aid in this distinction. In a thrombosed

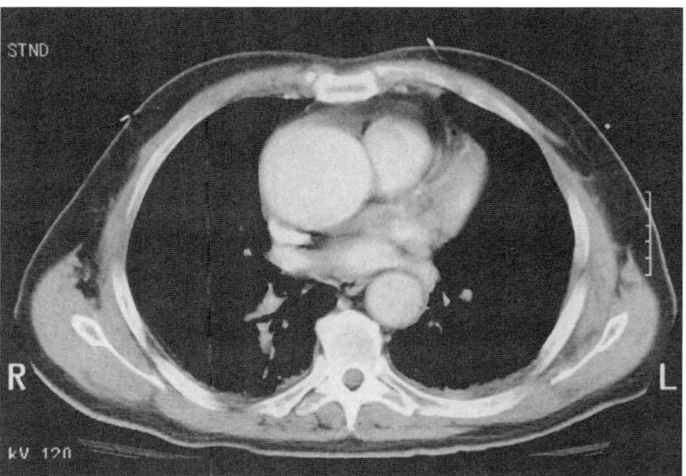

A

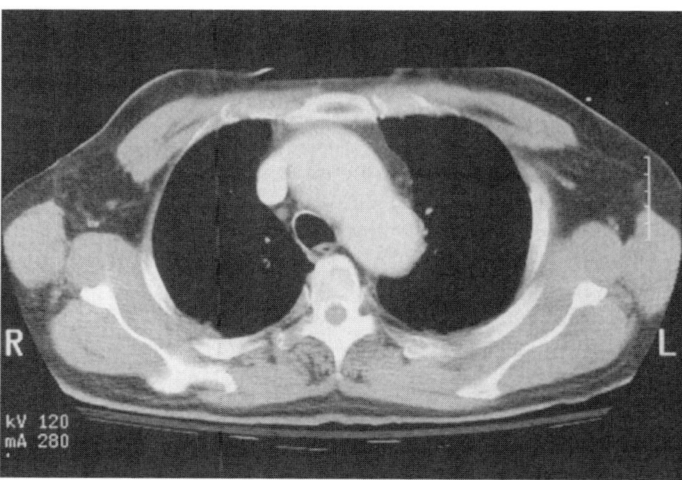

B

Figure 13 Ascending aortic and arch aneurysm. (A) Contrast-enhanced CT at the level of the top of the left atrium in a patient with Reiter's syndrome shows an ascending aortic aneurysm. (B) Scan at the level of the aortic arch shows mild aneurysmal dilatation of the arch that tapers distally.

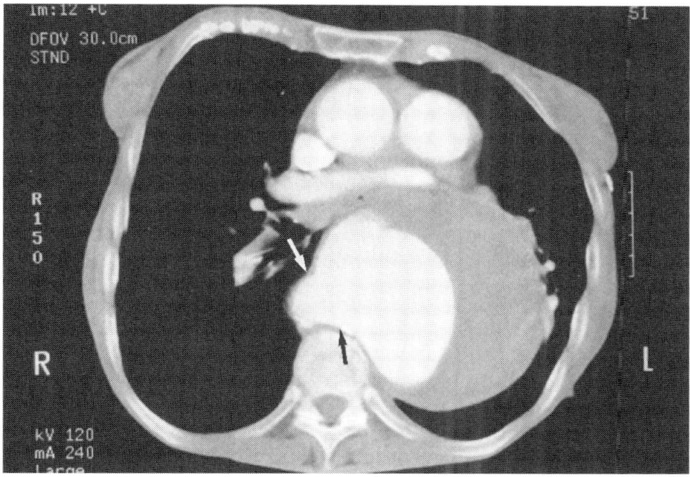

A

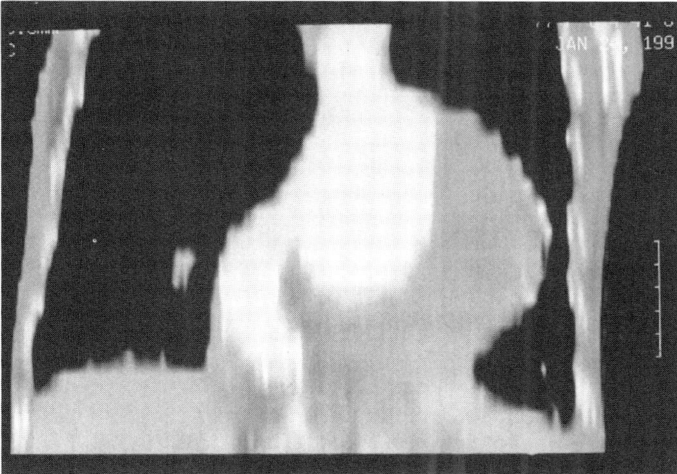

B

Figure 14 Pseudoaneurysm of the descending aorta. (A) Contrast-enhanced CT through the lower chest shows a large aneurysm of the descending aorta with a large amount of mural thrombus. Note the relatively narrow aneurysm neck (arrows). (B) Coronal reconstruction shows the aneurysm projecting into the left lung and a surgically confirmed pseudoaneurysm complicating a penetrating atherosclerotic ulcer.

aneurysm, the residual aortic lumen is generally smooth and the thrombus circumferential (Fig. 14), while IMH and thrombosed dissection produces a more irregular interface with the aortic lumen. When present, atherosclerotic intimal calcifications are seen at the peripheral edge of thrombus, whereas they are displaced medially by IMH and thrombosed dissection. Despite these characteristic features, the distinction between a thrombosed aneurysm and IMH or thrombosed dissection may be difficult in selected cases, particularly when the thrombus within an aneurysm is calcified [38,39].

While there is no direct relationship between the etiology of a TAA and its radiologic appearance, the appearance and location of a TAA as depicted on spiral CT should suggest specific etiologies. Patients with cystic medial necrosis typically have annuloaortic ectasia with dilated sinuses of Valsalva and the classic Marfanoid pear-shaped aneurysmal aorta with a smooth taper to a normal aortic arch. This appearance is best appreciated on coronal reformations through the ascending aorta. Atherosclerotic aneurysms appear as continuous fusiform dilatations of the descending aorta with smooth mural thrombus that can be either crescentic or concentric. Mycotic aneurysms arising from bacterial infection of a diseased aortic wall are most often saccular with focal dilatation and eccentric thrombus and mural calcification (Fig. 15) [40]. They have a propensity to affect the ascending aorta likely due to its proximity to the regions affected by endocarditis, which is often an associated condition [41]. Traumatic pseudoaneurysms following blunt trauma most often develop near the aortic isthmus and are usually saccular with mural calcification common. Aneurysms arising as a complication of penetrating atherosclerotic ulcers are most often seen as saccular aneurysms of the descending aorta. Aortitis due to noninfectious diseases, particularly connective tissue diseases such as rheumatoid arthritis; Reiter's syndrome; and ankylosing spondylitis usually produces fusiform aneurysms of the ascending aorta (Fig. 13).

As in other aortic diseases, the axial reconstructions provide the primary means of helical CT interpretation. However, there are advantages of specific types of reformations unique to the evaluation of aortic aneurysms that differ from those performed for aortic dissection and its variants. Multiplanar reformations (MPRs) of volumetric data provide a more accurate measurement of the diameter of a TAA than axial scans, particularly in the descending aorta where the dilated lumen may course oblique to the scan plane. MPRs also allow display of intraluminal contents, particularly mural thrombus and atherosclerotic changes [10]. In patients with aneurysms complicated by dissection, curved planar reformats (CPRs) best depict the relationship of the intimal flap to the great vessel ostia. Shaded surface displays, a three-dimensional volume-rendering technique, is useful in displaying complex relationships of aneu-

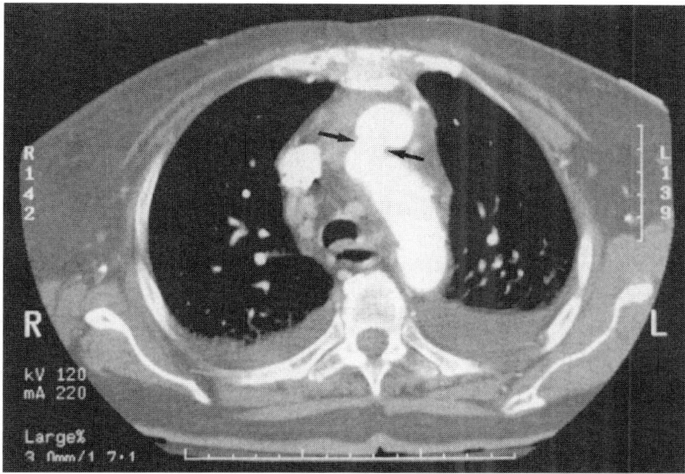

A

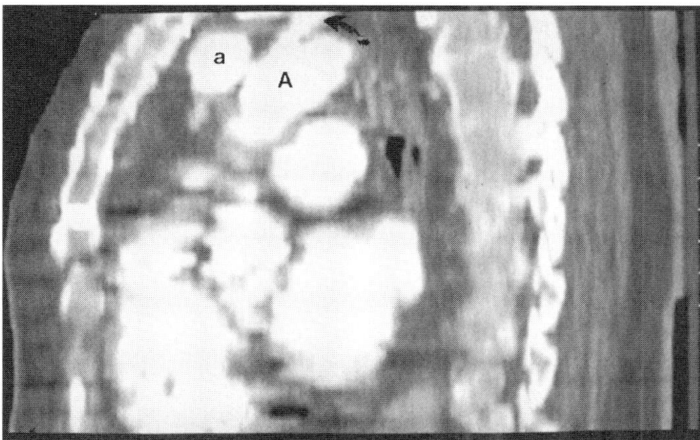

B

Figure 15 Mycotic aneurysm of the aorta. (A) Contrast-enhanced CT at the level of the aortic arch shows an aneurysm projecting anteriorly from the proximal arch. Note the narrow aneurysm neck (arrows) suggesting a pseudoaneurysm. (B) Sagittal reconstruction shows the aneurysm (a) with narrow neck projecting anteriorly from the arch (A) arising just proximal to the brachiocephalic artery (curved arrow). (C) Corresponding lateral digital subtraction confirms the findings in (B). Surgically confirmed mycotic aneurysm.

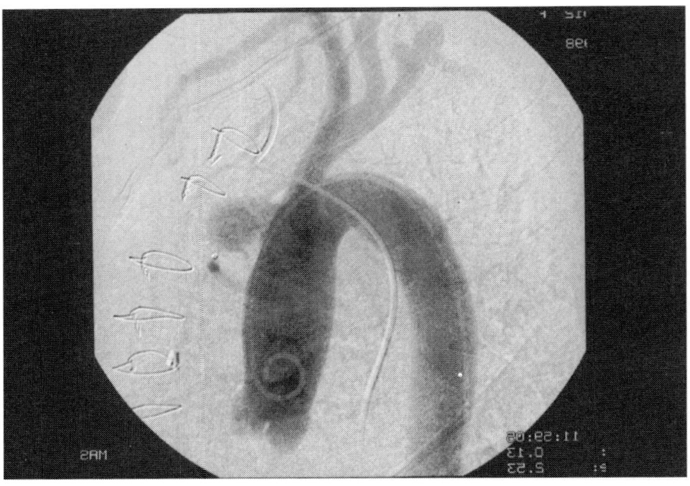

C

Figure 15 Continued

rysms to adjacent mediastinal vessels but does not provide visualization of aneurysmal contents.

Magnetic resonance using standard spin-echo techniques can provide information regarding TAAs analogous to spiral CT, though without the use of ionizing radiation or intravenous contrast. Magnetic resonance depicts mural thrombus as intermediate signal material on T1-weighted images but cannot detect calcification within the wall of an aneurysm. Oblique sagittal MR scans of the aorta allow simultaneous display of the entire length of the thoracic and upper abdominal aorta, which is beneficial in patients with thoracoabdominal aneurysms [42]. Magnetic resonance is particularly useful in the follow-up of patients with known TAAs and in those with contraindications to intravenous contrast administration.

Complications of TAA, including progressive dilatation, dissection, and hemorrhage, are easily assessed by CT. In particular, spiral CT is the modality of choice in the setting of suspected acute aortic rupture, as it can detect active contrast extravasation (Fig. 16) or high-attenuation hematoma within the pleural or pericardial space or mediastinum [43]. A crescent of high-attenuation material within the mural thrombus of a TAA represents acute or impending contained aneurysm rupture [44]. A contained rupture of the posterior aortic wall in close apposition to the spine may show a draped aorta sign, thought

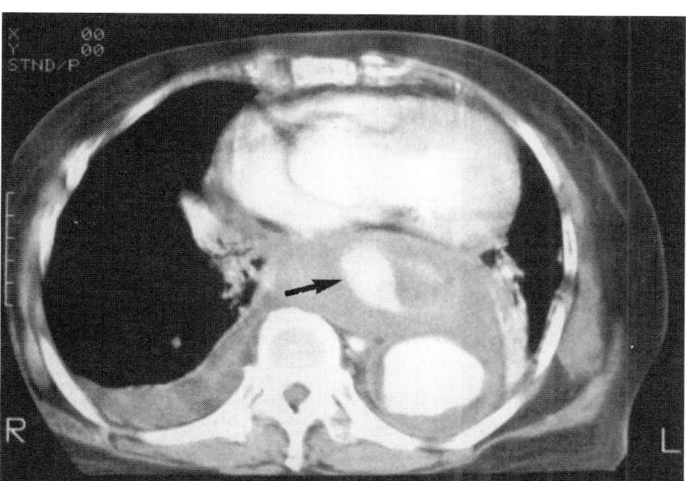

Figure 16 Ruptured aortic aneurysm. Contrast-enhanced scan through the lower chest in a patient with sudden onset of chest pain shows active extravasation of contrast (arrow) from a descending aortic aneurysm into a retrocardiac hematoma.

to be indicative of a deficient aortic wall [45]. Aortobronchial fistula results from communication between the aorta and bronchial tree and most often arises as a complication of an atherosclerotic TAA or as a postsurgical complication of aneurysm repair. The fistulous communication in an aortobronchial fistula is between the descending aorta and left bronchopulmonary tree in nearly 90% of cases [46]. Patients usually present with massive hemoptysis. Spiral CT does not often demonstrate the fistula itself but shows an aortic aneurysm adjacent to consolidated lung [47]. Management consists of surgical repair of the aortic and bronchial defects, with approximately three-fourths of patients successfully repaired. Similarly, aortoesophageal fistula is a catastrophic and often fatal complication of TAA, resulting from communication between the descending aorta and esophagus. Patients present with massive upper gastrointestinal hemorrhage with endoscopy, often failing to delineate the source of bleeding. Computed tomography may demonstrate the aneurysm and its intimate relationship to the esophagus; mediastinal hematoma or rarely contrast extravasation into the esophagus may be seen. Immediate surgical repair is mandatory [48].

The natural history of TAA is directly related to its size. While TAAs can present due to mass effect on adjacent mediastinal structures, the most serious complication is aortic rupture, which occurs in up to 70% of affected patients [49]. While aortic rupture usually results in exsanguinating hemorrhage into the mediastinum, lung, or pleural space, sometimes a communication will develop with the tracheobronchial tree or esophagus producing hemoptysis or hematemesis respectively. The risk of rupture increases with increasing size of the aneurysm, and TAAs have been observed to dilate at a mean rate of 0.12 cm/year [50]. Based on these data, elective surgical repair has been recommended for ascending aortic aneurysm diameters of 5–5.5 cm and descending aortic aneurysms of 5.5–6.5 cm [50]. Surgical treatment generally consists of the placement of a Dacron graft within the diseased aortic segment: Ascending aortic aneurysms that involve the aortic annulus and valve, most often seen in patients with annuloaortic ectasia due to Marfan's syndrome, usually require a composite graft (i.e., combined aortic valve with prosthetic ascending aortic graft) with reimplantation of the coronary arteries.

VI. AORTITIS

There are a number of autoimmune disorders that can produce aortitis. These noninfectious inflammatory processes include many of the connective tissue diseases such as rheumatoid arthritis, ankylosing spondylitis, Reiter's syndrome, giant cell arteritis, Behcet's disease, and relapsing polychondritis. These diseases weaken the aortic wall and predispose to aneurysm formation with a predilection for involvement of the ascending aorta (Fig. 13). The most common noninfectious cause of aortitis is Takayasu's arteritis, usually seen in young Asian women. This is a vasculitis of unknown etiology that primarily affects the thoracic aortic arch with variable involvement of the abdominal aorta and pulmonary arteries. This disease produces inflammation of the media and adventitia that most commonly results in arterial stenosis and occlusion, hence the use of the descriptor ''pulseless'' disease. Aneurysmal dilatation of the aorta is a less common manifestation of the disease [51].

Patients with thoracic aneurysms resulting from the aortitis associated with connective tissue disease usually have fusiform dilatation of the ascending aorta with variable involvement of the aortic valve annulus. Fine curvilinear calcification may be seen in the wall of the aneurysm. The CT features of Takayasu's arteritis of the aorta have been described [52]. Unenhanced CT demonstrates high attenuation of the thickened aortic wall and mural calcifications in the majority of affected patients. Mural enhancement during the arterial phase following contrast administration was seen in 75% of patients with active disease and was 100% specific. Aortic arch and branch vessel stenoses are present in the majority of patients. Aneurysm formation is uncommon, may be fusiform or saccular in shape, and is often difficult to distinguish from dilatation proximal to a hemodynamically significant stenosis.

VII. POSTOPERATIVE AORTA

An effective imaging evaluation of the postoperative aorta cannot be accomplished without an understanding of the surgical techniques utilized in aortic repair and the resultant alterations in aortic anatomy. A familiarity with those procedures most commonly employed at the specific institution and their imaging manifestations should allow for rapid distinction between a normal postoperative appearance and the development of a postoperative complication that requires intervention.

Two standard techniques are currently employed for the repair of aortic aneurysm and dissection [53]: (1) interposition graft and (2) inclusion graft. In interposition graft the diseased segment is excised and the graft is sewn end to end; tributary vessels are reimplanted. Inclusion graft consists of aortotomy and insertion of the graft within the diseased aortic lumen, leaving a potential space between the graft and the native aortic wall. This potential space may thrombose or may contain clot and persistent blood flow in combination. A Cabrol procedure, whereby the perigraft space is decompressed into the right atrial appendage, is thought to prevent progression of pseudoaneurysm formation [54]. For patients with involvement of the aortic root, a composite graft that includes a prosthetic aortic valve may be utilized.

Non-contrast-enhanced CT of aortic grafts shows the graft as a ring of high attenuation (Fig. 17). While this ring will form the outer boundaries of the aorta when the graft is interposed, inclusion grafts will appear as a ring within a larger circle representing the native aortic wall. Many patients with inclusion grafts demonstrate a peripheral thrombosed space between the graft and the native aortic wall. Occasionally there will be flow in the perigraft space, a finding readily demonstrated on spiral CT. The vast majority of patients with repairs of acute Type A dissections will demonstrate a persistent intimal flap distal to the graft site on spiral CT [55]. One of the complications of aortic inclusion graft is aneurysmal dilatation of the aorta, which is easily depicted on spiral CT or MR (Fig. 17).

Endoluminal repair of aortic aneurysm and dissections is now possible with the use of endovascular stent grafts. These are placed at most institutions in a collaborative effort by interventional radiology and cardiovascular surgery. This procedure for the management of TAAs is predominantly limited

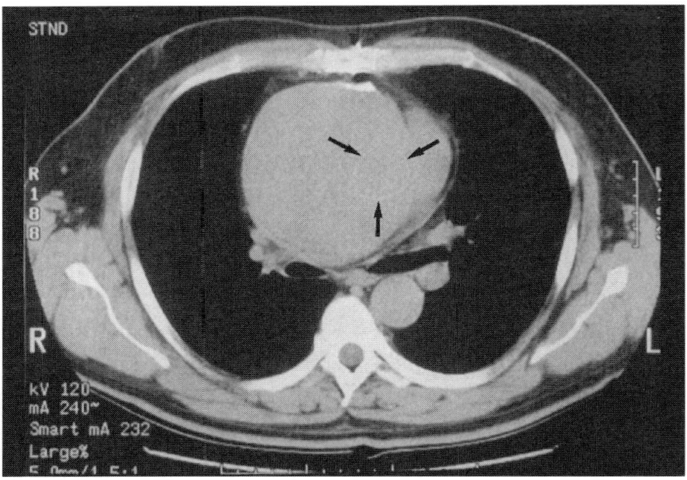

A

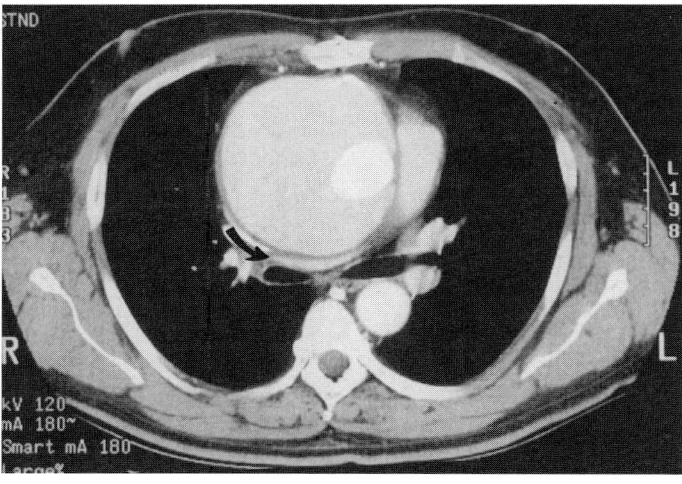

B

Figure 17 Aneurysm complicating aortic graft repair of ascending aortic aneurysm. (A) Unenhanced CT at level of main pulmonary artery shows an aortic graft (arrows) engulfed by a large amount of soft tissue. (B) Following contrast enhancement, the lumen of the graft is opacified with enhancement of the perigraft space, representing an aneurysm of the ascending aorta due to graft leakage. Note marked compression of the right pulmonary artery (curved arrow) by the aneurysm.

to patients who are poor operative candidates. Spiral CT has proven useful for both pre- and postoperative evaluation of stent graft repair of thoracic aortic aneurysms [56,57]. On spiral CT scans, the metallic portion of the stent-graft, most often a series of modified Z-stents, is easily identified [58]. Complications such as stent-graft migration, incomplete deployment or collapse, perigraft leakage, branch vessel occlusion, and progressive aneurysmal dilatation are more easily detected on spiral CT than with conventional aortography [59].

REFERENCES

1. Edwards JE. Anomalies of the derivatives of the aortic arch system. Med Clin North Am 1948; 32:925.
2. Kersting-Sommerhoff BA, Sechtem UP, Fisher MR, Higgins CB. MR imaging of congenital anomalies of the aortic arch. Am J Roentgenol 1987; 149:9–13.
3. Katz M, Konen E, Rozenman J, Szeinberg A, Itzchak Y. Spiral CT and 3D reconstruction of vascular rings and associated tracheobronchial anomalies. J Comput Assist Tomogr 1995; 19:564–568.
4. Levinson DC, Edmeades DT, Griffith GC. Dissecting aneurysm of the aorta: its clinical electrocardiographic and laboratory features: a report of fifty-eight autopsied cases. Circulation 1950; 1:360–387.
5. Prete R, Von Segesser LK. Aortic dissection. Lancet 1997; 349:1461–1464.
6. DeBakey ME, McCollum CH, Crawford ES, et al. Dissection and dissecting aneurysms of the aorta: Twenty-year follow-up of 527 patients treated surgically. Surgery 1982; 92:1118–1134.
7. Nienaber CA, von Kodolitsch Y, Nicholas V. The diagnosis of thoracic aortic dissection by noninvasive imaging procedures. N Engl J Med 1993; 328:1–9.
8. Sommer T, Fehske W, Holzknecht N, et al. Aortic dissection: A comparative study of diagnosis with spiral CT, multiplanar transesophageal echocardiography, and MR imaging. Radiology 1996; 199:347–352.
9. Demos TC, Posniak HV, Churchill RJ. Detection of the intimal flap of aortic dissection on unenhanced CT images. Am J Radiol 1986; 146:601–603.
10. Rubin GD. Helical CT angiography of the thoracic aorta. J Thorac Imaging 1997; 12:128–149.
11. Batra P, Bigoni B, Maning J, et al. Pitfalls in the diagnosis of thoracic aortic dissection at CT angiography. Radiographics 2000; 20:309–320.
12. Posniak HV, Olson MC, Demos TC. Aortic motion artifact simulating dissection on CT scans. Am J Radiol 1993; 161:557–558.
13. Loubeyre P, Angelie E, Grozel F, Albidi H, Minh VAT. Spiral CT artifact that simulates aortic dissection: image reconstruction with use of 180° and 360° linear interpolation algorithms. Radiology 1997; 205:153–157.
14. Yamada T, Takamiya M, Naito H, et al. Diagnosis of aortic dissection without

intimal rupture by x-ray computed tomography. Nippon Acta Radiol 1985; 45: 699–710.
15. Coady MA, Rizzo JA, Elefteriades JA. Pathologic variants of thoracic aortic dissections: penetrating atherosclerotic ulcers and intramural hematomas. Cardiol Clin 1999; 17:637–657.
16. Patrick TO, Roman WD. Acute aortic dissection and its variants: toward a common diagnostic and therapeutic approach. Circulation 1993; 88:1–10.
17. Murray JG, Manisali M, Flamm SD, et al. Intramural hematoma of the thoracic aorta: MR image findings and their prognostic implications. Radiology 1997; 204:349–355.
18. Bluemke DA. Definitive diagnosis of intramural hematoma of the aorta with MR imaging. Radiology 1997; 204:319–321.
19. Moriyama Y, Yotsumoto G, Kuriwaki K, et al. Intramural hematoma of the thoracic aorta. Eur J Cadiothoracic Surg 1998; 13:230–239.
20. Stanson AW, Kazmier FJ, Hollier LH, et al. Penetrating atherosclerotic ulcers of the thoracic aorta: natural history and clinicopathologic correlations. Ann Vasc Surg 1986; 1:15–23.
21. Hayashi H, Matsuoka Y, Sakamoto I, et al. Penetrating atherosclerotic ulcer of the aorta: imaging features and disease concept. Radiographics 2000; 20:995–1005.
22. Kazerooni EA, Bree RI, Williams DM. Penetrating atherosclerotic ulcers of the descending thoracic aorta: evaluation with CT and distinction from aortic dissection. Radiology 1992; 183:759–765.
23. Harris JA, Bis KG, Glover JL, Bendick PJ, Shetty A, Brown OW. Penetrating atherosclerotic ulcers of the aorta. J Vasc Surg 1994; 19:90–98.
24. Cooke JP, Kazmier FJ, Orszulak TA. Penetrating atherosclerotic ulcers of the aorta: pathologic manifestations, diagnosis, and management. Mayo Clin Proc 1988; 63:718–725.
25. Levy JR, Heiken JP, Gutierrez FR. Imaging of penetrating atherosclerotic ulcers of the aorta. Am J Radiol 1999; 173:151–154.
26. Parmley LF, Mattingly TW, Manion WC, Jahnke EJ. Nonpenetrating traumatic injury of the aorta. Circulation 1958; 17:1086–1101.
27. Mirvis SE, Bidwell, JK, Buddemeyer EU, et al. Value of chest radiography in excluding traumatic aortic rupture. Radiology 1987; 163:487–493.
28. Morgan PW, Goodman LR, Aprahamian C, Foley WD, Lipchik EO. Evaluation of traumatic aortic injury: does dynamic contrast-enhanced CT play a role? Radiology 1992; 182:661–666.
29. Raptopoulos V, Sheiman RG, Phillips DA, Davidoff A, Silva WE. Traumatic aortic tear: screening with chest CT. Radiology 1992; 182:667–673.
30. Gavant ML, Menke PG, Fabian T, Flick PA, Graney MJ, Gold RE. Blunt traumatic aortic rupture: detection with helical CT of the chest. Radiology 1995; 197: 125–133.
31. Gavant ML, Flick PA, Menke PG, Gold RE. CT aortography of thoracic aortic rupture. Am J Radiol 1996; 166:955–961.

32. Dyer DS, Moore EE, Mestek MF, et al. Can chest CT be used to exclude aortic injury? Radiology 1999; 213:195–202.
33. Gavant ML. Helical CT grading of traumatic aortic injuries. Radiol Clin North Am 1999; 37:553–574.
34. Aronberg DJ, Glazer HS, Madsen K, Sagel SS. Normal thoracic aorta diameters by computed tomography. J Comput Assist Tomogr 1984; 8:247–250.
35. Bickerstaff LK, Pairolero PC, Hollier LH, et al. Thoracic aortic aneurysms: a population-based study. Surgery 1982; 92:1103–1108.
36. Coady MA, Davies RR, Roberts M, et al. Familial patterns of thoracic aortic aneurysms. Arch Surg 1999; 134:361–367.
37. Quint LE, Francis IR, Williams DM, et al. Evaluation of thoracic aortic disease with the use of helical CT and multiplanar reconstructions: comparison with surgical findings. Radiology 1996; 201:37–41.
38. Heiberg E, Wolverson MK, Sundaram M, Shields JB. CT characteristics of atherosclerotic aneurysm versus aortic dissection. J Comput Assist Tomogr 1985; 9:78–83.
39. Torres WE, Maurer DE, Steinberg HV, Robbins, S, Bernadino ME. CT of aortic aneurysms: the distinction between mural and thrombus calcification. Am J Roentgenol 1988; 150:1317–1319.
40. Gonda RL, Gutierrez OH, Azodo MV. Mycotic aneurysms of the aorta: radiologic features. Radiology 1988; 168:343–346.
41. Posniak HV, Olson MC, Demos TC, Benjoya RA, Marsan RE. CT of thoracic aortic aneurysms. Radiographics 1990; 10:839–855.
42. Dinsmore RE, Liberthson RR, Wismer GL, et al. Magnetic resonance imaging of thoracic aortic aneurysms: comparison with other imaging methods. Am J Roentgenol 1986; 146:309–314.
43. Kucich VA, Vogelzang RL, Hartz RS, LoCicero J, Dalton D. Ruptured thoracic aneurysm: unusual manifestation and early diagnosis using CT. Radiology 1986; 160:87–89.
44. Mehard WB, Heiken JP, Sicard GA. High-attenuating crescent in abdominal aortic aneurysm wall at CT: a sign of acute or impending rupture. Radiology 1994; 192:359–362.
45. Halliday KE, Alkutoubi A. Draped aorta: CT sign of contained leak of aortic aneurysms. Radiology 1996; 199:41–43.
46. MacIntosh EL, Parrott JCW, Unruh HW. Fistulas between the aorta and tracheobronchial tree. Ann Thorac Surg 1991; 51:515–519.
47. Coblentz CL, Sallee DS, Chiles C. Aortobronchopulonary fistula complicating aortic aneurysm: diagnosis in four cases. Am J Roentgenol 1988; 150:535–538.
48. Amin S, Luketich J, Wald A. Aortoesophageal fistula: case report and review of the literature. Digest Dis Science 1998; 43:1665–1671.
49. Kouchoukos NT, Dougenis D. Medical progress: surgery of the thoracic aorta. N Engl J Med 1997; 336:1876–1888.
50. Coady MA, Rizzo JA, Hammond GL, et al. What is the appropriate size criterion

for resection of thoracic aneurysms? J Thoracic Cardiovasc Surg 1997; 113:476–491.
51. Sharma S, Sharma S, Taneja K, Gupta AK, Rajani M. Morphologic mural changes in the aorta revealed by CT in patients with nonspecific aortoarteritis (Takayasu's arteritis). Am J Roentgenol 1996; 167:1321–1325.
52. Park JH, Chung JW, Im JG, et al. Takayasu arteritis: evaluation of mural changes in the aorta and pulmonary artery with CT angiography. Radiology 1995; 196: 89–93.
53. Naidich DP, Webb WR, Muller NL, Krinsky GA, Zerhouni EA, Siegelman SS. Aorta, arch vessels, and great veins. In Computed Tomography and Magnetic Resonance Imaging of the Thorax. 3d ed. Philadelphia: Lippincott-Raven, 1999: 570–576.
54. Cabrol C, Pavie A, Mesnildrey P, et al. Long-term results with total replacement of the ascending aorta and reimplantation of the coronary arteries. J Thorac Cardiovasc Surg 1986; 91:17–25.
55. Mathieu D, Keta K, Loisance D. Post-operative CT follow-up of aortic dissection. J Comput Assist Tomogr 1986; 10:216–218.
56. Mitchell RS, Dake MD, Semba CP, et al. Endovascular stent-graft repair of thoracic aortic aneurysms. J Thorac Cardiovasc Surg 1996; 111:1054–1060.
57. Kato N, Dake MD, Miller DC, et al. Traumatic thoracic aortic aneurysm: treatment with endovascular stent-grafts. Radiology 1997; 205:657–662.
58. Fillinger MF. Postoperative imaging after endovascular AAA repair. Semin Vasc Surg 1999; 12:327–338.
59. Armerding MD, Rubin GD, Beaulieu CF, et al. Aortic aneurysmal disease: assessment of stent-graft treatment-CT versus conventional angiogaphy. Radiology 2000; 215:138–146.

9

Virtual Bronchoscopy

Suzanne L. Aquino
Harvard Medical School and
Massachusetts General Hospital
Boston, Massachusetts

I. INTRODUCTION

Helical computed tomography (CT) has revolutionized cross-sectional imaging with the introduction of rapid volumetric scanning. Patients are scanned at a much faster rate with a consequent decrease in motion artifact [1]. With the recent introduction of multidetector helical CT scanning, multiple sequential CT slices are acquired simultaneously. Not only are patients scanned even faster, there is now the added feature of reconstruction to thinner slices and space intervals.

The direct impact of helical and multidetector helical CT scan imaging is faster imaging, a decrease in motion artifact, and, in most instances, a decrease in dosage as compared to nonhelical scanning [2,3]. When this technology is used to its greatest advantage, images can be recreated to refine anatomic detail without further patient imaging [4]. Thinner slice intervals create better definition of small anatomic structures [5]. With multidetector helical CT, retrospective thinner slice reconstruction enables the radiologist to scan a patient faster at a thicker slice width and postprocess the data to thinner slices to improve resolution. Because multidetector imaging is associated with both improved 3D reformations and improved vascular conspicuity, this technology is most useful in vascular imaging [6,7]. However, this same technology can be applied to imaging the airways both in multiplanar imaging and three-dimensional virtual bronchoscopy [8–10].

Commercially available computer programs have been designed to automatically create a three-dimensional tracheobronchial tree model from CT scans of the thorax. This technology has the potential to revolutionize the diagnostic imaging of airways disease and diseases adjacent to the airways (e.g., mediastinal and hilar masses). In this chapter we discuss how virtual bronchoscopy (VB) images are generated, the feasibility of VB in the clinical setting today, and what future directions radiology and medicine can take with this noninvasive imaging tool.

II. TECHNICAL FEATURES

A. Computed Tomography Scan Images

Intravenous contrast is recommended to better define the surrounding mediastinal anatomy. With single-detector helical CT, the slice thickness normally ranges from 5 to 10 mm. The pitch, or the incremental table movement with respect to slice thickness as a patient is scanned, ranges from 1 to a maximum of 2. In other words, if the scan slice thickness is 5 mm and the pitch is 1, the CT scan table moves 5 mm for every 5-mm slice acquired.

With single-detector helical CT, the chest is usually imaged during three breath holds to insure an adequate breath hold during imaging of the trachea and proximal airways. Usually the patient is imaged from the thoracic inlet to the top of the aortic arch in the first breath hold, from the top of the aortic arch to the mid cardiac level in the second breath hold, and from the mid cardiac level to the lung bases during the third breath hold.

Computed tomography slice thickness for VB should range from 3 to 5 mm. The pitch or table feed should be 1 to 1.5 [11,12]. With single-detector CT, image slices cannot be reconstructed to thinner slices retrospectively. Therefore, it is necessary to scan the mid thorax at a preselected 3- to 5-mm slice thickness. The upper and lower chest is not included in the virtual bronchoscopy technique; therefore 5- to 7-mm slice thickness is usually applied to these regions.

With multidetector scanning, the entire chest is imaged in a fraction of the time needed for a single-detector helical CT to image the thorax. Therefore, the entire thorax can be imaged during a single breath hold at a constant slice thickness and table speed. We have implemented a standard protocol for scanning the thorax at 5-mm slice thickness at the Hi-Speed mode table speed, which is equivalent to a 6:1 pitch and allows for thinner reconstruction to

2.5-mm slice thickness (CT Lightspeed, General Electrics Medical Systems, Milwaukee, WI). For studies in which we plan to create three-dimensional or multiplanar images (e.g., virtual bronchoscopy or CT angiography to evaluate for pulmonary embolism), we use the same protocol for slice thickness and table speed. The only alteration is that we initiate scanning at the base of the chest to avoid beam-hardening artifact from intravenous contrast in the subclavian veins during the initial bolus. This approach also minimizes respiratory motion artifact from the diaphragms should the patient terminate the breath hold prematurely.

B. Reconstruction of Computed Tomography Images

In order to create a VB study, the CT images are modified or ''reconstructed.'' This step needs to be performed while the CT scanner still has the raw data available on the computer. The helical images, which are automatically acquired incrementally, are computer processed to overlap each other at smaller slice intervals. In other words, when 3-mm-slice-thickness images are reconstructed at 1-mm intervals, they are recreated to overlap each other every 1 mm rather than sequentially.

Reconstruction of images from the multidetector scan includes creating thinner slices as well as overlapping images. For instance, for a scan obtained with the GE Lightspeed CT scanner, images can be acquired at 5-mm slice thickness with the HS protocol and reconstructed to 2.5-mm slice thickness with 1-mm slice spacing (Table 1).

Table 1 Scanning Parameters for Virtual Bronchoscopy with Multidetector (GE Lightspeed) and Single-Detector (GE HiSpeed) CT Scanners

Parameters	Multidetector (one acquisition)	Single detector (three acquisitions)	
Level	Lung bases to apex	Mid cardiac to top of aortic arch	Base to midcardiac/ aortic arch to apex
Slice thickness	5 mm	3 mm	5 mm
Image spacing	5 mm	3 mm	5 mm
Table feed	15	—	—
Mode/pitch	HiSpeed	Pitch 1.5–1.7	Pitch 1.5–1.7
Slice reconstruct	2.5-mm slice	Not available	Not available
Space reconstruct	1-mm spacing	1-mm spacing	None

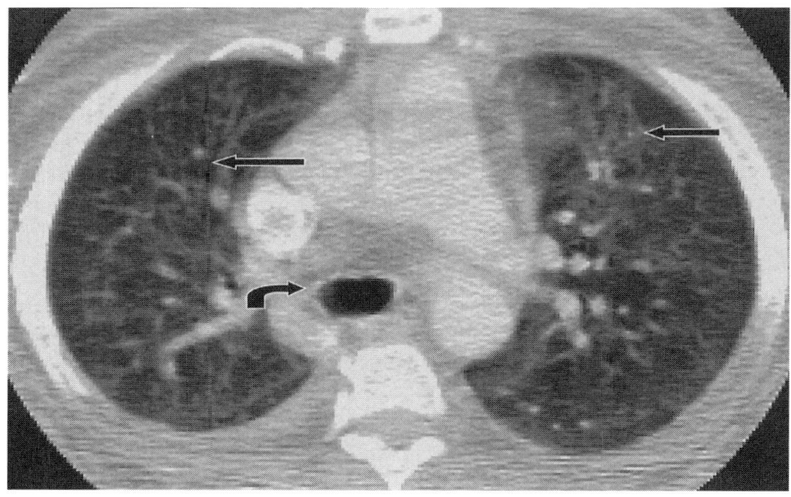

A

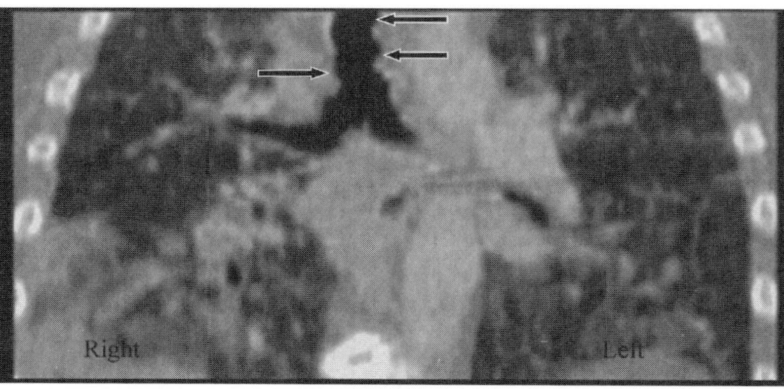

B

Figure 1 (A) Computed tomography scan of the thorax of a 60-year-old woman who was unable to completely hold her breath during acquisition of the CT scan. Image detail of the lungs are blurred (arrows). The trachea outline shows a double density (curved arrow). (B) Coronal planar reconstruction shows rippling (arrows) along the trachea, also referred to as stairstepping artifact. (C) Surface-rendered virtual bronchoscopy image at the level of the trachea shows numerous ridges or stairstepping artifact (arrows) along the airway that create artifactual narrowing.

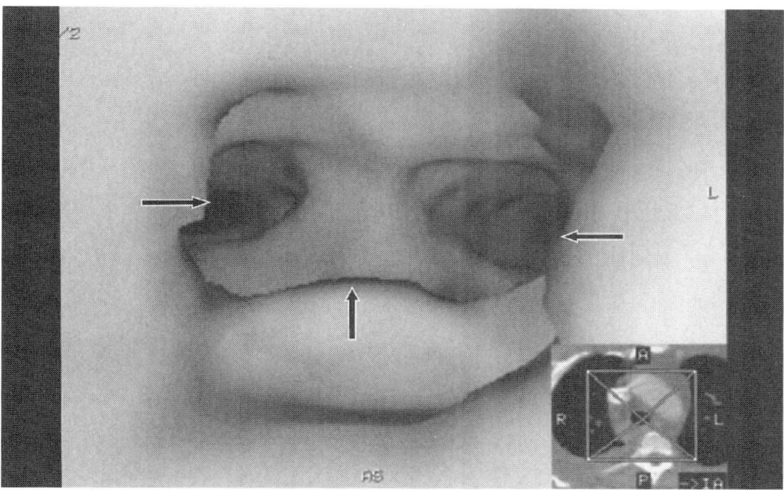

C

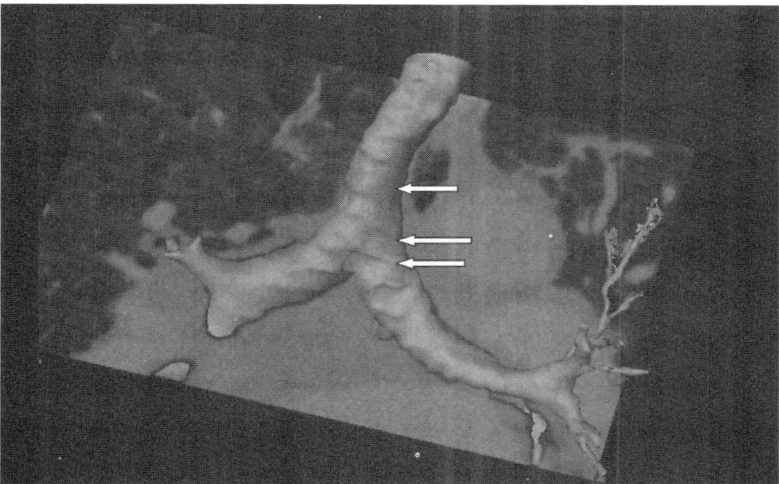

Figure 2 Surface-rendered 3D reconstruction of the trachea in the coronal view shows multiple stair-stepping artifacts (arrows), which can result from respiratory motion, slice thickness greater than 3 mm, or failure to reconstruct images at overlapping slices.

The reconstruction of CT slices at thinner intervals provides a smoothing feature to the three-dimensional generated structure. Normally reconstruction for three-dimensional imaging is performed at 1- to 2-mm overlap for 3- to 5-mm slice thickness. A thicker reconstruction interval leads to irregularity or rippling to the three-dimensional airway wall that is termed ''stairstepping'' (Figs. 1 and 2) [12,13]. Stairstepping not only creates an image that is distorted from the true anatomic airway, it also creates artifactual narrowing [14].

Once images are reconstructed, they are transferred to a separate and independent computer. There, the images are imported into a specific software program that creates the three-dimensional images of the airway with virtual bronchoscopy capabilities.

III. GENERATING VIRTUAL BRONCHOSCOPY IMAGES

Two techniques have been applied to create the virtual airway, surface rendering and volume rendering. To create a three-dimensional airway, a surface-rendering program uses the natural contrast between the air in the tracheobronchial tree and the soft tissue of the airway wall and mediastinum to establish a threshold plane or surface for generating the virtual airway outline. The

Figure 3 (A) Combined volumetric and surface rendering of a CT scan of the thorax of a 19-year-old woman with postpneumonectomy syndrome. The right and left sides are inverted as though one is viewing the airway in a simulated bronchoscopy. The right lung was resected and mediastinum has shifted to the right. The left bronchus (arrow) is compressed between the transverse aorta and the spine. (B) Surface-rendered 3D reconstruction of the trachea with superimposed axial planar image shows narrowing of the 3D bronchus (arrow) between the aorta (star) and spine. (C) Three-dimensional reconstruction of the trachea with superimposed sagittal planar image shows narrowing (arrow) of the 3D left bronchus between the aorta (star) and spine from a different perspective. (D) Volumetric rendering of the postoperative CT scan after repair. The right pneumonectomy space is filled (octagon) and the mediastinum is repositioned to the middle of the thorax. The intraluminal caliber of the left bronchus (arrow) increased from 4 to 8 mm in diameter (star marks the aorta). (E) A three-dimensional reconstruction of the postoperative airway with superimposed sagittal planar image shows improvement of left bronchial narrowing (arrow). (F) Virtual bronchoscopy view of the airways at the level of the distal carina. The right bronchus (black star) narrows consistent with resection. The left bronchus (white star) appears normal in caliber.

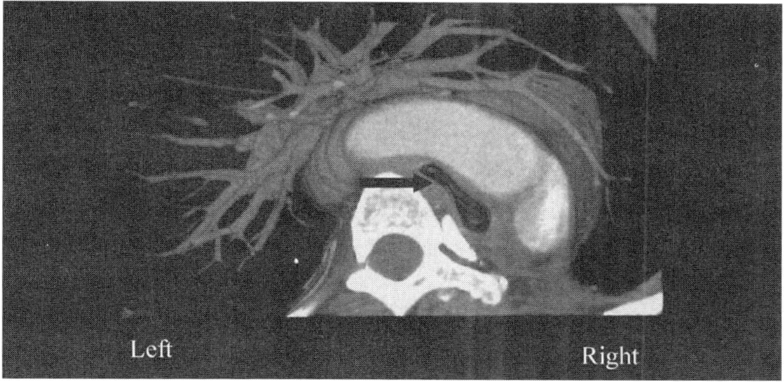

A

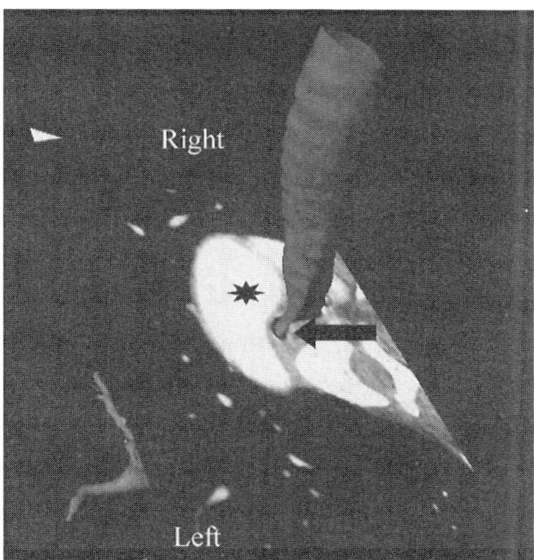

B

program takes this natural contrast and creates an airway "caste" along the lumen of the tracheobronchial tree. The caste is then generated into a three-dimensional airway (Figs. 2, 3B, and 3C), through which a fly-through can be performed in real time. Multiple planar CT images are viewed simultaneously either in separate view boxes on the same screen or superimposed on the three-dimensional airway to display the overlying mediastinal anatomy

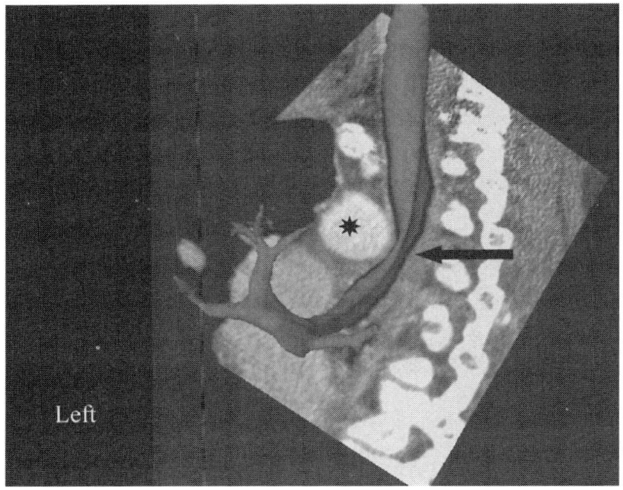

C

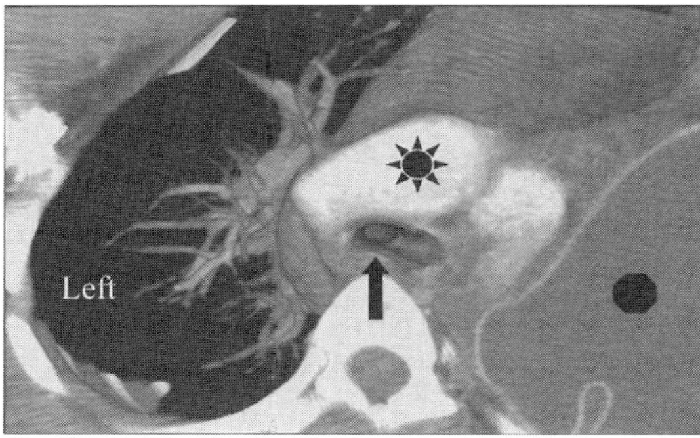

D

Figure 3 Continued

surrounding the three-dimensional airway. One of the disadvantages of surface-rendering is the need to set the proper window and level threshold for the program to create its 3D structure. If the window and level are slightly off, the tracheal wall may appear discontinuous or fragmented and small or stenotic airways may not be properly reconstructed.

The volume-rendering algorithm generates a three-dimensional recon-

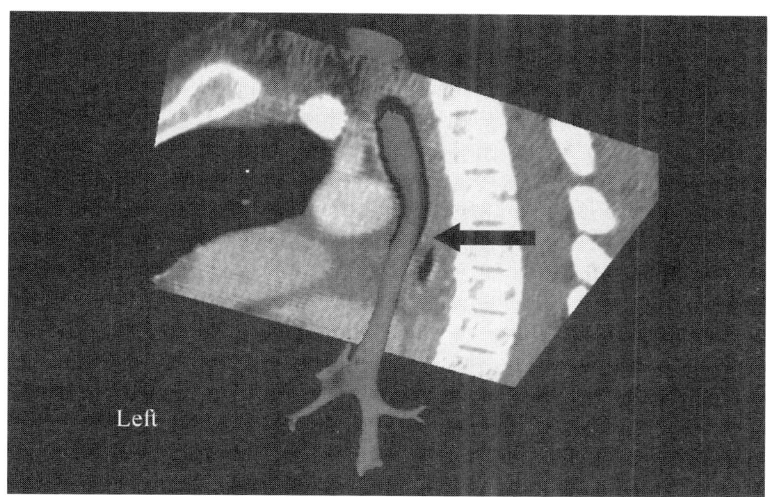

E

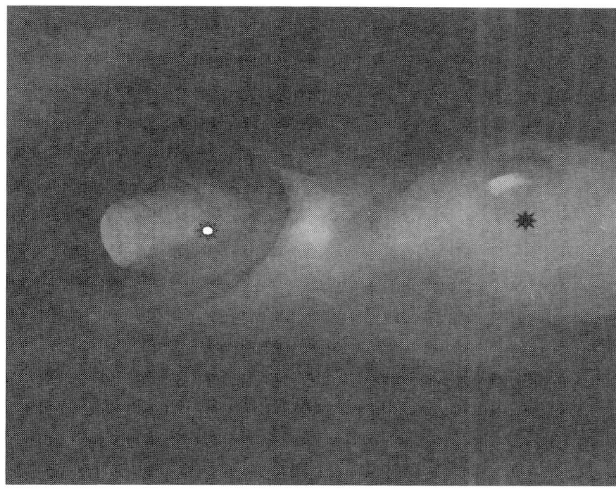

F

struction of the entire thorax from the CT data (Fig. 3). This technique does not depend on adjusting the threshold window and level prior to creating the images. The lumen of the trachea and bronchi is naturally constructed as a hollow column of air within the soft tissue volumetric dataset of the mediastinum. Unlike the surface-rendering algorithm, the airway is not a freestanding three-dimensional structure but is ''embedded'' in the three-dimensional mediastinum. Because images are created from standard CT images, the 3D structure needs to be rotated 180° to invert the left and right. This inversion is necessary in order for the viewer to visualize the airway as though one is truly performing bronchoscopy. Real-time fly-through is not available for this type of reconstruction at this time. A simulated fly-through of the airway can still be performed by the viewer, however, by manually selecting a travel path and replaying this path through a movie loop.

Commercial programs, which create VB using either of these algorithms, can be installed on independent work stations in the radiology department. Volume-rendering programs have the advantage of reconstructing multiaxial data sets from any part of the body into three-dimensional and multiplanar imaging. Such programs provide flexibility in the clinical radiology practice and can be applied to imaging of the brain, vasculature, and solid and hollow organs.

IV. IMAGING ADVANTAGES OF VIRTUAL BRONCHOSCOPY

Studies have shown that three-dimensional VB imaging adds valuable information to conventional helical CT imaging. Reconstruction of standard CT images to thinner intervals improves spatial resolution of CT data; i.e., smaller lesions are better resolved.

Currently, reports show that the ability to fly-through a CT-generated three-dimensional airway has been very successful in evaluating obstructive airway lesions [15,16]. By displaying the airway three-dimensionally, VB can display the level of obstruction and the extent to which the obstruction narrows the airway, thereby helping the user to determine any airway patency beyond the obstruction [9,10]. Additionally, measuring the width and length of airway stenosis can help the bronchoscopist determine whether a bronchoscope can be passed successfully through an area of narrowing. This information can be helpful in preoperative planning in a variety of settings, including resection of tracheobronchial tumors, treatment of postpneumonectomy syndrome

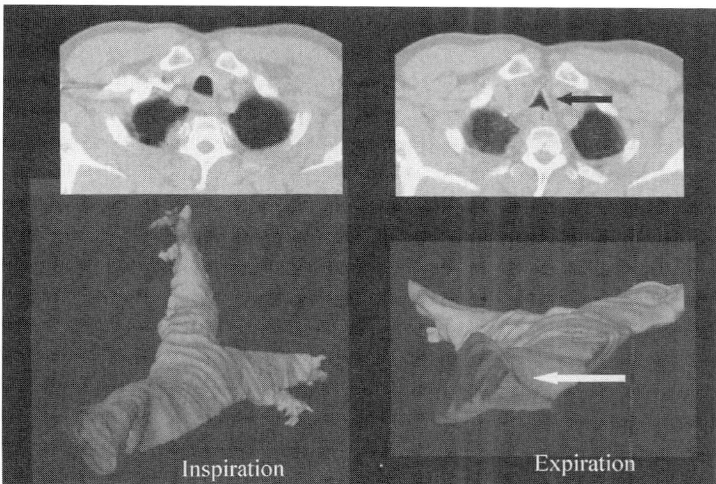

Figure 4 Surface-rendered three-dimensional reconstruction of the trachea of 57-year-old man with tracheobronchomalacia. Inspiratory CT (left-hand upper and lower images) shows that the trachea and proximal bronchi are widened and enlarged. Expiratory CT (right-hand upper and lower images) shows increased narrowing of the proximal trachea (arrow).

(Fig. 3), and palliative stent placement in airways constricted by tumor or scar or tracheomalacia (Fig. 4).

Imaging of the three-dimensional airway has improved the understanding and confidence of image interpretation for clinicians [16–18]. Three-dimensional images provide better orientation of both the airways and the adjacent mediastinal and hilar structures. The ''fly-through'' feature helps the bronchoscopist prepare for the actual procedure by providing a road map of a patient's airway anatomy, thereby limiting unanticipated findings. In this sense, VB has the potential value of decreasing bronchoscopy procedure time by guiding the bronchoscopist to an obstructing airway lesion, displaying abnormal lymph nodes and their location with respect to airway landmarks, and showing the best approach for transbronchial needle biopsy.

Another feature of VB is the ability to rotate images on the computer monitor. This interactive, ''hands-on'' ability to manipulate the images helps the physician visually grasp the relationship between the mediastinal structures and the airways from multiple angles. This interactive dimension of VB, plus the simultaneous use of multiplanar imaging, helps the imager reconfirm the anatomic landmarks seen on other views. Unlike the actual endoscopic procedure, the viewer can repeatedly navigate through the airway without any adverse consequences to the patient.

Virtual bronchoscopy will never supplant true endoscopy, especially in the evaluation of the airway mucosa or if a biopsy of a mediastinal lymph node or mass is needed for diagnosis. However, unlike the actual procedure, with VB, the imager is able to simultaneously view both the contents of the airway and the extraluminal mediastinal and hilar structures. The mediastinum and hila may be viewed either through the airway walls, which can be rendered semitransparent, or by superimposing multiplanar (coronal, sagittal, and axial) or three-dimensional-volume-rendered mediastinal images.

V. LIMITATIONS OF VIRTUAL BRONCHOSCOPY

In order to create a virtual bronchoscopy study, images need to be obtained on a prospective basis: Therefore, the clinician and radiologist have to be in direct communication for an appropriate study to be performed. This is critical since the collimation necessary may be thinner than what is routinely obtained in the radiology department. For example, 5- to 10-mm CT scan slices may be routinely obtained rather than the 3- to 5-mm slices required for VB. Without the appropriate slice thickness and reconstruction, the program may not be able to reconstruct the data into a satisfactory three-dimensional image. If images of 7- to 10-mm slice thickness were reconstructed retrospectively, they would be suboptimal due to stairstep artifacts.

A protocol for VB must be established in order to select the appropriate slice thickness and reconstruction algorithm. The reconstruction of images for VB formatting has to be performed while the original helical CT raw data is still available on the CT scanner's computer. Raw data requires a substantial amount of memory on a CT scanner's computers and unless the data is moved to a separate storage unit (e.g., disk or disk drive) it is discarded as new incoming scans of other patients are performed throughout the day.

Not all patients are candidates for VB imaging. Virtual bronchoscopy requires continuous scanning of the trachea and proximal airways during a single breath hold; in other words, a patient is required to hold his or her breath for up to 30 sec. With the multidetector CT scanners, this time can be shorted substantially and, unless a patient is in respiratory distress, a reasonable scan should be obtainable, especially if prescanning hyperventilation is applied.

Although VB has advantages over actual endoscopy in terms of simultaneously imaging extraluminal and endoluminal anatomy, it is not capable of evaluating the mucosa of the airways and small lesions such as ulcers or plaques. In addition, mucus in the airways may mimic an endobronchial lesion. In this sense, VB should be considered an imaging guide and bronchoscopy should still be performed on any patient with a suspected airway lesion.

Virtual bronchoscopy appears to be useful for imaging pediatric airways for disorders such as vascular rings, tracheomalacia, bronchomalacia, or congenital tracheoesophageal fistula [19]. However, respiratory motion is a significant limitation to its use with small children who are unable to hold their breaths on command [20]. Infants and the very young are unable to perform the breath holding necessary to avoid artifacts such as stairstepping and resultant pseudonarrowing of the airway. In addition, radiation dosage is a concern in this patient group. Although a single helical CT scan is standard for imaging a child with suspected or known thoracic disease, thin collimation inspiratory and expiratory CT images of the entire airway to diagnose disorders such as bronchomalacia and tracheomalacia exposes the patient to excess radiation. Even though multidetector CT scanners decrease scan time, a child still has to be able to comply with breath holding instructions, even if it is for less than 10 sec.

VI. THE FUTURE OF VIRTUAL BRONCHOSCOPY

As discussed above, the power of VB lies in its three-dimensional imaging of the airway with simultaneous imaging of the mediastinum. Three-dimensional VB creates images that a physician without formal image training can comfortably understand. It is noninvasive and can be readily reconstructed from clinically obtained CT scans. To date studies have shown that VB is useful as a preprocedure guide to bronchoscopy by providing excellent anatomy of the airway and demonstrating the presence of stenosis [21,22]. Preliminary studies show that VB can add to the confidence of the bronchoscopist performing transbronchial needle aspiration biopsy by mapping out mediastinal masses and locating lymph nodes.

Conventional CT scanning has significant limitations in detecting abnormal lymph nodes [23]. Contrast enhanced helical CT has provided finer resolution from thinner sliced and reconstructed images and as a result can better distinguish enhancing vascular structures from the hilar and mediastinal lymph nodes [24]. The juxtaposed hilar and paratracheal nodes are the most difficult lymph nodes to distinguish from one another. However, distinction of nodes

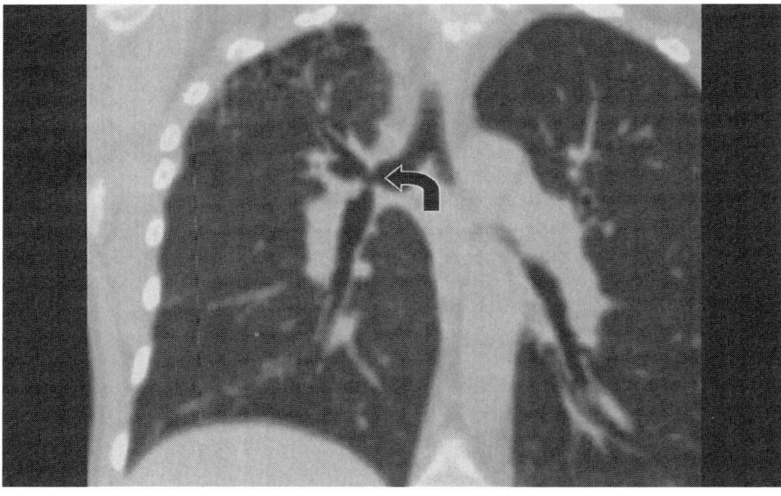

A

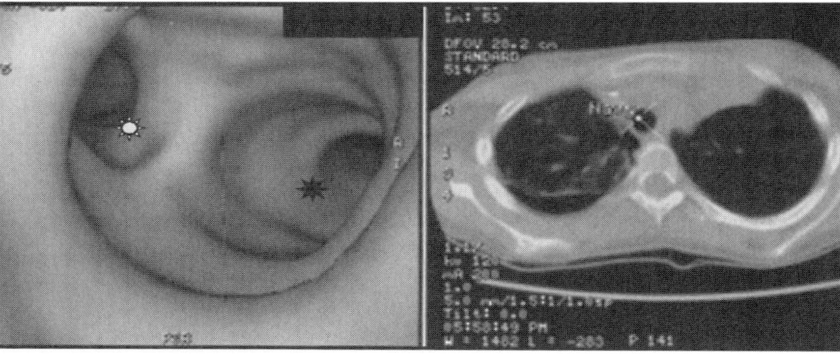

B

Figure 5 (A) Coronal reformation of thoracic CT scan of 40-year-old woman who received a double lung transplantation 10 months previously. She developed stenosis at the right bronchial anastomosis site (arrow). (B) Virtual bronchoscopy image created by surface rendering method shows the patent distal trachea and proximal right (black star) and left (white star) bronchi. Incidental note of pneumothorax on the left on corresponding axial CT image. The right and left sides are inverted as though one is viewing the airway in a simulated bronchoscopy. (C) Virtual bronchoscopy image through the narrowed upper lobe bronchus (curved arrow) shows patency of the segmental bronchi beyond the level of stenosis. (D) Virtual bronchoscopy view at the level of the bronchus intermedius shows the lower lobe superior segmental bronchus is angled inferiorly (arrow); the basal segmental bronchi (double arrow) are within normal limits.

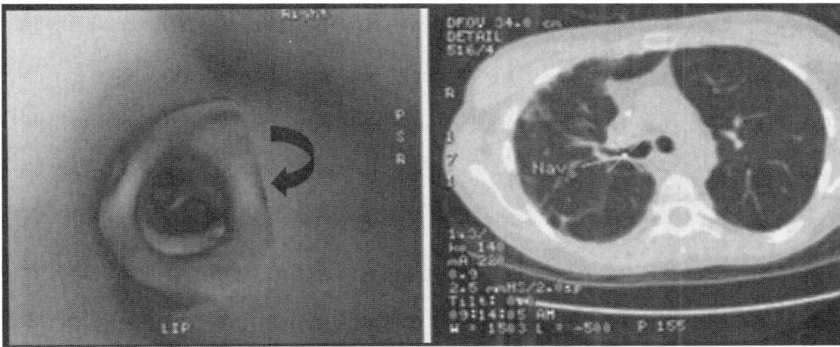

C

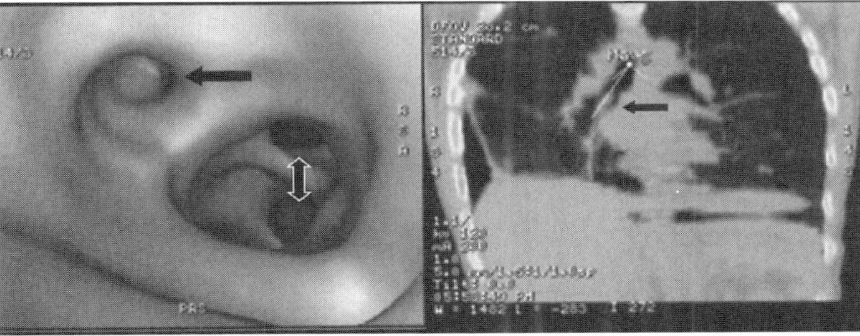

D

Figure 5 Continued

in the hila from those in the mediastinum is essential in staging patients with lung cancer and distinguishing those who have surgically resectable from nonresectable tumors. By rotating images and visualizing them in simultaneous three-dimensional and multiplanar formatting, VB can help radiologists better identify the exact location of enlarged lymph nodes. This ability to better map abnormal mediastinal and hilar nodes, as well as noninvasively guide the bronchoscopist or surgeon to biopsy these abnormal lymph nodes, is a feature which can have a significant impact in improving the radiologic evaluation of patients with lung cancer.

Other clinical uses for VB include the preoperative measurement of the airway caliber prior to the placement of special endobronchial tubes or stents [25,26] and assessing airway diameter in conditions such as stenosis, prior tracheal reconstruction, and lung transplantation (Fig. 5) [18].

In summary, recent advances in CT imaging technology have facilitated and popularized multiplanar and three-dimensional imaging of the body. In the thorax, three-dimensional VB has evolved into a useful imaging tool. The ability to navigate through the airway lumen in a simulated bronchoscopy provides the imager with a better appreciation of the presence and extent of airway disorders and their relationship to other mediastinal structures. As a means of displaying thoracic anatomy, VB is both an excellent teaching tool and an effective means of evaluating the airway prior to interventional procedures.

References

1. Kalender WA, Seissier W, Klotz E, Vock P. Spiral volumetric CT with single-breath-hold technique, continuous transport, and continuous scanner rotation. Radiology 1990; 176(1):181–183.
2. Heiken JP, Brink JA, Vannier MW. Spiral (helical) CT. Radiology 1993; 189(3): 647–656.
3. Zeman RK, Baron RL, Jeffrey RB Jr, Klein J, Siegel MJ, Silverman PM. Helical body CT: evolution of scanning protocols. Am J Roentgenol 1998; 170(6):1427–1438.
4. Kasales CJ, Hopper KD, Ariola DN, et al. Reconstructed helical CT scans: improvement in z-axis resolution compared with overlapped and nonoverlapped conventional CT scans. Am J Roentgenol 1995; 164:1281–1284.
5. Hopper KD, Pierantozzi D, Potok PS, et al. The quality of 3D reconstructions from 1.0 and 1.5 pitch helical and conventional CT. J Comput Assist Tomogr 1996; 20:841–847.
6. Dillon EH, van Leeuwen MS, Fernandez MA, Fernandez MA, Mali WPTM. Spiral CT angiography. Am J Roentgenol 1993; 160(6):1273–1281.
7. Napel S, Marks MP, Rubin GD, et al. CT angiography with spiral CT and maximum intensity projection. Radiology 1992; 185(2):607–610.
8. Vining DJ, Liu K, Choplin RH, Haponik EF. Virtual bronchoscopy: relationships of virtual reality endobronchial simulations to actual bronchoscopic findings. Chest 1996; 109(2):549–553.
9. Ferretti GR, Vining DJ, Knoplioch J, Coulomb M. Tracheobronchial tree: three-dimensional spiral CT with bronchoscopic perspective. J Comput Assist Tomogr 1996; 20(5):777–781.
10. Higgins WE, Ramaswamy K, Swift RD, McLennan G, Hoffman EA. Virtual bronchoscopy for three-dimensional pulmonary image assessment: state of the art and future needs. Radiographics 1998; 18(3):761–778.
11. Hopper KD, Iyriboz TA, Mahraj RP, et al. CT bronchoscopy: optimization of imaging parameters [In Process Citation]. Radiology 1998; 209(3):872–877.

12. Summers RM, Shaw DJ, Shelhamer JH. CT virtual bronchoscopy of simulated endobronchial lesions: effect of scanning, reconstruction, and display settings and potential pitfalls. Am J Roentgenol 1998; 170(4):947–950.
13. Fleischmann D, Rubin GD, Paik DS, et al. Stair-step artifacts with single versus multiple detector-row helical CT. Radiology 2000; 216:185–196.
14. Fleiter T, Merkle EM, Aschoff AJ, et al. Comparison of real-time virtual and fiberoptic bronchoscopy in patients with bronchial carcinoma: opportunities and limitations. Am J Roentgenol 1997; 169(6):1591–1595.
15. Kauczor HU, Wolcke B, Fischer B, Mildenberger P, Lorenz, Thelen M. Three-dimensional helical CT of the tracheobronchial tree: evaluation of imaging protocols and assessment of suspected stenoses with bronchoscopic correlation. Am J Roentgenol 1996; 167(2):419–424.
16. Remy-Jardin M, Remy J, Artaud D, Firbourg M, Duhamel A. Volume rendering of the tracheobronchial tree: clinical evaluation of bronchographic images. Radiology 1998; 208:761–770.
17. McAdams HP, Goodman PC, Kussin P. Virtual bronchoscopy for directing transbronchial needle aspiration of hilar and mediastinal lymph nodes: a pilot study. Am J Roentgenol 1998; 170(5):1361–1364.
18. Feretti GR, Thony F, Bosson JL, Pison C, Arbib F. Benign abnormalities and carcinoid tumors of the central airways: diagnostic impact of CT bronchography. Am J Roentgenol 2000; 174:1307–1313.
19. Konen E, Katz M, Rozenman J, Ben-Shlush A, Itzchak Y, Szeinberg A. Virtual bronchoscopy in children: early clinical experience [In Process Citation]. Am J Roentgenol 1998; 171(6):1699–1702.
20. Frush P, Donnelly LF. Helical CT in children: technical considerations and body applications. Radiology 1998; 209(1):37–48.
21. Haponik E, Aquino S, Vining D. Will virtual bronchoscopy have a real impact? American College of Chest Physicians: Pulmonary Perspectives, Sep 7–9, 1997.
22. Quint LE, Whyte RI, Kazerooni EA, et al. Stenosis of the central airways: evaluation by using helical CT with multiplanar reconstructions. Radiology 1995; 194: 871–877.
23. McLoud TC, Bourgouin PM, Greenberg RW. Bronchogenic carcinoma: analysis of staging in the mediastinum with CT by correlative lymph node mapping and sampling [see comments]. Radiology 1992; 182(2):319–23.
24. Remy-Jardin M, Duyck P, Remy J, et al. Hilar lymph nodes: identification with spiral CT and histologic correlation. Radiology 1995; 196:387–394.
25. Eberle B, Weiler N, Vogel N, Kauczor H, Heinrichs W. Computed tomography-based tracheobronchial image reconstruction allows selection of the individually appropriate double-lumen tube size. J Cardiothorac Vasc Anesth 1999; 13:532–537.
26. McAdams HP, Palmer SM, Erasmus JJ, et al. Bronchial anastomotic complications in lung transplant recipients: virtual bronchoscopy for noninvasive assessment [In Process Citation]. Radiology 1998; 209(3):689–695.

10
CT Quantification of Emphysema

Ella A. Kazerooni
University of Michigan Health System, Ann Arbor, Michigan

INTRODUCTION

Before the reintroduction of lung volume reduction surgery (LVRS) in the mid-1990s as a surgical treatment for advanced emphysema [1], the routine clinical use of medical imaging for emphysema was largely limited to the chest radiograph. Emphysema was commonly depicted on computerized tomography (CT) scans of the thorax performed for other reasons, such as lung cancer diagnosis or staging; however, there has been little reason to apply advanced imaging techniques routinely to the emphysema itself. While CT for the detection of emphysema has proven useful in the evaluation of dyspnea patients with an isolated reduction in diffusing capacity at pulmonary function testing in the setting of a normal chest radiograph [2,3], this is a fairly limited indication for performing chest CT.

Since the resurgence of LVRS, the imaging of emphysema with computerized tomography has received tremendous attention. Computerized tomography is the most accurate method in vivo for identifying and quantifying emphysema [4,5]. Many investigators have shown that the severity and distribution of emphysema within the lungs at CT are strong predictors of a successful outcome after LVRS, creating a new indication for the advanced imaging of emphysema [6–13]. Increasingly, the quantitative measurement of emphysema is being advocated and used to measure the effectiveness of medical therapies for emphysema and change in emphysema over time [14–16].

This chapter defines the appearance of emphysema on CT, describes methods for quantifying emphysema with CT, and presents the published data on use of CT to select candidates for LVRS.

DEFINITIONS AND PATHOLOGY

Emphysema is commonly included with asthma and chronic bronchitis in the group of diseases that together make up chronic obstructive pulmonary disease (COPD). ''The term 'COPD' is generally used in clinical discourse to describe individuals diagnosed with one or more of the following conditions: asthmatic bronchitis, chronic bronchitis, chronic obstructive bronchitis and emphysema,'' according to a National Heart, Lung and Blood Institute Workshop on the subject [17]. Airflow obstruction is common to all forms of COPD. In emphysema and chronic bronchitis, the airflow obstruction does not markedly change over months and is largely fixed or irreversible, while in asthma the airflow obstruction is largely reversible, except in chronic, long-standing asthma where airflow obstruction may also become fixed [18,19]. Of the approximately 15 million people in the United States with COPD, approximately 1.65 to 2 million have emphysema [18].

According to the American Thoracic Society, emphysema is defined as ''a condition of the lung characterized by abnormal, permanent enlargement of the air spaces distal to the terminal bronchiole, accompanied by destruction of their walls,'' and without obvious fibrosis [18]. In general, emphysema occurs due to an imbalance in the proteolytic activity in the lungs, resulting in destruction of alveolar tissue. This may be seen with an overabundance of proteolytic enzymes, a lack of antiproteases, or a combination of both.

The pathologic classification of emphysema is based on the anatomic unit of the lung known as the secondary pulmonary lobule, with a paired pulmonary artery branch and bronchiole at the center of each lobule. The four major categories of emphysema are centrilobular (centriacinar), panacinar (panlobular), paraseptal, and paracicatricial [20]. Centrilobular emphysema is the form of emphysema most commonly associated with cigarette smoking and is the most common form of emphysema overall. The destruction of alveolar walls begins in the central portion of the secondary pulmonary lobule; is heterogeneous, affecting adjacent lobules with varying degrees of severity; and is usually most severe in the upper lobes. The relatively greater ventilation–perfusion ratio in the upper portion of the lungs compared to the lung bases favors greater deposition of the particulate matter from cigarette smoke in the upper lungs. Activated macrophages release the proteolytic enzyme, elastase, and free radicals and oxidants in cigarette smoke inactivate the normally protective antiproteases, leading to greater destruction of the upper lobes that the lower lobes [20].

Panacinar emphysema typically occurs in patients with α-1-antiprotease deficiency and is accelerated by superimposed cigarette smoking. In contrast to centrilobular emphysema, panacinar emphysema is usually more severe in the lower lungs than the upper lungs, and homogeneously affects the entire lobule as well as adjacent lobules. The proteolytic enzyme, elastase, is found within neutrophils and macrophages in the lung. More circulating α-1-antiprotease is delivered to the lower lungs than the upper lungs due to the greater distribution of blood flow to the lower lungs. When α-1-antiprotease is deficient, the greatest deficiency from normal is therefore seen at the lung bases. With the lack of antiproteolytic activity, greater destruction of lung parenchyma occurs at the lung bases.

Paraseptal emphysema involves the peripheral or paraseptal portion of the secondary pulmonary lobules and the apices and paramediastinal portion of the upper lobes and may be related to aging, although this remains poorly understood. Paracicatricial emphysema occurs adjacent to areas of scarring, fibrosis, and granulomas. As an example, it may be seen in the periphery of the upper lungs in patients with silicosis and conglomerate masses.

COMPUTERIZED TOMOGRAPHY

Defining the Severity of Emphysema

Computerized tomography provides excellent anatomic detail for detecting, characterizing, and quantifying the severity of emphysema. Not surprisingly, high-resolution CT (HRCT) is more accurate than conventional CT at demonstrating the presence, severity and distribution of emphysema [21–23]. On CT, emphysema appears as areas of abnormally low attenuation pulmonary parenchyma, without definable walls, resulting in a decrease in the mean attenuation value of the lung parenchyma (Fig. 1) [24]. Several investigators have shown that CT is accurate for quantifying emphysema, using either visual scoring methods or attenuation threshold-based quantitative analysis [4,5,21,25–36]. It should be noted that both visual scoring methods and quantitative analysis of emphysema may fail to detect mild emphysema [5,22].

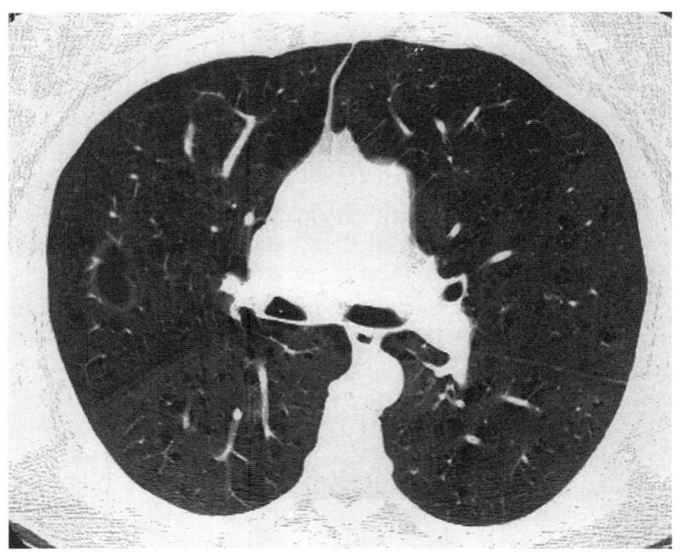

(A)

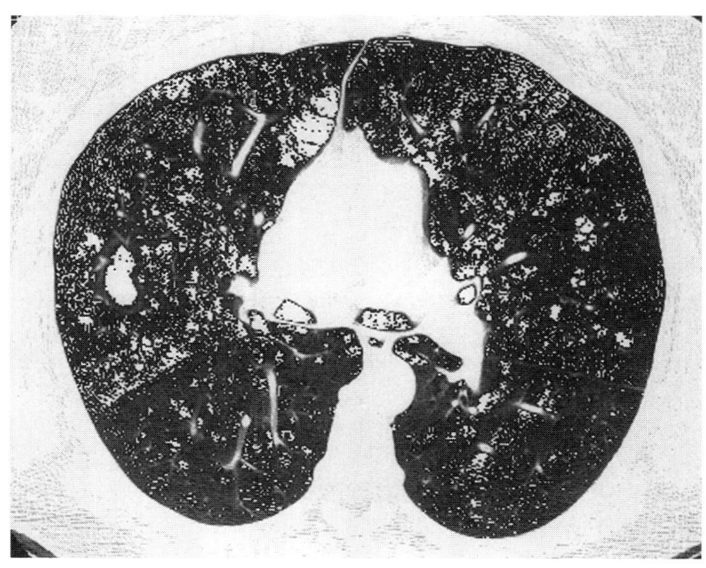

(B)

Visual Scoring and Quantitative Scoring of Emphysema with Pathologic Correlation

The severity of emphysema identified on HRCT and conventional CT has demonstrated excellent correlation with the pathologic severity of emphysema, using both visual scoring systems and quantitative analysis [4,5,22,30,37]. Radiologic–pathologic study by Hruban et al. using a visual estimation of emphysema on in vitro 2-mm collimation HRCT images of resected lung tissue compared to the severity of emphysema in the pathologic specimens demonstrated a correlation of $r = 0.91$ ($P < 0.005$) [26]. Subsequently, Müller et al compared a visual CT scoring system and the density mask technique (pixels between −910 and −1024 HU representing emphysema) applied to a single 10-mm collimation axial image of the lung to the inflation-fixed lung specimen pathology scores in patients undergoing thoracotomy for tumor resection. The density mask technique is performed by setting an attenuation threshold below which all pixel values represent emphysema. Histologic specimens were scored using a modification of the Thurlbeck picture-grading system, with scores ranging from 0 to 100 (0 representing no emphysema) [38]; 89% of the 28 patients had pathology scores less than or equal to 50. The visual score ($r = 0.9$; $P < 0.001$) and the density mask score ($r = 0.94$) demonstrated excellent correlation with the pathology score. Using the visual method, the two CT readers missed emphysema on CT in six patients and three patients each; all had mild emphysema by pathology score. Each reader called emphysema in one normal patient. The density mask technique missed three cases of mild emphysema and incorrectly called one normal case emphysema. This yielded sensitivities of 71, 86, and 86% for reader 1, reader 2, and the density mask technique, respectively, and a specificity of 86% for each.

Miller et al. later used a visual grid scoring system and compared 10-mm conventional CT and 1.5-mm HRCT images of patients undergoing lung resection for malignancy to the severity of emphysema in corresponding inflation-fixed lung pathologic specimens. The visual grid scoring method is performed by superimposing a crosshair grid on an image, with emphysema

---

Figure 1 Mild centrilobular emphysema. (A) Axial 1-mm collimation HRCT image through the midthorax demonstrates small focal areas of low attenuation without definable walls. (B) Axial density mask technique applied at an attenuation threshold of −950 HU demonstrates the emphysema in white. By knowing both the volume of the emphysema and the lung (using a density mask threshold of −700 HU and lower) the percentage of the lung replaced by emphysema can be measured.

scored in each box as present or absent. A correlation of $r = 0.81$ ($P < 0.001$) was found between the 10-mm CT visual grid score and the pathology score that improved slightly, $r = 0.85$ ($P < 0.001$), using the 1.5-mm HRCT images [22].

When performing quantitative analysis using an attenuation threshold technique, attention to regular calibration of the CT scanner to correct for any drift in CT numbers is critically important. Studies of third- and fourth-generation CT scanners from different vendors have demonstrated that scanner conformity is reproducible for lung densitometry measurements of attenuation and that measurement of the low-attenuation area of the lung with minimal variation can be obtained when appropriate calibration for water and air is performed [39,47,48]. The correct upper attenuation threshold to use for quantitative CT analysis varies with slice thickness and inspiration versus expiration. By using an inappropriately high threshold, emphysema will be overestimated, while using an inappropriately low threshold will underestimation emphysema. For example, the optimum threshold for 10-mm collimation inspiratory CT is −910 HU [5], while −950 HU is the optimum threshold for 1-mm collimation inspiratory CT [30]. The optimum threshold for 1-mm collimation expiratory CT [30] has been shown to be −820 HU.

Most quantitative analysis of emphysema is performed using CT obtained at inspiration. While some investigation has been performed on expiratory images, results are less accurate. For example, in a series of 89 patients undergoing lung resection undergoing both inspiratory and expiratory HRCT at 1-mm collimation, the quantification of emphysema was less accurate at expiration, which may in part be related to superimposed small airway disease resulting in air trapping and reduced lung attenuation [30]. In this study a computer-based method was used to determine the areas of macroscopic and microscopic emphysema [29]. With the use of spirometry gating, measurements are reproducible within the same patient, even in patients with severe respiratory insufficiency. These measurement are the most reproducible at 90% of vital capacity [40]. At end-expiration, reproducibility in the same study was worse by a factor of three.

Other quantitative measurements have been investigated, such as mean lung attenuation. However, these have demonstrated poorer correlation with the emphysema severity in pathologic specimens. For example, using 10-mm collimation images, the correlation between mean lung density and the visual score with pathology scores was only moderate, $r = 0.44$, $P < 0.01$, and $r = 0.46$, $P < 0.01$, respectively [5]. A sliding thin-slab, minimum-intensity projection technique has recently been demonstrated to be more accurate at the detection of mild emphysema than HRCT, when evaluating images for the presence or absence of emphysema only [25].

The quantitative analysis of the severity of emphysema referred to as the density mask technique was initially performed on selected axial two-dimensional images [5], with a region of interest drawn around the lungs on the image or images of interest. To perform this technique on the entire lungs is cumbersome. The same technique can be applied to a three-dimensional volume of the entire lungs acquired during a single inspiration using helical CT (Fig. 2–4) [13,41,42]. These analyses can be performed on commercially available scanner consoles or workstations from all CT scanner manufacturers.

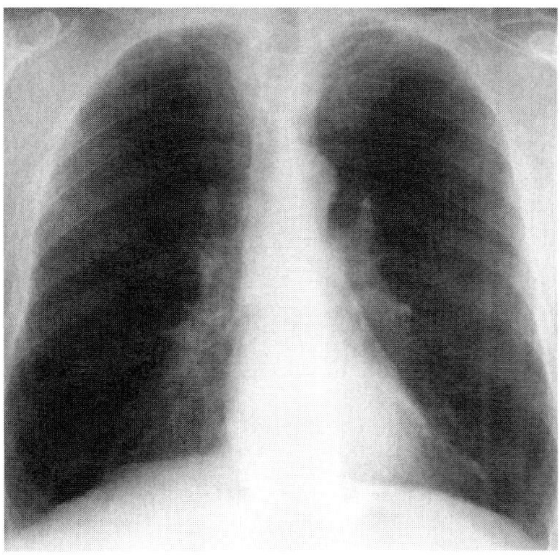

(A)

Figure 2 Upper lobe predominant emphysema in a 64-year-old man. Posteroanterior (A) and lateral (B) chest radiographs demonstrate pulmonary hyperinflation with flattened hemidiaphragms, increased anteroposterior chest dimension and an enlarged retrosternal clear space, increased lung height; less evident is the disparity between the fewer and smaller upper lobe pulmonary vessels compared to the lower lobes. Axial HRCT images through the upper lobes (C) and lower lungs (D) demonstrate more severe anatomic destruction in the upper lobes compared to the lung bases, with greater separation and thinning of pulmonary blood vessels at the lung apices. (E and F) Helical CT shaded surface display reconstructions of the lung in the anterior and lateral projections, with the emphysema displayed in white (all pixels less than −900 HU) on the background total lung volume (all pixels less than −700 HU), shown in gray. Using CT, the total lung volume was 6.6 L, compared to a total lung capacity of 6.9 L using pulmonary function testing. The emphysema volume was 3.6 L, or 54% of the total lung volume. Seventy-three percent of the upper half of the lungs and 37% of the lower half of the lungs is emphysema, for a CT ratio of 1.95.

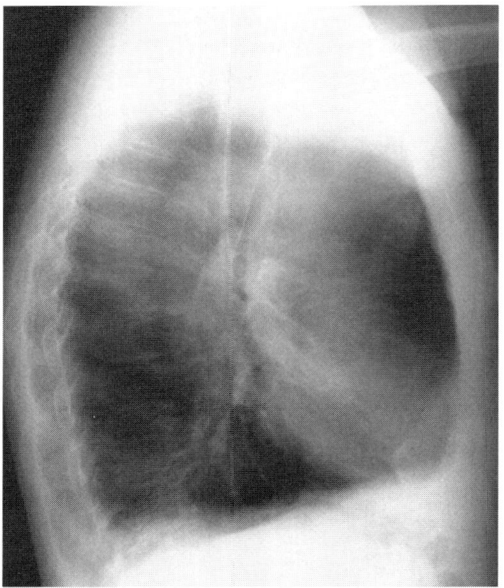

(B)

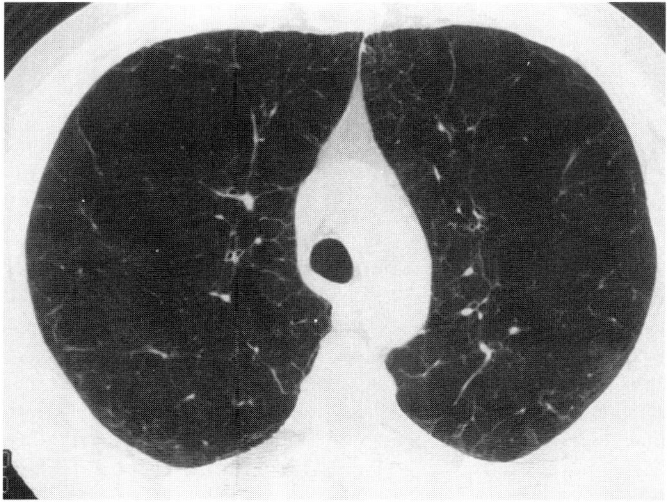

(C)

Figure 2 Continued

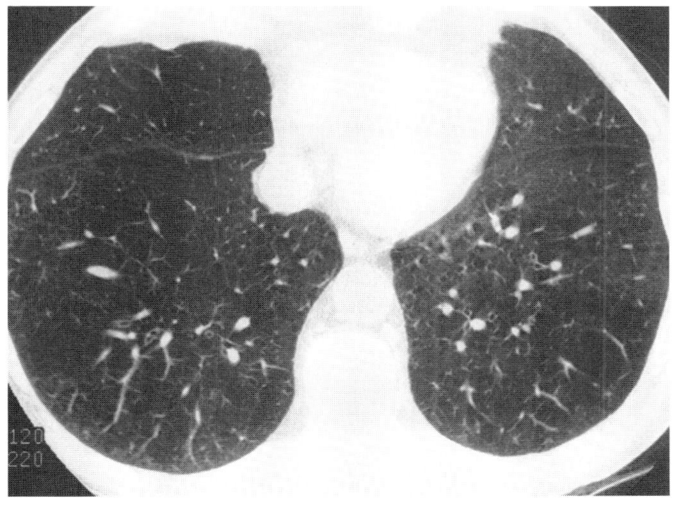

(D)

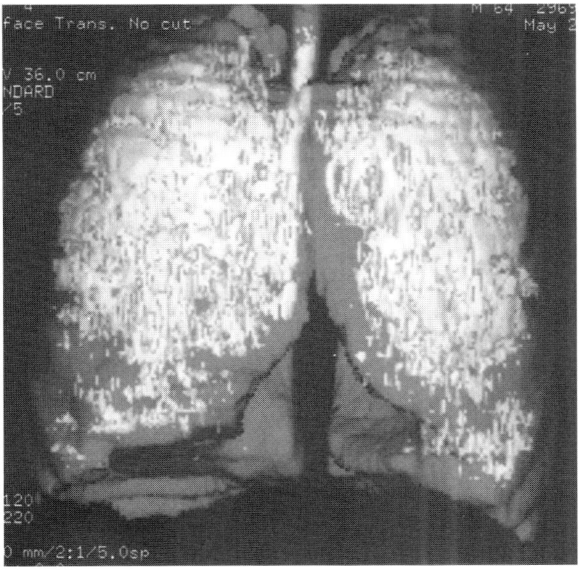

(E)

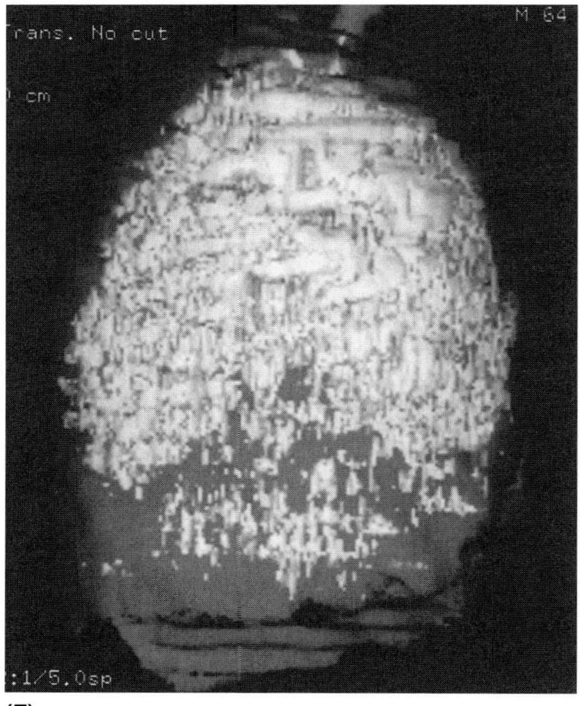

(F)

Figure 2 Continued

In conventional CT, individual axial images or clusters of axial images are obtained in a single breath hold, with the patient allowed to breathe before scanning of the next individual image or cluster of images. However, with variation in the level of each breath hold, portions of the thorax are inevitably missed or overlapped. The fast acquisition times of helical CT almost completely eliminate this error. Lung volumes, including total lung capacity (TLC) and residual volume (RV), can also be calculated from inspiratory and expiratory helical CT data with excellent correlation to static lung volumes [43]. Other quantitative tools have been applied to the evaluation of data obtained from CT in patients with emphysema, including a texture-based adaptive multiple feature method (AMFM) incorporating multiple statistical and fractal texture features, but have not yet demonstrated clinically applicable uses [44,45].

Correlation with Pulmonary Function

The CT methods for quantifying emphysema have shown excellent correlation with diffusing capacity and pulmonary capillary blood volume, but only correlate moderately with measures of airflow obstruction, such as the forced expiratory volume in 1 sec (FEV1), forced vital capacity (FVC), and the FEV1/FVC ratio [46,47]. Some have therefore speculated that the severity of expiratory airway obstruction in emphysema is not related to the severity of alveolar wall destruction [36,46–49]. In one study in which patients with emphysema underwent both inspiratory and expiratory CT, the visual emphysema score correlated well with the severity of emphysema, but not with air trapping. In contrast, the ratio of the CT attenuation number at expiration to inspiration (the E/I ratio) correlated well with air trapping and less well with emphysema severity [50].

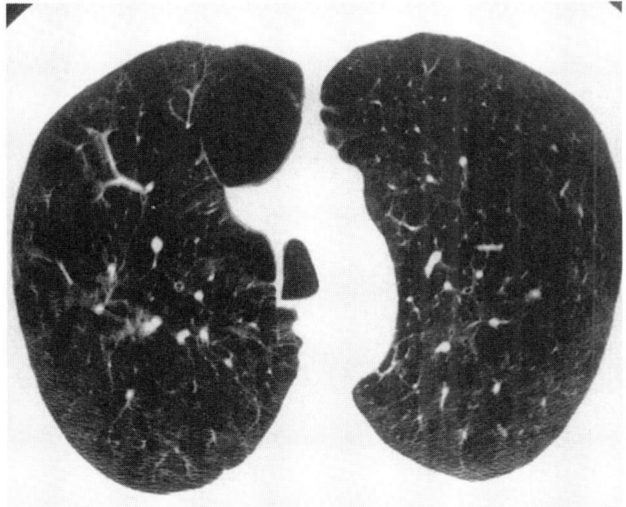

(A)

Figure 3 Diffuse emphysema in a 53-year-old man. Axial HRCT images through the upper lobes (A) and lower (B) lungs demonstrate more uniform anatomic destruction throughout the lungs. Anterior (C) three-dimensional shaded surface display reconstructions shows diffuse emphysema. Using quantitative CT analysis, the total lung volume was 6.8 L, emphysema volume 3.6 L, with 54% of the volume representing emphysema. Fifty-five and a half percent of the upper half of the lungs and 52.4% of the lower half of the lungs represented emphysema, for a CT ratio of 1.06.

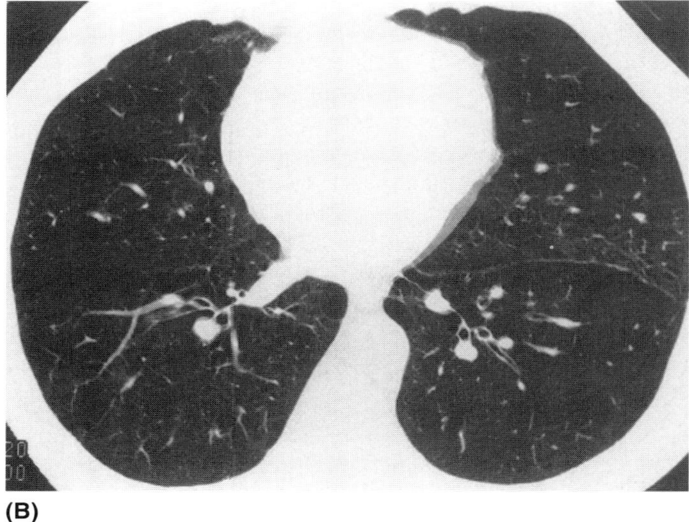

(B)

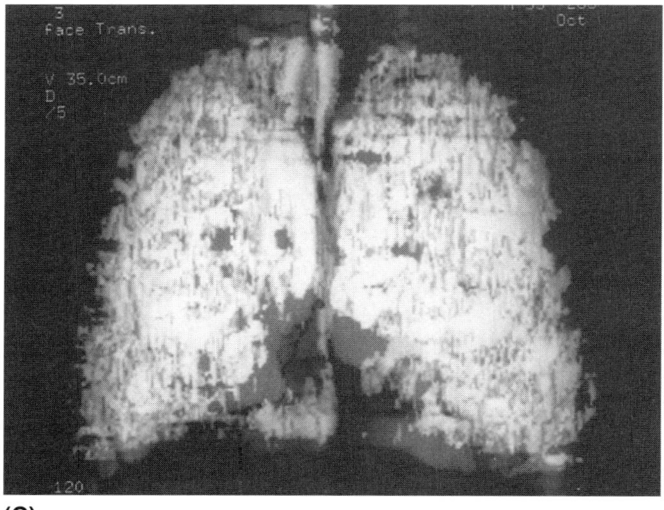

(C)

Figure 3 Continued

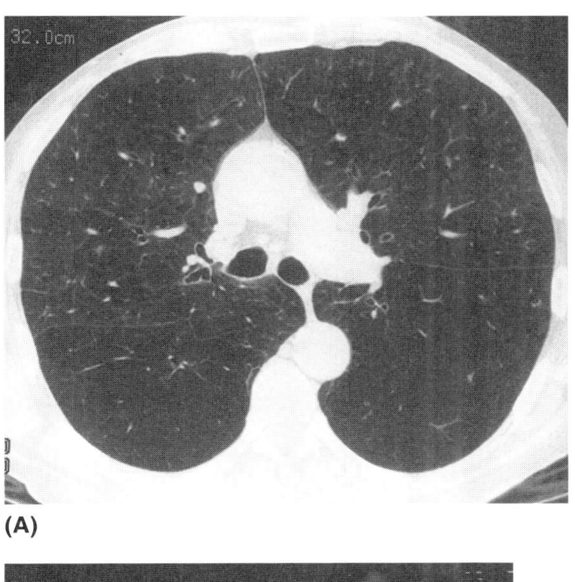

(A)

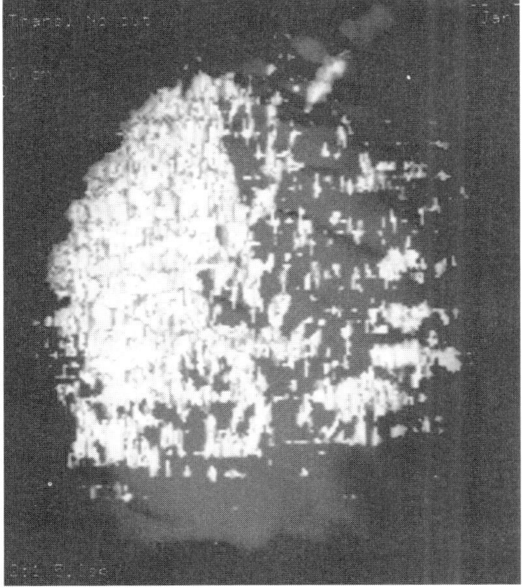

(B)

Figure 4 Lower lobe predominant panacinar emphysema in a 66-year-old woman. Axial HRCT image through the midlungs (A) demonstrate more uniform anatomic destruction posterior to the major fissures in the lower lobes than in the upper lobes. Lateral (B) three-dimensional shaded surface display reconstruction shows most of the emphysema posterior to the expected location of the major fissures.

The anatomic distribution of emphysema in the lungs may also have differential impact on pulmonary function. For example, a greater severity of emphysema in the central portion of the lung has a greater correlation with pulmonary function impairment than peripheral emphysema, and the more uniform the emphysema between the upper and lower lung, or the central and peripheral lung, the more severe the airway obstruction [51,52].

SELECTION FOR LUNG VOLUME REDUCTION SURGERY

Computerized Tomography Distribution and Severity

Many investigators have now shown that the anatomic distribution of emphysema within the lungs demonstrated on CT is an excellent predictor of patient outcome after LVRS [6,8,9,13,53–58]. This has been shown for both visual semiquantitative or qualitative emphysema scoring systems [53–55,58] and quantitative analysis methods [6,8,9,13,56,57]. The more homogeneous the emphysema from lung apices to bases, the poorer the outcome after surgery. Patients with upper lobe or lower lobe predominant emphysema, referred to as target areas for resection, with large areas of normal lung remaining, experience the greatest improvements after LVRS. The advantages of a visual semiquantitative scoring system are both ease of application and that a computer workstation is not required for analysis. An advantage of quantitative analysis is the reproducibility of the technique across individuals of varying expertise, and across institutions, allowing more accurate comparison of results between different centers. While qualitative scoring systems for emphysema have reported excellent inter- and intraobserver agreement, the investigators have largely been experts in thoracic radiology, and whether such systems are effective among practitioners of varying expertise is unknown [59]. Furthermore, a dominant method for the quantification of emphysema for LVRS selection has not yet arisen.

Some examples of the use of qualitative and quantitative CT measurements of emphysema in the selection of LVRS candidates are as follows. In a series of 50 consecutive patients by Weder et al. undergoing bilateral LVRS with video-assisted thoracoscopy, a qualitative assessment of emphysema was made using preoperative HRCT and spiral CT images. Patients with markedly heterogeneous pulmonary emphysema had significantly greater improvement in FEV1 3 months after surgery compared to preoperative measurements (81% ± 17%) versus patients with intermediately heterogeneous emphysema (44% ± 10%) and patients with homogeneous emphysema (34% ± 6%) [54].

Wisser et al. in a study of 47 patients undergoing bilateral LVRS by median sternotomy ($n = 15$) or video-assisted thoracoscopy ($n = 32$), used a 4-point grading scheme for emphysema heterogeneity and a 48-point scale for severity of lung parenchymal destruction on HRCT and helical CT images. The heterogeneity of emphysema correlated with postoperative improvements in FEV1 3 months after surgery, and all 4 patients who died within 30 days of LVRS had significantly greater parenchymal destruction scores (28.4 vs. 21.3; $P = 0.003$), and [53].

Similar results have been demonstrated for quantitative analysis. Gierada et al. reported a series of 46 patients undergoing bilateral LVRS demonstrating postoperative improvements measured 6 months postoperatively in FEV1, PaO_2 and 6-min walk distance that were greater in patients with mean total lung attenuation values greater than −900 HU, an emphysema index with 75% or greater of the upper half of the lung representing emphysema (threshold −900 to −1024 HU), a greater volume of normal-attenuation lung (−701 to −850 HU), and a ratio of upper to lower lung emphysema indices of greater than 1.5, indicating greater regional heterogeneity of emphysema [9]. In this study the CT scanning technique was 8- or 10-mm collimation in incremental mode; one scan was performed in helical mode. Our work has demonstrated similar results with the three-dimensional density mask technique applied to a single breath hold acquisition at 10-mm collimation, pitch 2 : 1 [13,60]. While thinner collimation is more desirable, it would require several breath-holds due to increased scan acquisition time on single-detector helical CT scanners, which the currently available analysis packages cannot readily evaluate as a single volume. Multidetector helical CT scanners with faster scan times make scanning of the entire lungs at 2.5-mm collimation possible in 15 sec., and scanning at 1.25-mm collimation possible in 30 sec. The emphysema ratio (percentage emphysema in upper lungs divided by percentage emphysema in the lower lungs) has been the single, best predictor of improvements in FEV1 and 6-min walk distance 3, 6, 12, 18, and 24 months after bilateral apical LVRS performed through a median sternotomy, as demonstrated using ROC analysis. Our results extend the published CT outcome data from 3–6 months after LVRS to 2 years after LVRS. The CT emphysema ratio has demonstrated a better correlation with outcomes than measures of pulmonary hyperinflation (RV, TLC, and RV/TLC), baseline FEV1, diffusing capacity, and other quantitative CT measures, such as the percentage of normal lower lung and the percentage of emphysema in the entire lungs. The prediction of outcome with the CT ratio is slightly improved when combining the CT ratio with the RV, TLC, or RV/TLC. Newer, multidetector helical CT scanners allow faster scanning at thinner collimation, acquiring images between 0.5- and 1.25-mm colli-

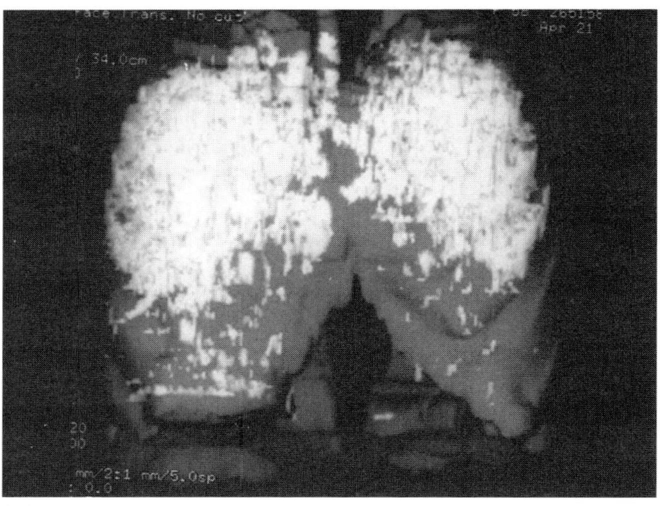

(A)

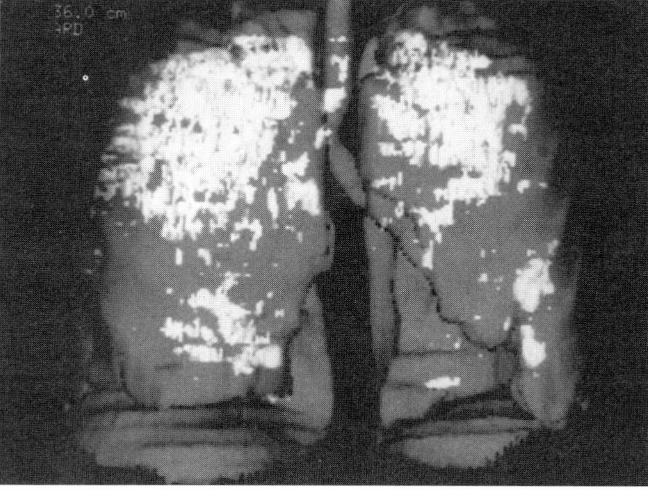

(B)

Figure 5 Reduction in target zones of upper lobe emphysema after bilateral apical lung volume reduction surgery through a median sternotomy in a 59-year-old woman. Three-dimensional shaded surface display reconstructions before (A) and after lung volume reduction surgery demonstrate larger target areas of emphysema before surgery than after surgery. Prior to surgery, 65% of the upper half of the lungs represented emphysema using quantitative CT. After surgery, this number was reduced to 30%.

mation of the entire lungs. These should improve the accuracy of helical CT quantitative assessment and potentially the accuracy of predicting outcome after LVRS. Quantitative helical CT performed before and after surgery can be used to measure the anatomic changes that occur due to surgery and evaluate for progression of emphysema in the remaining lung over time (Fig. 5).

Pulmonary Nodules and Incidental Lung Cancer

Patients with emphysema are at risk for developing lung cancer. Three separate investigations of severe emphysema patients being evaluated for LVRS or lung transplantation have demonstrated a 5% incidence of bronchogenic carcinoma at the time of initial patient evaluation [61–63]. These results have been reported despite different scanning techniques, ranging from 10-mm contiguous axial images in two reports [61,63] to HRCT with 1 to 1.5-mm collimation at 10-mm intervals in the third series [62]. A greater percentage of patients, 11–26%, had one or more noncalcified pulmonary nodules identified during evaluation that raised the suspicion of bronchogenic carcinoma (Fig. 6) [61–65]. While the majority of these nodules are benign, further evaluation

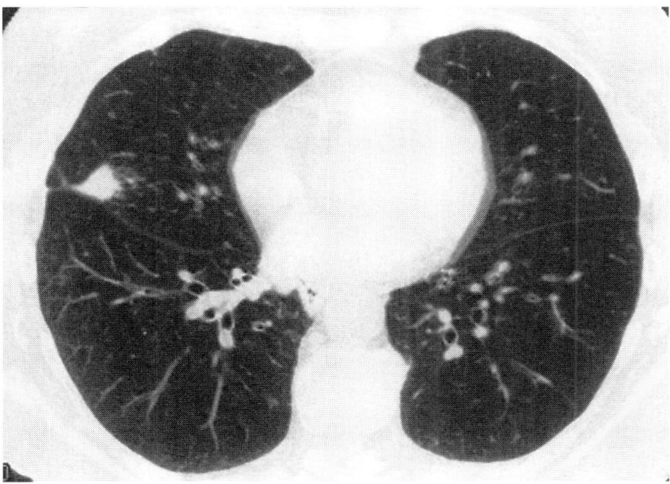

Figure 6 Incidental 14-mm noncalcified right middle lobe pulmonary nodule in a 72-year-old woman with emphysema undergoing CT as part of the evaluation for lung-volume-reduction surgery. The nodule is suspicious for bronchogenic carcinoma. To date, no tissue diagnosis or follow-up CT scan has been obtained.

with close follow-up serial CT, biopsy, or resection is warranted to identify the malignant nodules. Unfortunately, PET scanning is not an option for most of these cases because of the small size of the nodules. Noncalcified lung nodules in one series were identified in 113 of 442 patients with severe emphysema being evaluated for LVRS, with only 22% of the nodules measuring greater than 1 cm in diameter [64].

When a nodule is identified in an LVRS candidate, it is important to note whether the nodule is within the portion of lung that can be resected during LVRS, as some patients with insufficient pulmonary function to tolerate conventional lung cancer surgery with lobectomy may be eligible for resection of the nodule during a combined LVRS procedure, with the potential to improve pulmonary function and dyspnea as well as resect the malignancy [65]. The combined surgery can be performed successfully, with little morbidity and mortality [65,66]. However, during such a combined procedure the LVRS procedure may be altered or compromised in order to completely resect the nodule, with some investigators reporting that the post-LVRS outcomes in patients undergoing combined nodule resection and LVRS are less substantial than patients undergoing LVRS alone [66].

SUMMARY

Lung volume reduction surgery has created an opportunity for the advanced imaging of emphysema. Patients with CT demonstrating an upper or lower lobe predominant pattern of emphysema have better patient outcomes after LVRS than patients with diffuse, homogeneously distributed emphysema throughout the lungs. While some patients with diffuse or homogeneous emphysema may have improved function or dyspnea after surgery, the magnitude of the improvement seen is less than in patients with heterogeneous emphysema. Given that emphysema patients are at risk for bronchogenic carcinoma, care should be taken to identify and anatomically describe the location of noncalcified pulmonary nodules in patients that are candidates for LVRS.

REFERENCES

1. JD Cooper, EP Trulock, AN Triantafillou, et al. Bilateral pneumectomy (volume reduction) for chronic obstructive pulmonary disease. J Thorac Cardiovasc Surg 1995; 109:106–119.

2. JS Klein, G Gamsu, WR Webb, JA Golden, NL Müller. High-resolution CT diagnosis of emphysema in symptomatic patients with normal chest radiographs and isolated low diffusing capacity. Radiology 1992; 182:817–821.
3. NK Chin, TK Lim. A 39-year-old smoker with effort dyspnea, normal spirometry results, and low diffusing capacity. Chest 1998; 113:231–233.
4. PA Gevenois, V de Maertelaer, P De Vuyst, J Zanen, JC Yernault. Comparison of computed density and macroscopic morphometry in pulmonary emphysema. Am J Respir Crit Care Med 1995; 152:653–657.
5. NL Müller, CA Staples, RR Miller, RT Abboud. ''Density mask'': An objective method to quantitate emphysema using computed tomography. Chest 1988; 94: 782–787.
6. K Bae, R Slone, D Gierada, R Yusen, J Cooper. Patients with emphysema: quantitative CT analysis before and after lung volume reduction surgery–work in progress. Radiology 1997; 203:705–714.
7. RM Slone, DS Gierada. Radiology of pulmonary emphysema and lung volume reduction surgery. Semin Thorac Cardiovasc Surg 1996; 8:61–82.
8. RM Slone, TK Pilgram, DS Gierada, et al. Lung volume reduction surgery: comparison of preoperative radiologic features and clinical outcome [see comments]. Radiology 1997; 204:685–693.
9. DS Gierada, RM Slone, KT Bae, RD Yusen, SS Lefrak, JD Cooper. Pulmonary emphysema: comparison of preoperative quantitative CT and physiologic index values with clinical outcome after lung-volume reduction surgery. Radiology 1997; 205:235–242.
10. K Suga, K Nishigauchi, N Matsunaga, et al. Three-dimensional surface displays of perfusion SPECT in the evaluation of patients with pulmonary emphysema for thoracoscopic lung volume reduction surgery. Nucl Med Commun 1997; 18: 719–727.
11. K Suga, K Nishigauchi, N Matsunaga, et al. Preliminary application of dynamic pulmonary xenon-133 single-photon emission tomography in the evaluation of patients with pulmonary emphysema for thoracoscopic lung volume reduction surgery. Eur J Nucl Med 1998; 25:410–416.
12. K Sugi, T Matsuoka, T Tanaka, et al. Lung volume reduction surgery for pulmonary emphysema using dynamic Xenon-133 and Tc-99m-MAA SPECT images. Ann Thorac Cardiovasc Surg 1998; 4:149–153.
13. KR Flaherty, EA Kazerooni, JL Curtis, et al. Emphysema gradient and the severity of hyperinflation predict outcome after bilateral lung volume reduction surgery for emphysema. Chest 2001; 119:1337–1346.
14. A Dirksen, JH Dijkman, F Madsen, et al. A randomized clinical trial of alpha(1)-antitrypsin augmentation therapy. Am J Respir Crit Care Med 1999; 160:1468–1472.
15. HO Coxson, RM Rogers, KP Whittall, et al. A quantification of the lung surface area in emphysema using computed tomography. Am J Respir Crit Care Med 1999; 159:851–856.
16. M Mishima, H Itoh, H Sakai, et al. Optimized scanning conditions of high resolu-

tion CT in the follow-up of pulmonary emphysema. J Comput Assist Tomogr 1999; 23:380–384.
17. TL Petty, GG Weinmann. Building a national strategy for the prevention and managament of and research in chronic obstructive pulmonary disease. National Heart, Lung and Blood Institute Workshop Summary. Bethesda, Maryland, August 29–31, 1995. J Am Med Assoc 1997; 277:246–253.
18. AT Society. Standards for the diagnosis and care of patients with chronic obstructive pulmonary disease. Am J Respir Crit Care Med 1995; 152:S77–S121.
19. R Senior, N Anthonisen. Chronic obstructive pulmonary diseae (COPD). Am J Respir Crit Care Med 1998; 157:S139–S147.
20. P Pratt. Emphysema and chronic airways disease. In: D Dail, S Hammar, eds. Pulmonary Pathology. New York: Springer-Verlag, 1988, pp 654–659.
21. C Bergin, N Müller, DM Nichols, et al. The diagnosis of emphysema: A computed tomographic-pathologic correlation. Am Rev Respir Dis 1986; 133:541–546.
22. RR Miller, NL Müller, S Vedal, NJ Morrison, CA Staples. Limitations of computed tomography in the assessment of emphysema. Am Rev Respir Dis 1989; 139:980–983.
23. M Tanino, M Nishimura, T Betsuyaku, et al. [A comparative study of computed tomographic techniques for the detection of emphysema in middle-aged and older patient populations]. Nihon Kokyuki Gakkai Zasshi 2000; 38:368–372.
24. WR Webb. Radiology of obstructive pulmonary disease. Am J Roentgenol 1997; 169:637–647.
25. Remy-Jardin M, J Remy, B Gosselin, MC Copin, A Wurtz, A Duhamel. Sliding thin slab, minimum intensity projection technique in the diagnosis of emphysema: histopathologic–CT correlation. Radiology 1996; 200:665–671.
26. RH Hruban, MA Meziane, EA Zerhouni, et al. High resolution computed tomography of inflation-fixed lungs: pathologic–radiologic correlation of centrilobular emphysema. Am Rev Respir Dis 1987; 136:935–940.
27. D Spouge, JR Mayo, W Cardoso, NL Müller. Panacinar emphysema: CT and pathologic findings. J Comput Assist Tomogr 1993; 17:710–713.
28. PA Gevenois, JC Yernault. Can computed tomography quantify pulmonary emphysema? Eur Respir J 1995; 8:843–848.
29. PA Gevenois, J Zanen, V de Maertelaer, P De Vuyst, P Dumortier, JC Yernault. Macroscopic assessment of pulmonary emphysema by image analysis. J Clin Pathol 1995; 48:318–322.
30. PA Gevenois, P De Vuyst, M Sy, et al. Pulmonary emphysema: quantitative CT during expiration. Radiology 1996; 199:825–829.
31. F Sakai, G Gamsu, JG Im, CS Ray. Pulmonary function abnormalities in patients with CT-determined emphysema. J Comput Assist Tomogr 1987; 11:963–968.
32. N Sakai, M Mishima, K Nishimura, H Itoh, K Kuno. An automated method to assess the distribution of low attenuation areas on chest CT scans in chronic pulmonary emphysema patients. Chest 1994; 106:1319–1325.

33. C Sanders, PH Nath, WC Bailey. Detection of emphysema with computed tomography. Correlation with pulmonary function tests and chest radiography. Invest Radiol 1988; 23:262–266.
34. WL Foster, Jr, PC Pratt, VL Roggli, JD Godwin, RA Halvorsen, Jr, CE Putman. Centrilobular emphysema: CT-pathologic correlation. Radiology 1986; 159:27–32.
35. K Nishimura, K Murata, M Yamagishi, et al. Comparison of different computed tomography scanning methods for quantifying emphysema. J Thoracic Imaging 1998; 13:193–198.
36. NL Müller, WM Thurlbeck. Thin-section CT, emphysema, air trapping, and airway obstruction [editorial; comment]. Radiology 1996; 199:621–622.
37. K Kuwano, K Matsuba, T Ikeda, et al. The diagnosis of mild emphysema: correlation of computed tomography and pathology scores. Am Rev Respir Dis 1990; 141:169–178.
38. WM Thurlbeck, MS Dunnill, W Hartung, BE Heard, AG Hepplestn, RC Ryder. A comparison of three methods of measuring emphysema. Human Pathol 1972; 1:215–226.
39. M Mishima, T Hirai, Z Jin, et al. Standardization of low attenuation area versus total lung area in chest X-ray CT as an indicator of chronic pulmonary emphysema. Front Med Biol Eng 1997; 8:79–86.
40. RJ Lamers, GJ Kemerink, M Drent, van JM Engelshoven. Reproducibility of spirometrically controlled CT lung densitometry in a clinical setting. Eur Respir J 1998; 11:942–945.
41. EA Kazerooni, RI Whyte, A Flint, FJ Martinez. Imaging of emphysema and lung volume reduction surgery. Radiographics 1997; 17:1023–1036.
42. KJ Park, CJ Bergin, JL Clausen. Quantitation of emphysema with three-dimensional CT densitometry: comparison with two-dimensional analysis, visual emphysema scores, and pulmonary function test results. Radiology 1999; 211:541–547.
43. HU Kauczor, CP Heussel, B Fischer, R Klamm, P Mildenberger, M Thelen. Assessment of lung volumes using helical CT at inspiration and expiration: comparison with pulmonary function tests. Am J. Roentgenol 1998; 171:1091–1095.
44. R Uppaluri, T Mitsa, M Sonka, EA Hoffman, G McLennan. Quantification of pulmonary emphysema from lung computed tomography images. Am J Respir Crit Care Med 1997; 156:248–254.
45. EA Hoffman, G McLennan. Assessment of the pulmonary structure-function relationship and clinical outcomes measures: quantitative volumetric CT of the lung. Acad Radiol 1997; 4:758–776.
46. NJ Morrison, R Abboud, F Ramadan, et al. Comparison of single breath carbon monoxide diffusing capacity and pressure–volume curves in detecting emphysema. Am Rev Respir Dis 1989; 139:1179–1187.
47. NJ Morrison, RT Abboud, Müller NL, et al. Pulmonary capillary blood volume in emphysema. Am Rev Respir Dis 1990; 141:53–61.
48. AF Gelb, M Schein, J Kuei, et al. Limited contribution of emphysema in ad-

vanced chronic obstructive pulmonary disease. Am Rev Respir Dis 1993; 147: 1157–1161.
49. AF Gelb, JC Hogg, NL Muller, et al. Contribution of emphysema and small airways in COPD. Chest 1996; 109:353–359.
50. S Eda, K Kubo, K Fujimoto, Y Matsuzawa, M Sekiguchi, Sakai F. The relations between expiratory chest CT using helical CT and pulmonary function tests in emphysema. Am J Respir Crit Care Med 1997; 155:1290–1294.
51. M Haraguchi, S Shimura, W Hida, K Shirato. Pulmonary function and regional distribution of emphysema as determined by high-resolution computed tomography. Respiration 1998; 65:125–129.
52. Y Nakano, H Sakai, S Muro, et al. Comparison of low attenuation areas on computed tomographic scans between inner and outer segments of the lung in patients with chronic obstructive pulmonary disease: incidence and contribution to lung function. Thorax 1999; 54:384–389.
53. W Wisser, W Klepetko, M Kontrus, et al. Morphologic grading of the emphysematous lung and its relation to improvement after lung volume reduction surgery. Ann Thorac Surg 1998; 65:793–799.
54. W Weder, R Thurnheer, U Stammberger, M Burge, EW Russi, KE Bloch. Radiologic emphysema morphology is associated with outcome after surgical lung volume reduction. Ann Thorac Surg 1997; 64:313–319; discussion 319–320.
55. R Thurnheer, E Hermann, W Weder, et al. Role of lung perfusion scintigraphy in relation to chest computed tomography and pulmonary function in the evaluation of candidates for lung volume reduction surgery. Am J Respir Crit Care Med 1999; 159:301–310.
56. MD Becker, YM Berkmen, JH Austin, et al. Lung volumes before and after lung volume reduction surgery: quantitative CT analysis. Am J Respir Crit Care Med 1998; 157:1593–1599.
57. E Kazerooni, F Martinez, L Quint, R Whyte. Quantitative helical CT indices of emphysema as predictors of outcome after lung volume reduction surgery. Radiology 1996; 201(P):298.
58. E Pompeo, G Sergiacomi, I Nofroni, W Roscetti, G Simonetti, TC Mineo. Morphologic grading of emphysema is useful in the selection of candidates for unilateral or bilateral reduction pneumoplasty. European Journal of Cardio-Thorac Surg 2000; 17:680–686.
59. WM Thurlbeck, NL Müller. Emphysema: definition, imaging, and quantification. Am J Roentgenol 1994; 163:1017–1025.
60. EA Kazerooni, JL Curtis, R Paine, MD Iannettoni, P Lewis, FJ Martinez. Long-term outcome after bilateral apical lung volume reduction surgery (LVRS) via median sternotomy: predictive value of quantitative helical CT analysis (QCT) and physiologic severity of hyperinflation. Radiology 1998; 209(P):257.
61. A Rozenshtein, CS White, JH Austin, BM Romney, Z Protopapas, MJ Krasna. Incidental lung carcinoma detected at CT in patients selected for lung volume reduction surgery to treat severe pulmonary emphysema. Radiology 1998; 207: 487–490.

62. EA Kazerooni, LC Chow, RI Whyte, FJ Martinez, JP Lynch. Preoperative examination of lung transplant candidates: value of chest CT compared with chest radiography. AJR Am J Roentgenol 1995; 165:1343–1348.
63. R Slone, D Gierada, T Lopes. Unsuspected bronchogenic carcinoma in patients with severe pulmonary emphysema being evaluated for lung volume reduction surgery. AJR 1997; 168(A):112.
64. S Adusumilli, E Kazerooni, T Ojo. Screening CT for lung cancer: a study of emphysema patients being evaluated for lung volume reduction surgery. Radiology 1998; 209(P):222–223.
65. RJ McKenna, Jr., RJ Fischel, M Brenner, AF Gelb. Combined operations for lung volume reduction surgery and lung cancer. Chest 1996; 110:885–888.
66. TC Ojo, F Martinez, R Paine, 3rd et al. Lung volume reduction surgery alters management of pulmonary nodules in patients with severe COPD. Chest 1997; 112:1494–1500.

11
Hyperpolarized Gas-Enhanced Magnetic Resonance Imaging of the Lung

Holman Page McAdams
Duke University Medical Center
Durham, North Carolina

Lane F. Donnelly
University of Cincinnati and
Children's Hospital Medical Center
Cincinnati, Ohio

James R. MacFall
Duke University Medical Center
Durham, North Carolina

I. INTRODUCTION

The role of conventional hydrogen magnetic resonance imaging (MRI) for evaluation of the lung parenchyma remains limited, despite advances in instrumentation and pulse-sequence design [1–4]. This is because (1) the concentration of hydrogen protons in lung tissue is low, (2) only a small fraction of these hydrogen protons becomes polarized when an external magnetic field is applied, (3) local magnetic-field gradients around the air-filled alveoli rapidly dephase transverse magnetization (magnetic susceptibility), and (4) respiratory and cardiac motion can result in significant artifacts that obscure the lung parenchyma [1–3,5]. To overcome these difficulties, novel techniques for MRI of pulmonary parenchyma have been proposed, including hyperpolarized gas [6] and 100% molecular oxygen enhanced [7] MRI. Early results with these techniques have been promising. This chapter reviews the basic principles of, and preliminary results with, hyperpolarized gas-enhanced MRI of the lungs.

II. BASIC PRINCIPLES

Previous work has shown that the noble gases Helium-3 (^{3}He) and Xenon-129 (^{129}Xe-129) can be polarized using high-intensity laser illumination. This process results in an increased MR signal that is five orders of magnitude greater than thermal equilibrium [6,8–12]. When a conventional MR imaging system is tuned to the resonant frequency of the hyperpolarized gas, high signal can be imaged within the airspaces after inhalation of the agent. Because the signal is generated by the gas and is not related to T1 recovery time, very short repetition times (TRs) can be used, and complete sets of lung images can be generated in a short breath hold [10].

A. The Gases

Helium-3 and Xenon-129 are the noble gases most commonly used in hyperpolarized gas-enhanced MR imaging experiments. Both isotopes have an unpaired electron and have important advantages and disadvantages for MR imaging.

Helium is a nontoxic gas that can be inhaled in high concentrations when mixed with oxygen (80% helium/20% oxygen) without adverse effects on tissue oxygenation [13]. Because helium is insoluble in blood, adverse systemic effects do not occur. Unfortunately, the natural abundance of ^{3}He is negligible, so the only available source of ^{3}He is from tritium decay. Thus, the overall supply of the gas is quite limited and consequently, the gas is quite expensive. If hyperpolarized ^{3}He proves to be useful for medical imaging, gas recovery after use will probably be required.

Xenon-129 is naturally abundant as a mixture (26%) with other xenon isotopes and is therefore relatively inexpensive, compared to ^{3}He. Unlike helium, xenon is soluble in blood and is lipophilic. Its solubility and lipophilia account, in part, for its anesthetic effects following inhalation in high concentration (30% xenon). As a pulmonary MR imaging agent, ^{129}Xe has several disadvantages when compared to ^{3}He. First, ^{129}Xe has a lower gyromagnetic ratio than ^{3}He, which results in a decreased signal compared to ^{3}He (approximately three times less). Second, the levels of polarization of ^{129}Xe, thus far, have not been as high as those achieved with ^{3}He. Thus, the signal-to-noise ratio for imaging with ^{129}Xe is considerably less than that for imaging with ^{3}He for a similar quantity of inhaled gas. Third, because the ^{129}Xe atom is larger and heavier than the ^{3}He atom, ^{129}Xe may not distribute homogeneously but might preferentially accumulate in dependent portions of lung.

Although hyperpolarized ^{3}He, at this point, appears to be a better agent for pulmonary imaging than ^{129}Xe, the latter gas has some attractive features for nonpulmonary imaging. Because xenon is rapidly absorbed into blood, it may be useful as an agent for quantifying blood flow, both within the lungs and elsewhere in the body. In particular, it may be useful for measuring cerebral perfusion. And, because its resonant frequency is changed (chemical-shift effect) when it is absorbed into blood, it may be possible to separate gas and blood fractions in vivo, leading to novel methods of quantification. Using spectroscopic methods, hyperpolarized ^{129}Xe may prove useful as a noninvasive probe for measuring tissue and blood oxygenation [14].

For these reasons, most early investigators have used ^{3}He for pulmonary MR imaging experiments, although experience with ^{129}Xe enhanced MR imaging is growing [6,12,15,16]. The authors' experience in human imaging has been with ^{3}He, and most of the following discussion focuses on this agent.

B. Oxygen Effects

The paramagnetic effects of oxygen shorten the T1 relaxation time of hyperpolarized ^{3}He. This potentially results in rapid loss of signal in areas of lung with high oxygen concentration and raises concerns regarding coadministration of oxygen and hyperpolarized gas (see ''Safety Issues'' below). Some investigators have advocated prerinsing the lungs with either the noble gas or nitrogen to decrease this effect. However, as noted below, such techniques may result in potentially dangerous arterial desaturation. Although the T1 shortening effect of oxygen can result in substantial loss of ^{3}He signal in vitro, it is not clear that this is a significant problem in vivo. For instance, Hedlund and colleagues found that mixing inhaled hyperpolarized ^{3}He with equal parts of 100% oxygen, administered by ventilator to anesthetized rats, resulted in only a net 5% signal loss [17].

On the other hand, the T1 shortening effect of oxygen can also be used to some advantage. For instance, because the T1 of ^{3}He decreases in proportion to oxygen concentration in vitro, the loss of signal can be used to noninvasively measure local oxygen concentrations [18]. This technique could be very useful for mapping local oxygen partial pressures (an indirect indicator of pulmonary perfusion) in patients with various lung diseases [19].

C. Gas Polarization

Currently, there are two principal techniques for polarizing ^{3}He and ^{129}Xe: spin exchange and metastability exchange. The technical aspects of these techniques are beyond the scope of this article and are only summarized here. Further discussion can be found in a recent review [13]. Common to both techniques is the use of circularly polarized laser light to polarize a mixture of noble gas and either an alkali metal vapor (spin exchange) or metastable atoms (metastability exchange). In the spin-exchange technique, rubidium atoms are polarized and used to transfer their polarization to the noble gas (either ^{3}He or ^{129}Xe) by a process known as *collisional spin exchange* (Fig. 1). In the metastability-exchange technique, a layer of metastable ^{3}He atoms is created by laser illumination and used to polarize the remaining ^{3}He atoms by collisional spin exchange. The metastability-exchange technique has, thus far, only been successfully used to polarize ^{3}He.

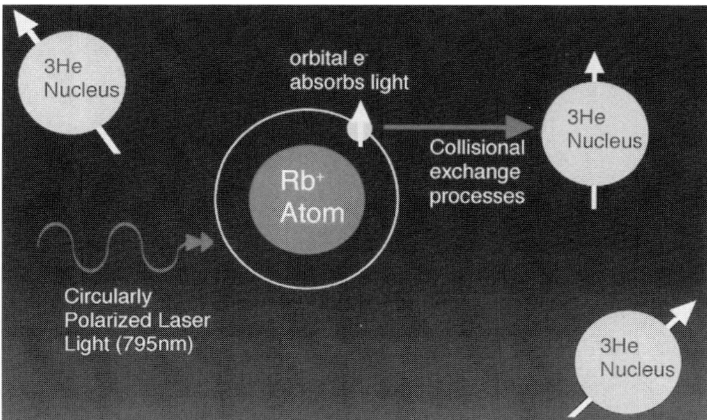

Figure 1 Hyperpolarization of ^{3}He by laser irradiation and collisional spin exchange with rubidium atoms. (From Ref. 63.)

Each technique has important advantages and disadvantages for hyperpolarized gas production. The spin-exchange technique uses commercially available laser diode arrays and can be used to polarize either ^{3}He or ^{129}Xe. A relatively compact spin-exchange polarizer is now commercially available and can produce up to 2.0 L of ^{3}He at a polarization level of 25% in approximately 6 to 8 hr. Higher polarization levels for ^{3}He (in excess of 50%) should soon be attainable with the spin-exchange technique in the near future. Polarization levels for ^{129}Xe using the spin-exchange technique are typically lower, between 4 and 10%, but with technological advances, polarization levels may be increased to the 40% range.

The metastability exchange technique requires a specialized laser to optically pump ^{3}He—a laser not yet commercially available. This technique also requires pressurization of the gas, which, in the past, required a fairly large compression chamber. However, a more compact metastability exchange polarizer has been recently developed [20]. An important advantage of the metastability exchange technique is that it can produce larger quantities of gas at higher levels of polarization and at a faster rate than can be produced with the spin-exchange technique. An important disadvantage of this technique is that it cannot be used to polarize ^{129}Xe.

III. MAGNETIC RESONANCE INSTRUMENTATION AND IMAGING TECHNIQUES

There are numerous differences between MR imaging with hyperpolarized gases and conventional MR imaging of hydrogen protons. First, the MR imaging instrument must be equipped with a broadband radiofrequency (RF) system and a special-purpose RF coil tuned to the appropriate frequencies for imaging ^{1}H, ^{3}He or ^{129}Xe. Most MR spectroscopy equipment works well for this purpose. Second, because the gas is polarized outside the magnet, the level of polarization is independent of field strength. Thus, although most investigators have used 1.5-T magnets, it may be possible to image these gases with lower field strength systems. Third, because there is no recoverable polarization, there is no need to consider T1 recovery in pulse-sequence design. Thus, very short TRs can be used to image the lungs in a short breath hold. Fourth, magnetization of the gas decreases irreversibly during imaging. In fact, a single excitation pulse destroys all gas polarization. Automatic calibration protocols, therefore, cannot be used, and multiple sequences of images cannot be obtained during the same inhalation.

For these reasons, most investigators have used gradient-echo sequences with low flip angles and short echo and repetition times to image the gas during a single breath hold. These techniques result in a set of static images that depict gas distribution immediately after inhalation. Dynamic, functional images that depict gas distribution throughout the respiratory cycle can also be obtained at a single level using such techniques. Echo-planar imaging sequences [21,22] or ultrafast gradient-echo sequences [23] may eventually prove useful for dynamic imaging at multiple levels.

We typically image hyperpolarized ^{3}He with a 1.5-T scanner (Signa, revision 5.6, GE Medical Systems, Milwaukee, WI) equipped with a broadband receiver and a specially designed transmit-receive torso surface coil (26 cm long). After positioning the patient in the magnet, fast spin-echo proton MR images of the thorax are obtained in the coronal plane using the following parameters: TR of 3000 ms, TE of 80 ms, 6-mm section thickness, 2-mm gap, 128 × 256 matrix, 32-cm field of view, one signal acquired, and respiratory gating. Following completion of these images, the machine is readjusted for ^{3}He imaging. After the ^{3}He is polarized, it is placed in a plastic bag with an attached tube and an on/off valve. The patient is instructed to inhale the gas and hold his or her breath. Gradient echo images are then obtained in the coronal plane using a TR of 9.5 ms, TE of 3.0 ms, an 8° flip angle, 6-mm section thickness, 2-mm gap, 128 × 256 matrix, 32-cm field of view, one signal acquired. Respiratory and pulse rates, blood pressure, and blood oxygenation levels by pulse oximetry are monitored. Using this technique, a complete set of coronal images is acquired in 12 to 14 sec.

A. Gas Delivery and Dosing

Methods for delivery of gas to the MR imaging instrument have not been systematically investigated. In our work, we have used a 1.0-L plastic bag with an attached tube and on/off valve to deliver the gas without significant loss of polarization. This rather simple technique works well because we image patients once during a single breath hold, as have most previous human studies. Studies in anesthetized animals, however, are often performed using either continuous or intermittent gas inhalation, requiring the use of specially designed ventilator systems for gas delivery [17,24,25].

The optimal dose of hyperpolarized gas is also not standardized. Doses administered to patients have ranged on 300 cc [26] to 2.0 L [27]. The optimal dose likely depends on a number of factors, including clinical indication and gas polarization level. For instance, patients with asthma may require less gas for adequate evaluation of the lungs than do patients with severe emphysema. And, as gas polarization levels increase, the total amount of inhaled gas needed to produce high-quality MR images decreases.

Clearly, if hyperpolarized gas-enhanced MR imaging of the lungs proves to be an economically viable and clinically useful tool, more standardized dosing and gas delivery techniques will need to be developed.

B. Safety Issues

Studies in patients have thus far suggested that inhalation of up to 2.0 L of ^{3}He is well tolerated and does not cause a significant reduction in blood oxygenation. However, a recent animal study has raised some concerns in this regard. In this study, Ramirez and colleagues evaluated the effects of various gas administration protocols on arterial oxygen saturation in anesthetized, ventilated rats [25]. They found that alternate breath protocols (alternating pure oxygen and noble gas) and single-breath-hold protocols of up to 25 sec did not cause significant decreases in arterial oxygen saturation. However, breath-hold protocols longer than 30 sec, continuous breathing of noble gas, or breath holds of 10 sec or more after a double prerinse (two inspirations of pure noble gas prior to inhalation of the hyperpolarized gas) resulted in deleterious effects on arterial saturation (reduced below 90%). While it is unlikely that patients will be imaged during mechanical ventilation with pure noble gas or even alternating noble gas with oxygen protocols, prerinsing has been advocated to decrease signal loss due to the paramagnetic effects of oxygen (see above). This study suggests, however, that such a technique could well be dangerous, particularly when used with a breath hold of longer than 10 sec and in individuals with impaired pulmonary function.

C. Quantitative Measurements

Hyperpolarized gas-enhanced MR imaging has opened the door for various new quantitative measurements of lung function. As noted above, when a controlled amount of polarized ^{3}He gas is administered at known levels of polarization, it is possible to compute maps of local oxygen concentration [18]. Also as noted above, it may eventually be possible to measure blood and tissue oxygenation using polarized ^{129}Xe and spectroscopy methods [14]. Because both ^{3}He and ^{129}Xe have relatively high coefficients of diffusion, these compounds may be suitable for diffusion-weighted imaging techniques. Since in vivo diffusion is restricted by the size of airways and airspaces, such techniques may allow computation of the size of peripheral airways and airspaces.

Diffusion-weighted imaging techniques could thus prove useful for detection of abnormalities that increase the size of alveoli, such as early emphysema [19].

D. Animal Studies

An extensive body of literature is accumulating regarding animal studies with hyperpolarized gases. Most of these investigations have been concerned with (1) development of improved techniques for MR imaging and gas delivery [9,17,24,28–33], (2) safety issues [25], and (3) improved depiction of fine anatomic details. More recently, however, investigators are beginning to use these techniques in animal models of various pulmonary diseases such as emphysema and pulmonary embolism [34,35]. The following is a limited sampling of current work in this regard.

Shattuck and colleagues used hyperpolarized ^{3}He to produce isotropic three-dimensional MR images of lung in live laboratory animals at a spatial resolution of 0.013 mm^{3} [32]. Viallon and colleagues developed techniques to produce functional magnetic resonance images of the lung in small animals at microscopic resolution using hyperpolarized ^{3}He [33]. These investigators, using spiral scan techniques, obtained a dynamic series (up to 40 images) of high-resolution ^{3}He ventilation images in small animals using a single gas bolus [36]. Moller and colleagues recently demonstrated the feasibility of three-dimensional magnetic resonance imaging of the guinea pig lung using hyperpolarized (HP) noble gases. They obtained high-quality images at a voxel size of 17 μL using ^{3}He; airway structures down to the fifth or sixth generation were demonstrated (Fig. 2). Using ^{129}Xe, the same investigators imaged guinea pig lungs with a voxel size of 40 μL. They concluded on the basis of their studies that in vivo visualization of alveolar clusters distal to respiratory bronchioles may be possible in guinea pig lungs using hyperpolarized gas MR microscopy of the lungs [31].

Chen and colleagues, in a series of ^{3}He experiments with guinea pigs, showed that larger flip angles (50–90°) destroy magnetization before it reaches the smaller airways. However, when moderate angles (20–40°) were used, airway branching down to the fourth and fifth orders were seen [9]. This work suggests that selective airway imaging with hyperpolarized gases may be feasible.

Cremillieux and colleagues showed that combined magnetic resonance lung ventilation and perfusion imaging was feasible in rat lungs [35]. They used hyperpolarized ^{3}He to assess ventilation and then performed proton MR imaging after contrast agent injection to assess pulmonary perfusion in an experimental rat model of pulmonary embolism.

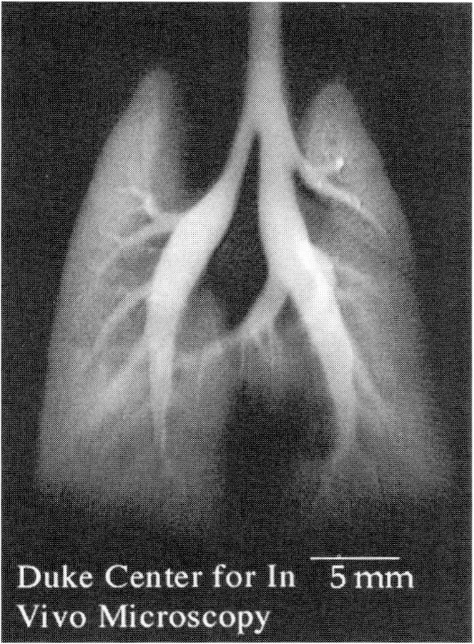

Figure 2 Projection-encoded MR image of a live Fisher 344 rat obtained during a single breath hold of hyperpolarized ^{3}He. In-plane resolution is ~120μ. Note visualization of distal airways and fine structure of lung. (Courtesy of G. Allan Johnson, and Duke Center for In Vivo Microscopy, Durham, North Carolina.)

Chen and colleagues also investigated the ability of high-resolution hyperpolarized ^{3}He MR imaging to diagnose early changes of emphysema in an animal model (elastase-treated rats) by measuring the apparent diffusion coefficient (ADC) of the gas following inhalation. Their data showed that the ADC was significantly larger in elastase-treated rats, indicating alveolar expansion—findings confirmed at histologic examination. These results suggest that measurement of the ADC of hyperpolarized ^{3}He could be a valuable research tool and has potential application in the evaluation of early emphysema [34].

E. Human Studies

Compared with conventional scintigraphic techniques for imaging pulmonary ventilation, hyperpolarized ^{3}He-enhanced MR imaging offers several advantages: increased spatial resolution, ability to perform cross-sectional imaging, postprocessing capabilities (including three-dimensional analysis and quantification), and absence of ionizing radiation [13]. Most work with hyperpolarized gas-enhanced MR imaging has involved patients with parenchymal lung diseases that affect ventilation, including cystic fibrosis (CF) [37], bronchiolitis obliterans syndrome (BOS) [38], and emphysema [27,39,40].

Imaging of Normal Volunteers

Our experience imaging normal human volunteers (Fig. 3) with hyperpolarized ^{3}He has shown the following:

1. Polarization is not delicate; the gas can be hand-carried over a long pathway to the imaging system.
2. Imaging is easily completed in a reasonable breath hold.
3. Very good images are achieved by inhalation of 0.75 to 1.0 L of ^{3}He at 5 to 15% polarization (Fig. 1).
4. Helium-3 rapidly distributes to all regions of healthy lung (Fig. 1).
5. Helium-3 is restricted to the air spaces and does not penetrate the pleura, trachea, or mediastinum or into the blood vessels (Fig. 1).
6. Helium-3-enhanced MR images are remarkably consistent in quality and are reproducible.

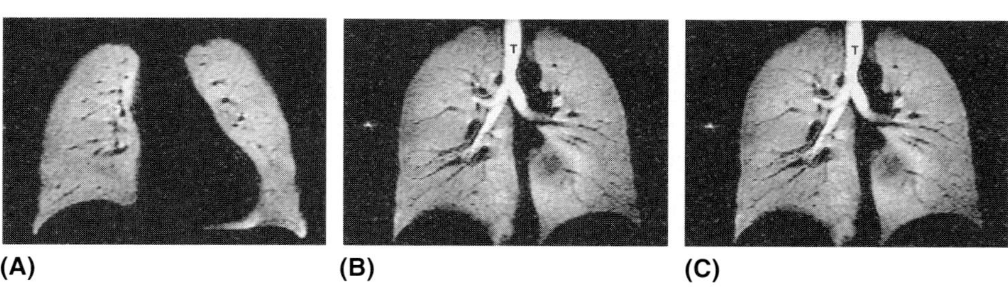

Figure 3 Hyperpolarized ^{3}He enhanced MR imaging of healthy volunteer. (A–C). Coronal ^{3}He-enhanced MR images obtained during a 15-sec breath hold, shown anterior (A) to posterior (C). Note that immediately following inhalation, gas rapidly distributes to all regions of healthy lung. Note also that the gas is restricted to airspaces and does not penetrate pleura, mediastinum, or into blood vessels. Gas is also identified within the trachea (T).

Guenther et al. imaged asymptomatic smokers and compared the results to a group of healthy controls. They demonstrated that, although there was no significant difference in forced expiratory volume in 1 sec (FEV_1) between the two groups, more ventilation defects were seen in the smoking group. These findings suggest that ^{3}He MR imaging may be a sensitive means for measuring regional airflow abnormalities in patients with early lung disease due to smoking [41].

Imaging of Lung Transplant Recipients with Bronchiolitis Obliterans Syndrome

Bronchiolitis obliterans syndrome, a manifestation of chronic rejection, is now the greatest limitation to long-term survival after lung transplantation [42–44]. The syndrome manifests histologically with dense submucosal scar tissue that partially or totally obliterates the lumen of small bronchi and bronchioles. Patients with BOS typically present with worsening dyspnea and have physiologic evidence of progressive small-airway obstruction [45,46]. Histologic diagnosis is problematic in initial stages because transbronchial biopsy is often negative until disease is quite advanced [47,48]. Thus, BOS is often diagnosed clinically and graded using the ratio of the current FEV_1, to the best posttransplant FEV_1 (FEV_1 ratio) [49]. Although thin-section CT scanning has proven useful for evaluating lung transplant recipients with advanced BOS [50–56], CT scans can be normal in patients with early disease [57,58]. Because BOS may be at least partially reversible if diagnosed and treated early, the authors are investigating the ability of hyperpolarized ^{3}He-enhanced MR imaging to diagnose BOS.

Preliminary work has shown that ventilation defects on ^{3}He-enhanced MR imaging are common in lung-transplant recipients and that these defects are more numerous and extensive in recipients with BOS than in those without BOS (Figs. 4 and 5) [38]. These data also suggest that the extent of ventilation defects correlates with severity of pulmonary dysfunction as measured by the FEV_1 ratio or by clinical BOS scores. Thus, the extent of ventilation defects seen on ^{3}He MR images may correlate with the presence and severity of BOS in lung-transplant recipients. More data are needed, however, to determine if (1) ventilation defects seen in patients without clinical BOS are indicative of early disease; (2) ^{3}He MR imaging is more sensitive than currently available diagnostic techniques such as thin-section CT scanning, transbronchial biopsy, or serial PFT evaluation; and (3) serial ^{3}He MR examinations can identify patients with BOS before significant declines in pulmonary function occur.

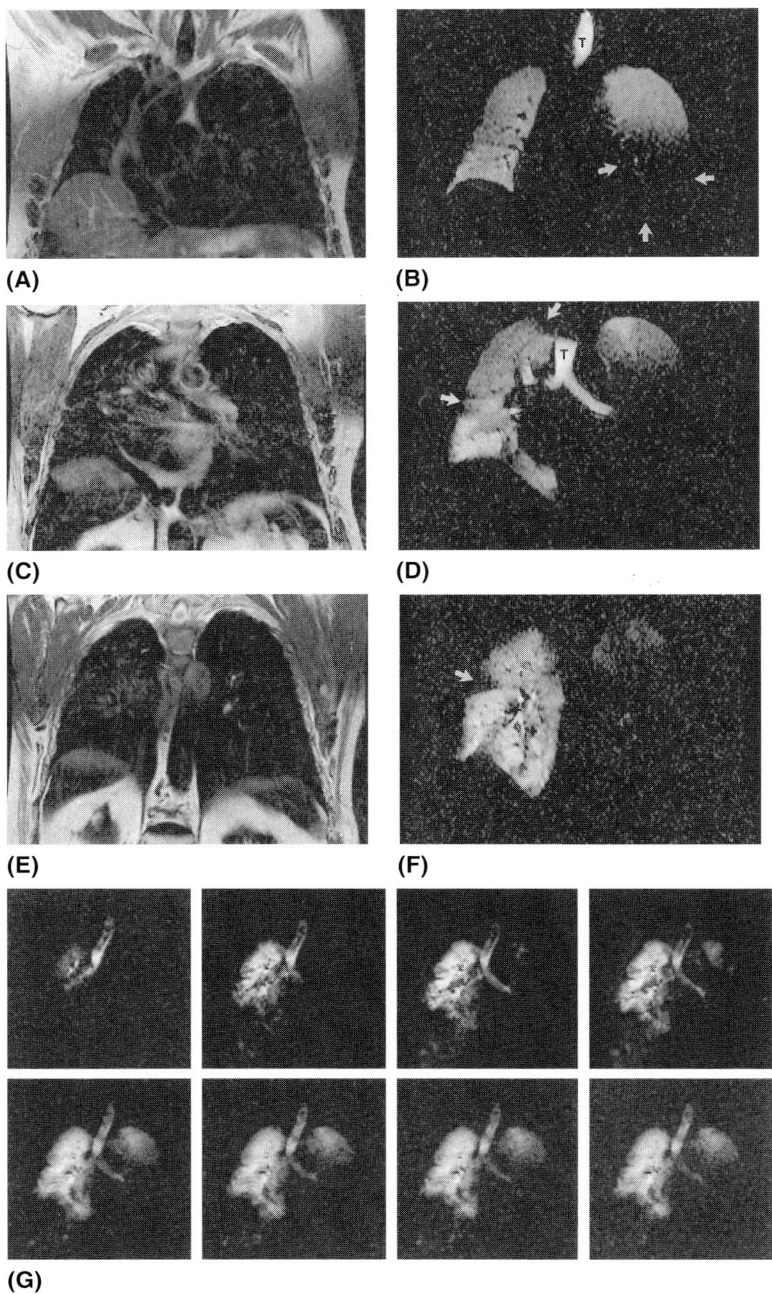
T
T
(A)
(B)
(C)
(D)
(E)
(F)
(G)

Imaging of Patients with Emphysema

Imaging of emphysema, particularly in regard to distribution and severity, has become an important clinical concern with the advent of lung-volume-reduction surgery (LVRS). Preliminary data indicate that patients with heterogeneous disease show greater improvement, both subjectively and objectively, after LVRS than do patients with diffuse, homogeneous emphysema. Imaging research has thus focused on methods to quantify and categorize emphysema in patients being considered for LVRS. Thin-section CT scanning is currently considered the single best test for assessment, although important ancillary information can be gained from radionuclide ventilation/perfusion scintigraphy. MRI with hyperpolarized gases, by showing focal or diffuse ventilation defects in patients with emphysema [19,27,39,40], may also prove to be a valuable selection tool for LVRS. The technique may also prove useful for early detection of obstructive lung diseases and emphysema.

Preliminary investigations have shown that focal ventilation defects are commonly identified in areas of lung destruction or airway obstruction (Fig. 4). In many cases, these defects are larger than the corresponding abnormalities seen on chest radiographs or CT scan [39,40,59]. It should be remembered, however, that focal regions of absent signal, although probably caused by impaired ventilation, could also be caused by other factors, including gas diffu-

Figure 4 Helium-3-enhanced MR imaging of 55-year-old man 1 year after unilateral right lung transplantation for emphysema. Patient is clinically well without significant reduction in FEV_1 (BOS-0). (A) Coronal FSE proton MR image at anterior level for reference. (B) Coronal ^{3}He-enhanced MR image obtained with 6-mm slice thickness and 2-mm gap during a 12-sec breath hold at same level as in A. Note homogeneous gas distribution in small right lung (allograft) and absence of ventilation in lower half of native emphysematous left lung (arrows). T = trachea. (C) Coronal FSE proton MR image at midthorax level for reference. (D) Coronal ^{3}He-enhanced MR image obtained at same level as in C. Note few, scattered ventilation defects in allograft (arrows) and near-complete absence of ventilation in lower two-thirds of native emphysematous left lung. T = trachea. (E) Coronal FSE proton MR image at posterior level for reference. (F) Coronal ^{3}He-enhanced MR image obtained at same level as in E. Note single wedge-shaped ventilation defect in allograft (arrow) and near-complete absence of ventilation in native emphysematous left lung. (G) Coronal ^{3}He-enhanced MR images obtained every 1 sec at single midthorax level during inhalation. Note filling of right lung (allograft) first, with few scattered peripheral ventilation defects. Note complete absence of filling of native emphysematous left lower lung and delayed filling of left upper lung.

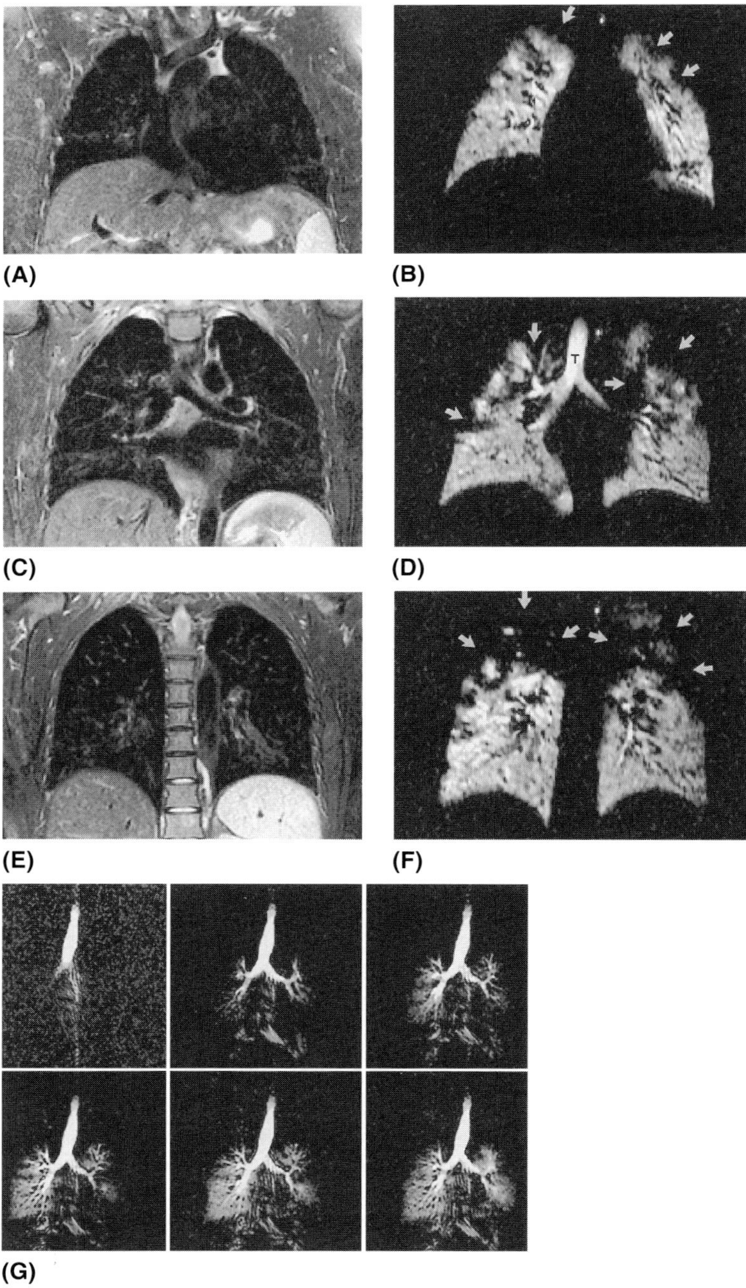
(A)
(B)
T
(C)
(D)
(E)
(F)
(G)

sion or loss of polarization due to the T1 shortening effect of oxygen. Investigators have identified two types of defects in patients with air-flow obstruction: wedge shaped and oval [27,40]. Although pathologic correlation is lacking, these investigators have suggested that the wedge-shaped defects probably indicate obstruction at the level of the distal bronchi and that oval defects indicate bronchiolar-level obstruction.

Gierada et al. [21] studied a group of patients with severe emphysema who were being evaluated for possible LVRS. They used an echo-planar sequence to dynamically image the lungs after inhalation of ^{3}He. They found delayed filling of portions of lung that were far larger than corresponding areas of emphysema on thin-section CT scans. However, because of the rapid loss of gas polarization during imaging, they were unable to image equilibrium or washout characteristics of the gas. Their data suggest that hyperpolarized gas-enhanced MR imaging, particularly with dynamic imaging, may be more sensitive to changes of early emphysema than thin-section CT.

Imaging of Patients with Cystic Fibrosis

Image-scoring systems are used clinically and as research tools to assess progression of lung disease in patients with CF [60,61]. These systems are necessary to evaluate existing and newly developed therapeutic regimens, such as gene therapy or mucolytic agents, objectively. Because CF can cause focal nonuniform lung injury, pulmonary function tests, which measure global pulmonary function, may not accurately assess patients with early CF. For this

Figure 5 Helium-3-enhanced MR imaging of 26-year-old woman 2 years after bilateral lung transplantation for cystic fibrosis. Patient complains of mild dyspnea and has moderate reduction in FEV_1 (BOS-1). (A) Coronal FSE proton MR image at anterior level for reference. (B) Coronal ^{3}He-enhanced MR image obtained with 6-mm slice thickness and 2-mm gap during a 12-sec breath hold at same level as in A. Note generally homogeneous gas distribution, with a few, scattered, peripheral ventilation defects in both lungs (arrows). (C) Coronal FSE proton MR image at midthorax level for reference. (D) Coronal ^{3}He enhanced MR image obtained at same level as in C. Note increasing size and number of ventilation defects (arrows). T = trachea. (E) Coronal FSE proton MR image at posterior level for reference. (F) Coronal ^{3}He-enhanced MR image obtained at same level as in E. Note near-complete absence of ventilation in upper lung zones (arrows). (G) Coronal ^{3}He-enhanced MR images obtained every 1 sec at single midthorax level during inhalation. Note delayed filling of left lung compared to right as well as peripheral ventilation defects in upper lungs.

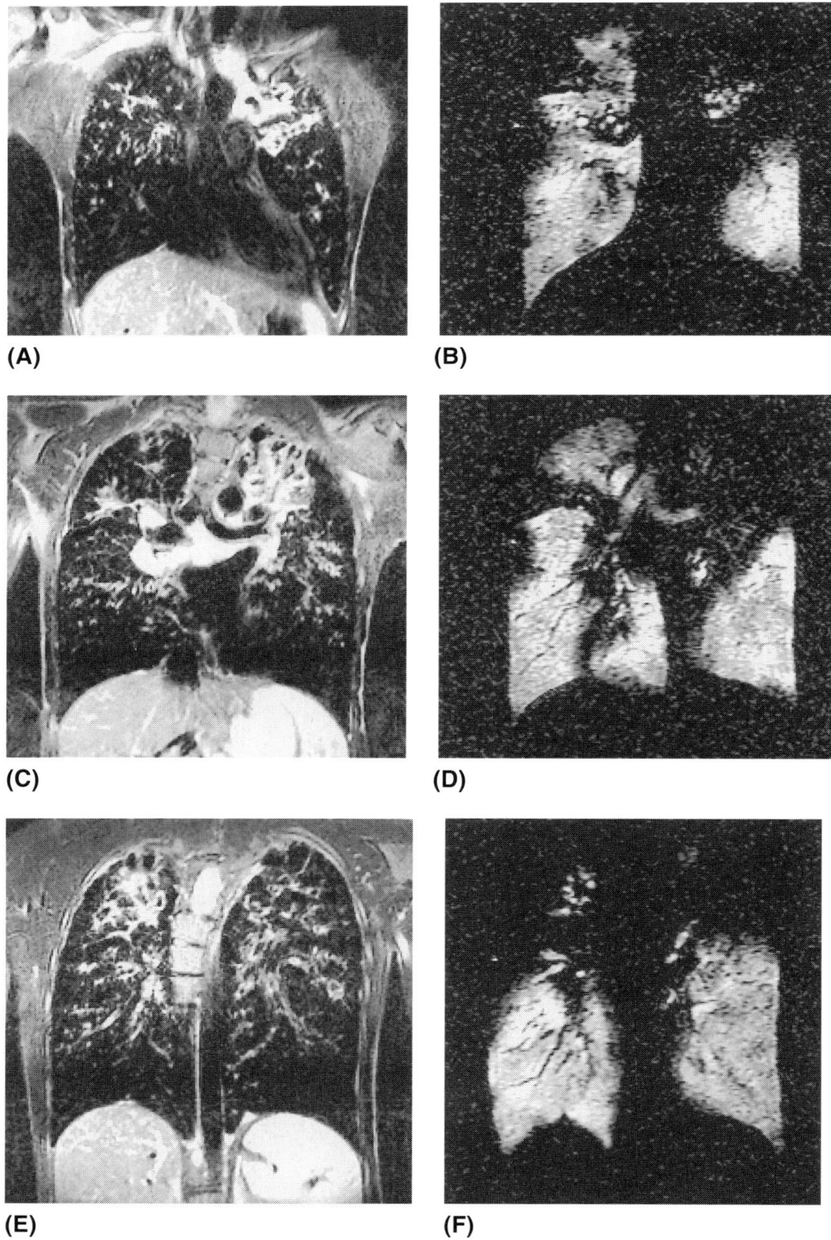
(A)
(B)
(C)
(D)
(E)
(F)

reason, scoring systems that monitor disease progression using chest radiography or thin-section CT scanning have been developed and applied. There is also concern, however, that chest radiographs or thin-section CT scanning may not accurately detect early disease [62]. Detection of early lung changes in CF is critical because many protocols evaluating new therapies involve young children with minimal or no lung disease. Thus, the optimal imaging modality for grading disease progression in CF patients should provide both morphologic and functional information, should be very sensitive for early disease, and, because serial examinations are required, should minimize or eliminate radiation exposure.

Preliminary work in patients with CF has shown that multiple areas of absent lung ventilation may be seen on ^{3}He-enhanced MR images (Figs. 6 and 7) [37]. These areas of absent ventilation range from wedge-shaped peripheral defects to entire lung zones. Combined scores based on the ventilation defects seen on ^{3}He MR images and the morphologic changes (bronchiectasis, mucus plugging, and peribronchial thickening) seen on proton MR images correlate well with clinical and radiographic assessments of disease severity. The severity of ventilation defects on ^{3}He MR images is often much greater than would have been predicted based upon the morphologic changes seen on proton MR images. This finding suggests that ^{3}He ventilation imaging may be more sensitive to the early changes of CF and may show abnormalities before morphologic changes are seen on chest radiographs or thin-section CT scans. Although these preliminary results are encouraging, further investigation in young patients with CF and minimal lung disease is necessary.

Figure 6 Helium-3-enhanced MR imaging of 20-year-old man with cystic fibrosis. (A) Coronal FSE proton MR image at anterior level for reference. Note morphologic changes of upper lobe bronchiectasis and mucoid impaction as well as left upper lobe volume loss. (B) Coronal ^{3}He-enhanced MR image obtained with 6-mm slice thickness and 2-mm gap during a 12-sec breath hold at same level as in A. Note multiple upper lobe ventilation defects corresponding to morphologic changes seen in A. (C) Coronal FSE proton MR image at midthorax level for reference. Note similar morphologic changes as seen in A as well as extensive mediastinal adenopathy. (D) Coronal ^{3}He-enhanced MR image obtained at same level as in C shows corresponding ventilation defects. (E) Coronal FSE proton MR image at posterior level for reference. Note extensive bronchiectasis. (F) Coronal ^{3}He-enhanced MR image obtained at same level as in E shows corresponding ventilation defects.

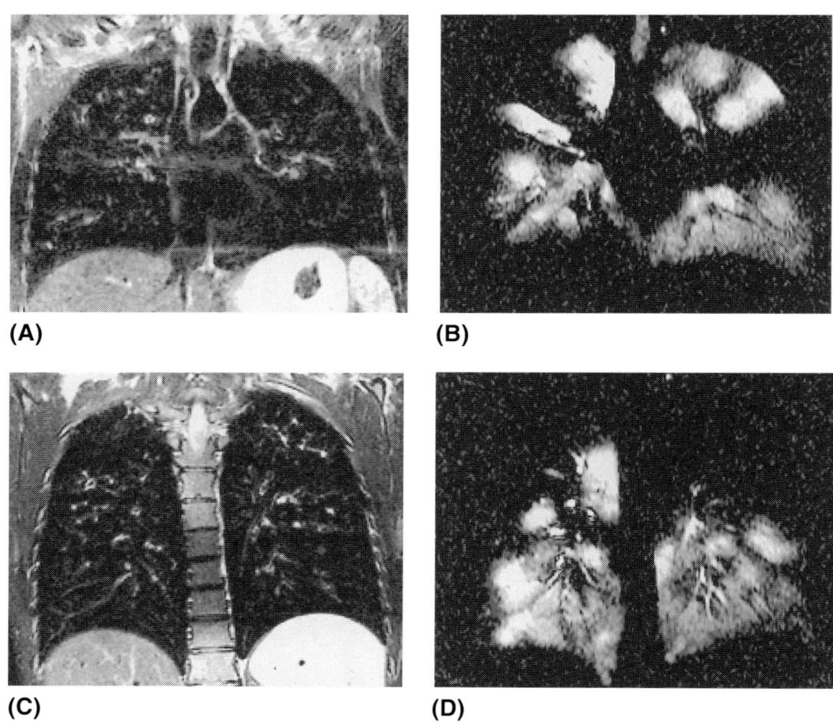

Figure 7 Helium-3-enhanced MR imaging of 19-year-old woman with cystic fibrosis. (A) Coronal FSE proton MR image at midthorax level for reference. Note morphologic changes of upper lobe bronchiectasis and mucoid impaction. (B) Coronal ^{3}He-enhanced MR image obtained with 6-mm slice thickness and 2-mm gap during a 12-sec breath hold at same level as in A. Note multiple large ventilation defects that are more extensive than would be expected based on morphologic abnomalities seen in A. (C) Coronal FSE proton MR image at posterior level for reference. Note morphologic changes of bronchiectasis and mucoid impaction. (D) Coronal ^{3}He-enhanced MR image obtained at same level as in C. Note extensive ventilation defects out of proportion to morphologic abnomalities seen in C.

IV. SUMMARY

Hyperpolarized gas-enhanced MR imaging is a new, promising technique for high-resolution MR imaging of pulmonary airspaces. Helium-3 and ^{129}Xe are the gases most commonly used for ventilation imaging. At present, the greatest clinical experience is with hyperpolarized ^{3}He. This technique is limited, however, by the limited availability of ^{3}He, its polarization requirements, and the need to tune the MR system to the resonant frequency of the gas. There is less clinical experience with ^{129}Xe. Because morphologic and functional information is obtained, and radiation is not used, hyperpolarized gas-enhanced MR imaging may prove ideal for serially evaluating patients with a variety of lung diseases that affect pulmonary ventilation, such as cystic fibrosis, emphysema, asthma, or bronchiolitis obliterans syndrome in lung transplant recipients.

REFERENCES

1. Bergin CJ, Glover GM, Pauly J. Magnetic resonance imaging of lung parenchyma. J Thorac Imag 1993; 8:12–17.
2. Bergin CJ, Glover GH, Pauly JM. Lung parenchyma: magnetic susceptibility in MR imaging. Radiology 1991; 180:845–848.
3. Bergin CJ, Noll DC, Pauly JM, Glover GH, Macovski A. MR imaging of lung parenchyma: a solution to susceptibility. Radiology 1992; 183:673–676.
4. Mayo JR. Magnetic resonance imaging of the chest: where we stand. Radiol Clin North Am 1994; 32:795–809.
5. Hatabu H, Chen Q, Stock KW, Gefter WB, Itoh H. Fast magnetic resonance imaging of the lung. Eur J Radiol 1999; 29:114–132.
6. Albert MS, Cates GD, Driehuys B, et al. Biological magnetic resonance imaging using laser-polarized 129Xe. Nature 1994; 370:199–201.
7. Chen Q, Jakob PM, Griswold MA, Levin DL, Hatabu H, Edelman RR. Oxygen enhanced MR ventilation imaging of the lung. Magma 1998; 7:153–161.
8. Black RD, Middleton HL, Cates GD, et al. In vivo He-3 MR images of guinea pig lungs. Radiology 1996; 199:867–870.
9. Chen XJ, Chawla MS, Hedlund LW, Moller HE, MacFall JR, Johnson GA. MR microscopy of lung airways with hyperpolarized 3He. Magn Reson Med 1998; 39:79–84.
10. MacFall JR, Charles HC, Black RD, et al. Human lung air spaces: potential for MR imaging with hyperpolarized He-3. Radiology 1996; 200:553–558.
11. Middleton H, Black RD, Saam B, et al. MR imaging with hyperpolarized 3He gas. Magn Reson Med 1995; 33:271–275.

12. Mugler JP III, Driehuys B, Brookeman JR, et al. MR imaging and spectroscopy using hyperpolarized 129Xe gas: preliminary human results. Magn Reson Med 1997; 37:809–815.
13. Kauczor H, Surkau R, Roberts T. MRI using hyperpolarized noble gases. Eur J Radiol 1998; 8:820–827.
14. Wolber J, Cherubini A, Leach MO, Bifone A. Hyperpolarized 129Xe NMR as a probe for blood oxygenation. Magn Reson Med 2000; 43:491–496.
15. Wagshul ME, Button TM, Li HF, et al. In vivo MR imaging and spectroscopy using hyperpolarized 129Xe. Magn Reson Med 1996; 36:183–191.
16. Ruppert K, Brookeman JR, Hagspiel KD, Driehuys B, Mugler JP III. NMR of hyperpolarized (129)Xe in the canine chest: spectral dynamics during a breath-hold. Nucl Magn Reson Biomed 2000; 13:220–228.
17. Hedlund LW, Moller HE, Chen XJ, Chawla MS, Cofer GP, Johnson GA. Mixing oxygen with hyperpolarized (3)He for small-animal lung studies. Nucl Magn Reson Biomed 2000; 13:202–206.
18. Eberle B, Weiler N, Markstaller K, et al. Analysis of intrapulmonary O(2) concentration by MR imaging of inhaled hyperpolarized helium-3. J Appl Physiol 1999; 87:2043–2052.
19. Kauczor HU. Current issues in hyperpolarized gases in MRI: biomedical investigations and clinical applications [editorial]. Nucl Magn Reson Biomed 2000; 13: 173–175.
20. Gentile TR, Jones GL, Thompson AK, et al. Demonstration of a compact compressor for application of metastability-exchange optical pumping of 3He to human lung imaging. Magn Reson Med 2000; 43:290–294.
21. Gierada DS, Saam B, Yablonskiy D, Cooper JD, Lefrak SS, Conradi MS. Dynamic echo planar MR imaging of lung ventilation with hyperpolarized (3)He in normal subjects and patients with severe emphysema. Nucl Magn Reson Biomed 2000; 13:176–181.
22. Yablonskiy DA, Gierada DS, Saam BT, et al. High speed dynamic MRI of lung ventilation with hyperpolarized 3He and EPI. Radiology 1998; 209(P):449–450.
23. Schreiber WG, Weiler N, Kauczor HU, et al. [Ultrafast MRI of lung ventilation using hyperpolarized helium-3]. Rofo Fortschr Geb Rontgenstr Neuen Bildgeb Verfahr 2000; 172:129–133.
24. Hedlund LW, Cofer GP, Owen SJ, Allan Johnson G. MR-compatible ventilator for small animals: computer-controlled ventilation for proton and noble gas imaging. Magn Reson Imaging 2000; 18:753–759.
25. Ramirez MP, Sigaloff KC, Kubatina LV, Donahue MA, Venkatesh AK, Albert MS. Physiological response of rats to delivery of helium and xenon: implications for hyperpolarized noble gas imaging. Nucl Magn Reson Biomed 2000; 13:253–264.
26. Kauczor HU, Kreitner KF. MRI of the pulmonary parenchyma. Eur Radiol 1999; 9:1755–1764.
27. de Lange EE, Mugler JP III, Brookeman JR, et al. Lung air spaces: MR imaging evaluation with hyperpolarized 3He gas. Radiology 1999; 210:851–857.

28. Christman RA, Ailion DC, Case TA, et al. Comparison of calculated and experimental NMR spectral broadening for lung tissue. Magn Reson Med 1996; 35: 6–13.
29. Johnson GA, Cates G, Chen XJ, et al. Dynamics of magnetization in hyperpolarized gas MRI of the lung. Magn Reson Med 1997; 38:66–71.
30. Moller HE, Chen XJ, Chawla MS, Driehuys B, Hedlund LW, Johnson GA. Signal dynamics in magnetic resonance imaging of the lung with hyperpolarized noble gases. J Magn Reson 1998; 135:133–143.
31. Moller HE, Chen XJ, Chawla MS, et al. Sensitivity and resolution in 3D NMR microscopy of the lung with hyperpolarized noble gases. Magn Reson Med 1999; 41:800–808.
32. Shattuck MD, Gewalt SL, Glover GH, Hedlund LW, Johnson GA. MR microimaging of the lung using volume projection encoding. Magn Reson Med 1997; 38:938–942.
33. Viallon M, Cofer GP, Suddarth SA, et al. Functional MR microscopy of the lung using hyperpolarized 3He. Magn Reson Med 1999; 41:787–792.
34. Chen XJ, Hedlund LW, Moller HE, Chawla MS, Maronpot RR, Johnson GA. Detection of emphysema in rat lungs by using magnetic resonance measurements of 3He diffusion. Proc Natl Acad Sci USA 2000; 97:11478–11481.
35. Cremillieux Y, Berthezene Y, Humblot H, et al. A combined 1H perfusion/3He ventilation NMR study in rat lungs. Magn Reson Med 1999; 41:645–648.
36. Viallon M, Berthezene Y, Callot V, et al. Dynamic imaging of hyperpolarized (3)He distribution in rat lungs using interleaved-spiral scans. Nucl Magn Reson Biomed 2000; 13:207–213.
37. Donnelly LF, MacFall JR, McAdams HP, et al. Cystic fibrosis: combined hyperpolarized 3He-enhanced and conventional proton MR imaging in the lung—preliminary observations. Radiology 1999; 212:885–889.
38. McAdams HP, Palmer SM, Donnelly LF, Charles HC, Tapson VF, MacFall JR. Hyperpolarized 3He-enhanced MR imaging of lung transplant recipients: preliminary results. Am J Roentgenol 1999; 173:955–959.
39. Kauczor HU, Hofmann D, Kreitner KF, et al. Normal and abnormal pulmonary ventilation: visualization at hyperpolarized He-3 MR imaging. Radiology 1996; 201:564–568.
40. Kauczor HU, Ebert M, Kreitner KF, et al. Imaging of the lungs using ^{3}He MRI: preliminary clinical experience in 18 patients with and without lung disease. J Magn Reson Imag 1997; 7:538–543.
41. Guenther D, Eberle B, Hast J, et al. (3)He MRI in healthy volunteers: preliminary correlation with smoking history and lung volumes. Nucl Magn Reson Biomed 2000; 13:182–189.
42. Kroshus TJ, Kshettry VR, Savik K, John R, Hertz MI, Bolman RM, III. Risk factors for the development of bronchiolitis obliterans syndrome after lung transplantation. J Thorac Cardiovasc Surg 1997; 114:195–202.
43. Paradis I. Bronchiolitis obliterans: pathogenesis, prevention, and management. Am J Med Sci 1998; 315:161–178.

44. Sundaresan S. The impact of bronchiolitis obliterans on late morbidity and mortality after single and bilateral lung transplantation for pulmonary hypertension. Semin Thorac Cardiovasc Surg 1998; 10:152–159.
45. Scott JP, Peters SG, McDougall JC, Beck KC, Midthun DE. Posttransplantation physiologic features of the lung and obliterative bronchiolitis. Mayo Clin Proc 1997; 72:170–174.
46. Patterson GM, Wilson S, Whang JL, et al. Physiologic definitions of obliterative bronchiolitis in heart-lung and double lung transplantation: a comparison of the forced expiratory flow between 25% and 75% of the forced vital capacity and forced expiratory volume in one second. J Heart Lung Transplant 1996; 15:175–181.
47. Cagle PT, Brown RW, Frost A, Kellar C, Yousem SA. Diagnosis of chronic lung transplant rejection by transbronchial biopsy. Mod Pathol 1995; 8:137–142.
48. Chamberlain D, Maurer J, Chaparro C, Idolor L. Evaluation of transbronchial lung biopsy specimens in the diagnosis of bronchiolitis obliterans after lung transplantation. J Heart Lung Transplant 1994; 13:963–971.
49. Cooper JD, Billingham M, Egan T, et al. A working formulation for the standardization of nomenclature and for clinical staging of chronic dysfunction in lung allografts. International Society for Heart and Lung Transplantation. J Heart Lung Transplant 1993; 12:713–716.
50. Ikonen T, Kivisaari L, Harjula AL, et al. Value of high-resolution computed tomography in routine evaluation of lung transplantation recipients during development of bronchiolitis obliterans syndrome. J Heart Lung Transplant 1996; 15: 587–595.
51. Ikonen T, Kivisaari L, Taskinen E, Piilonen A, Harjula AL. High-resolution CT in long-term follow-up after lung transplantation. Chest 1997; 111:370–376.
52. Lau DM, Siegel MJ, Hildebolt CF, Cohen AH. Bronchiolitis obliterans syndrome: thin-section CT diagnosis of obstructive changes in infants and young children after lung transplantation. Radiology 1998; 208:783–788.
53. Leung AN, Fisher K, Valentine V, et al. Bronchiolitis obliterans after lung transplantation: detection using expiratory HRCT. Chest 1998; 113:365–370.
54. Loubeyre P, Revel D, Delignette A, Loire R, Mornex JF. High-resolution computed tomographic findings associated with histologically diagnosed acute lung rejection in heart-lung transplant recipients. Chest 1995; 107:132–138.
55. Loubeyre P, Revel D, Delignette A, et al. Bronchiectasis detected with thin-section CT as a predictor of chronic lung allograft rejection [see comments]. Radiology 1995; 194:213–216.
56. Worthy SA, Park CS, Kim JS, Muller NL. Bronchiolitis obliterans after lung transplantation: high-resolution CT findings in 15 patients. Am J Roentgenol 1997; 169:673–677.
57. Lee ES, Gotway MB, Reddy GP, Golden JA, Keith FM, Webb WR. Early bronchiolitis obliterans following lung transplantation: accuracy of expiratory thin-section CT for diagnosis. Radiology 2000; 216:472–477.
58. Wittram C, Rappaport DC. Bronchiolitis obliterans after lung transplantation:

appearance on expiratory minimum intensity projection images. Can Assoc Radiol J 2000; 51:103–106.

59. Kauczor HU, Ebert M, Kreitner KF, et al. [The helium-3 MRT of pulmonary ventilation: the initial clinical applications]. Rofo Fortschr Geb Rontgenstr Neuen Bildgeb Verfahr 1997; 166:192–198.
60. Brasfield D, Hicks G, Soong S, Peters J, Tiller R. Evaluation of scoring system of the chest radiograph in cystic fibrosis: a collaborative study. Am J Roentgenol 1980; 134:1195–1198.
61. Bhalla M, Turcios N, Aponte V, et al. Cystic fibrosis: scoring system with thin-section CT. Radiology 1991; 179:783–788.
62. Donnelly LF, Gelfand MJ, Brody AS, Wilmott RW. Comparison between morphologic changes seen on high-resolution CT and regional pulmonary perfusion seen on SPECT in patients with cystic fibrosis. Pediatr Radiol 1997; 27:920–925.
63. McAdams HP, Hatabu H, Donnelly LF, Chen Q, Tadamura E, MacFall JR. Novel techniques for MR imaging of pulmonary airspaces. Magn Reson Imaging Clin North Am 2000; 8:205–219.

12

Magnetic Resonance Imaging Techniques for the Assessment of Pulmonary Emboli

Michael A. Blake
Harvard Medical School and
Massachusetts General Hospital
Boston, Massachusetts

Qun Chen and Vu Ming Mai
Northwestern University Medical School and
Evanston Northwestern Healthcare
Evanston, Illinois

Hiroto Hatabu
Hospital of the University of Pennsylvania
Philadelphia, Pennsylvania

I. INTRODUCTION

Pulmonary embolism (PE) is a serious and potentially fatal condition that is estimated to affect around 650,000 patients per year in the United States [1]. Pulmonary embolism is notoriously difficult to diagnose, and deaths related to untreated PE are estimated at 120,000/year. These statistics emphasize the difficulties in both suspecting and confirming the diagnosis of PE. A noninvasive method for evaluating PE has long been sought. Conventional angiography remains the gold standard for evaluation of pulmonary vascular anatomy, but its invasive nature is a drawback which avers most physicians from commonly requesting it. Radionuclide ventilation-perfusion (V/P) scanning and, more recently, computed tomography angiography (CTA) are more commonly used as first-line investigations for the diagnosis of PE. Scintigraphy has limited spatial resolution for the diagnosis of perfusion abnormalities and does not directly image arterial anatomy. Computed tomography angiography is gaining popularity as a screening technique for PE [2–9] and its ready accessibility and impressive record in recent studies have already gained it widespread acceptance. Furthermore, the recent development of multidetector systems may improve the conspicuity of the peripheral pulmonary vasculature and increase the sensitivity for detection of subsegmental pulmonary emboli. Recent studies have also demonstrated the use of CT for combined evaluation of the pulmonary arteries and the pelvic veins in one examination [9].

However, disadvantages of CT include the need for large intravenous injections of potentially nephrotoxic contrast medium and exposure to ionizing radiation [10]. Although CT has already gained wide acceptance as the primary cross-sectional technique to evaluate PE, many patients cannot have a CT examination because of an allergy to iodinated contrast media or severe renal insufficiency. These are not, however, contraindications to magnetic resonance imaging (MRI) evaluation.

MRI is a particularly appealing modality for diagnosing pulmonary embolism as it does not require radiation or iodinated contrast medium, can also evaluate the pulmonary vasculature and deep veins in one study, and can assess pulmonary perfusion and ventilation as well as the pulmonary vasculature. This chapter reviews the state-of-the-art development of pulmonary MR imaging for PE, the current clinical applications of the technique, and the prospects for future development.

II. BACKGROUND

Diagnosis of PE with radionuclide imaging is based on ventilation-perfusion mismatching and is expressed on a semiquantitative probability scale. In 1990, the multicenter Prospective Investigation of Pulmonary Embolism Diagnosis (PIOPED), sponsored by the National Institutes of Health, compared V/Q scans with conventional pulmonary angiography for the diagnosis of PE [11]. Seventy-eight percent of V/Q scans in the PIOPED study were read as intermediate, indeterminate, or low probability and therefore provided no firm diagnostic information. Other limitations of this exam include a relatively lengthy duration, the injection of a radioisotope, low-resolution images, and lack of direct arterial anatomic information.

A better screening tool is clearly needed. Since the early 1990s several promising new modalities have emerged for evaluation of patients with suspected PE. The D-dimer assay, a marker of fibrin lysis, is an emerging screening test with a high negative predictive value for PE. The long time required for this assay and its low specificity, however, limit its clinical usefulness [12]. Transesophageal echocardiography can image pulmonary embolism in central pulmonary arteries, but preliminary tests suggest that it has a low negative predictive value and cannot be used to exclude pulmonary embolism.

Pulmonary angiography is widely accepted as the gold standard for evaluation of arterial anatomy. However, the procedure is invasive and is associated with a small but definite morbidity and mortality (0.9% major complication rate), which is increased in the setting of pulmonary hypertension [13]. Although regarded as the ''gold standard'' for diagnosing PE, there is a 30% interobserver variation at the subsegmental level and many other interpretative difficulties.

Helical CT angiography has emerged as a popular new technique for assessment of the pulmonary circulation [2–9]. It has proved extremely useful for the detection of PE with reported sensitivities and specificities of 53–92% and 95–100% respectively, particularly in the central vessels [3–6]. Although lower sensitivities (45–60%) have been reported for segmental and subsegmental emboli using older systems [2,7], optimization of scanning protocols [14] and newer multidetector systems have the potential to improve this.

To date, CTA has performed far less well in diagnosing PE in subsegmental vessels. The significance of these peripheral emboli, is unclear, however, and it is not known if they herald larger emboli. Subsegmental emboli appear to have no significant effect in patients with good cardiopulmonary reserve but may be fatal in a compromised patient: 8 of 77 compromised patients with low probability V/Q scans (and not treated) died of PE (at postmortem). Their frequency in isolation is also not clear; Oser et al. found that 23 of 76 consecutive positive angiograms (30%) had subsegmental emboli only and 19 of the 76 (25%) patients had a single embolus [15]. The significance and isolated occurrence of subsegmental emboli is an important issue as the CT interpretative difficulty at this level is mirrored at MR imaging.

It is clear that the ideal diagnostic test for PE is still being sought. As PE disrupts the gas exchange between the airways and the blood, a test that would incorporate both high-resolution imaging and functional pulmonary information would be welcome. V/Q scanning can evaluate regional ventilation and perfusion, but is limited by poor spatial and temporal resolution. While CT is an accurate method for the detection of regional morphologic abnormalities, it does not provide a direct functional assessment of the lung. Magnetic resonance has the attractive potential to provide both functional and morphological information and thus elicit both direct and indirect evidence of embolism.

III. GENERAL TECHNIQUES OF THORACIC MAGNETIC RESONANCE IMAGING

The use of MRI for the evaluation of pulmonary embolism has thus far been rather limited. The unique composition of lung tissue makes it one of the most difficult organs to evaluate with MRI. Its low proton density means little signal can be detected using conventional spin-echo (SE) or gradient echo sequences. Additionally, the air-filled alveolar subunits of the lung create local magnetic field gradients which rapidly dephase transverse magnetization producing further signal loss [16]. Cardiac and respiratory-motion-induced artifacts are also difficult to avoid using conventional MRI techniques. Limited patient-breath-holding capability and difficulties monitoring patients in the scanning environment are further obstacles to successful pulmonary MR imaging. The underlying approach to help overcome these problems and acquire satisfactory lung signal is to rapidly acquire the signal before it decays by using a minimal effective echo delay (TE).

Early studies using electrocardiogram- (ECG) gated SE MRI demonstrated emboli as intraluminal foci of intermediate to high signal but slow-flowing blood often could not be differentiated from emboli [17,18]. Gradient-echo imaging, including cinegradient recalled acquisition in the steady state, is sensitive to flow and can demonstrate the embolus as a low-signal filling defect [19]. The introduction of a new generation of MR systems with enhanced gradient performance has helped promote the application of fast MRI techniques to the thorax. Hatabu et al. described a multislice-interleaved sub-millisecond TE gradient-echo sequence which allowed complete coverage of the lungs in a single breathhold [20]. High-performance gradients permitted TE values of 700 msec. This technique used fractional echo sampling, high bandwidth, and a truncated RF pulse to minimize the TE and has demonstrated a variety of parenchymal lung disorders to good advantage.

Half-Fourier acquisition single-shot turbo spin-echo (HASTE) has also proved valuable in providing a reliable and rapid platform for thoracic imaging. An echo spacing of 4.2 msec can be used, and the resulting acquisition time for a 128×256 matrix is just 302 msec. The brief acquisition time renders the sequence insensitive to motion, and the short echo spacing makes it resistant to the heterogeneous magnetic susceptibility of lung parenchyma. A centrically reordered phase encoding scheme can be used for the single-shot turbo spin-echo sequence to make the effective echo time extremely short, thereby further reducing signal losses from short T2 tissues and providing higher signal-to-noise ratio (SNR). Furthermore, T1 weighting can be produced by applying an inversion recovery pulse to the HASTE sequence (Fig.

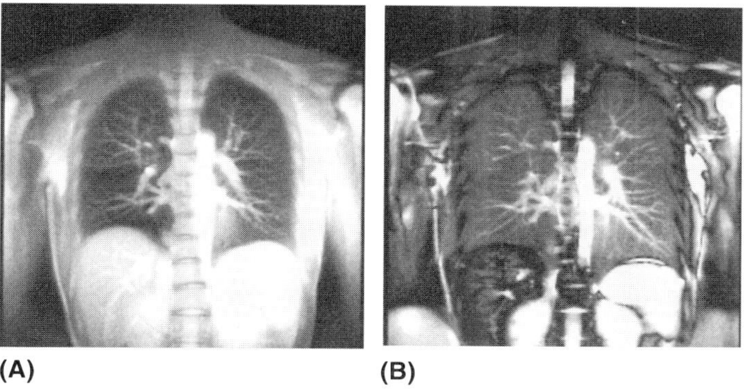

Figure 1 Coronal half-Fourier acquisition single-shot turbo spin-echo (HASTE) (A) and inversion recovery HASTE (B) MR images demonstrating thoracic anatomy.

1). A double inversion recovery sequence can also be used with suppression of signal from muscle and fat to enhance the visibility of the lung parenchyma (Fig. 2). Spatial modulation of magnetization (SPAMM) techniques produce tagging stripes which allow assessment of mechanical tissue deformation (Fig.3) and can help distinguish slow-flow-related signal from that of embo-

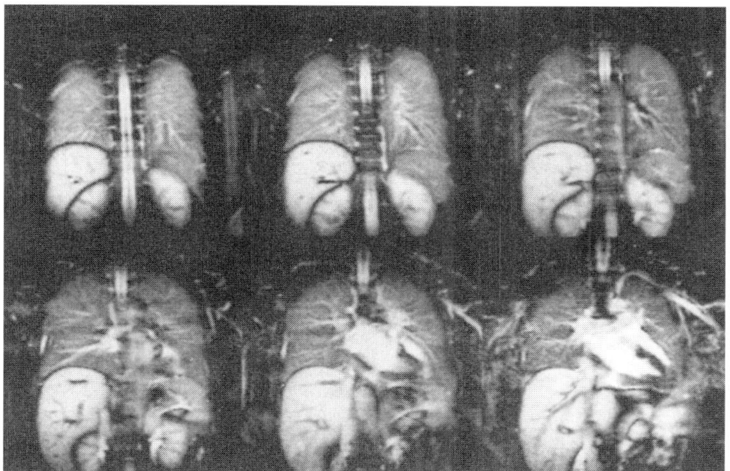

Figure 2 Multiple inversion recovery (MIR) HASTE MRI with six sequential coronal images of lungs showing anatomical detail.

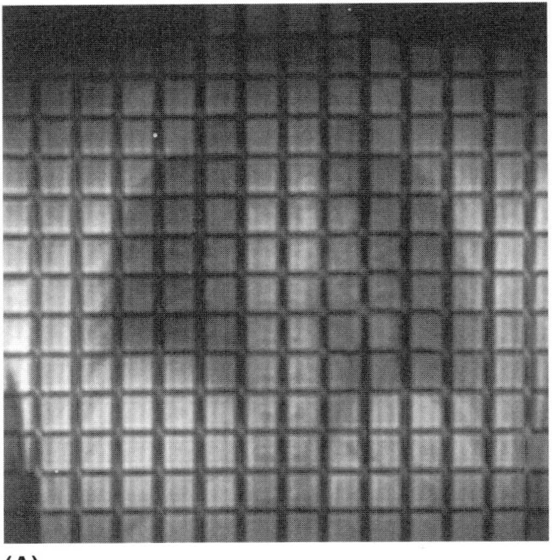

(A)

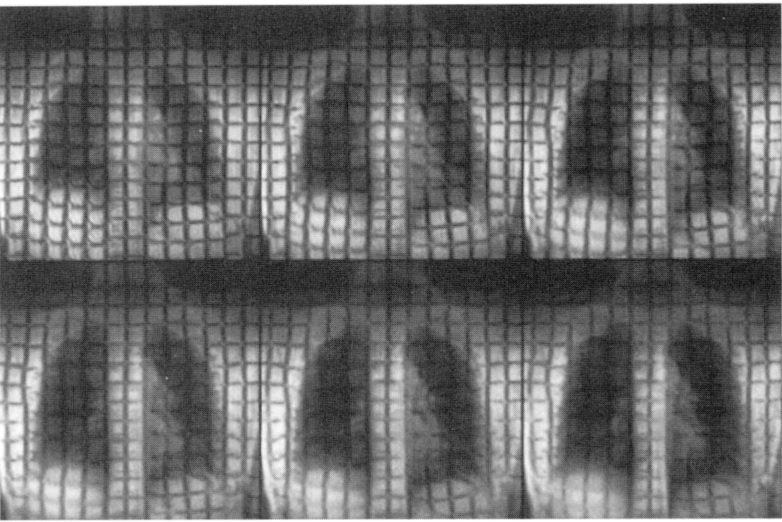

(B)

Figure 3 Coronal SPAMM (spatial modulation of magnetization) lung images with reference image at end of expiration (A) and consecutive images at 100-msec intervals (B). Grid tagging facilitates recognition of mechanical deformation over time.

lism. Hatabu and colleagues ntegrated the SPAMM technique into a conventional cardiac-synchronized spin-echo sequence [20]. Areas of persistent stripes were identified in central pulmonary arteries with thromboemboli, whereas the intraluminal stripes disappeared in normal pulmonary arteries.

IV. MAGNETIC RESONANCE PERFUSION/ VENTILATION TECHNIQUES AND MAGNETIC RESONANCE PULMONARY ANGIOGRAPHY

The new generation of MR scanners with high-performance gradients has greatly advanced the role of MR in imaging of the pulmonary vasculature. Improvements in gradient performance have made very short repetition and echo times on clinical scanners standard, thus enabling subsecond image acquisition. State-of-the-art capabilities now include functional imaging such as perfusion and ventilation and time-resolved 3D angiography. We now concentrate on some of these major advances in MR perfusion/ventilation techniques and MR pulmonary angiography.

A. Pulmonary Magnetic Resonance Angiography

Time-of-Flight Techniques

Pulmonary MR angiography (MRA) has evolved over the years. Initially time-of-flight imaging (TOF) was employed [21–24]. Several breath holds were generally necessary to cover the lungs, and scans suffered from misregistration and in-plane saturation signal loss effects, which mimicked the filling defects of emboli. McFall et al. used a single 4-cm slab acquired in the sagittal plane to image each lung separately [25]. This allowed short scan times and suppression of venous flow, but poor spatial resolution and slow flowing blood artifact limited this technique. Wielopolski et al. devised a 3D TOF technique for imaging the pulmonary vessels but imaging times were very long, approaching 13 min [24].

Dynamic Gadolinium Magnetic Resonance Imaging

More recent advances in MRA have involved 3D GRE imaging following intravenous injection of gadolinium [26,27]. This has been probably the greatest single recent advance in clinical MR angiography throughout the body. It offers many advantages over conventional MR angiographic techniques and is free from the risks of iodinated contrast material injection and arterial puncture associated with conventional angiography. The technique relies on the T1 shortening technique of the gadolinium agent, and images can be acquired in a single breath hold, making the approach ideal for imaging of the pulmonary vasculature (Fig. 4). The administration of gadolinium allows the use of very short TR times (made possible by the advances in gradient performance), which facilitate the acquisition of a 3D imaging volume with a reasonable number of slices within a single breath hold. This 3D technique may be viewed in cinematic fashion to depict hemodynamic changes associated with the cardiac cycle or reconstituted to create a three-dimensional display of the pulmonary vasculature. Two-dimensional and 3D pulmonary parenchymal perfusion imaging is also feasible and this subject is discussed below.

Several workers have described techniques for contrast enhanced pulmonary MRA [28–31]. Most authors have used 0.2–0.3 mmol/kg of gadolinium and have tailored the injection rate and scan delay time so that the central lines of K space are acquired during peak arterial enhancement. A 3D fast spoiled gradient-echo sequence is generally employed and the phase order can be either linear or centric if bolus detection techniques are used. The slice thickness (2–3mm) and number of slices per volume thickness (50/10 cm) are tailored for each individual patient.

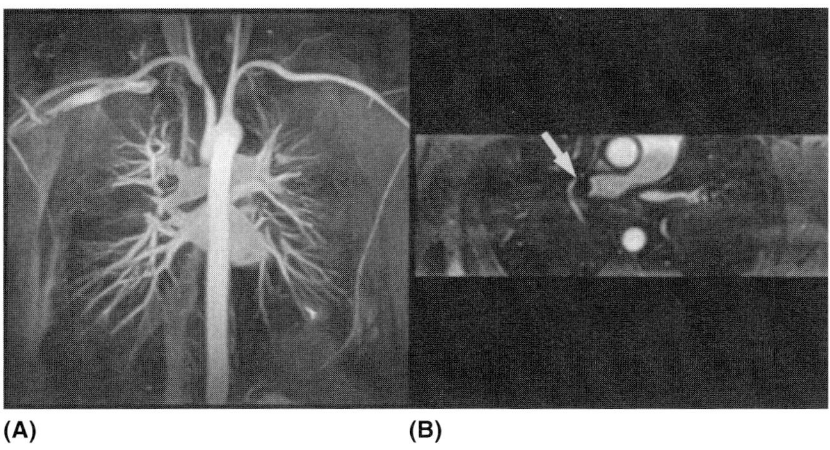

(A) (B)

Figure 4 Dynamic gadolinium MR pulmonary angiography MIP reconstruction (A) and single axial section demonstrating embolus in right pulmonary artery (B).

Table 1 Sensitivity and Specificity in Detection of Pulmonary Embolism in Comparison with Pulmonary Angiography or Scintigraphy

First author	Year	Ref.	n	Sensitivity%	Specificity%
Loubeyre	1994	28	23	70	100
Meaney	1997	29	30	87	97
Gupta	1999	30	36	85	96

In the first clinical study describing dynamic gadolinium MRA for the diagnosis of acute pulmonary embolism ($n = 23$ patients) spatial resolution was limited (slice thickness 20 mm, in-plane resolution 2.7 mm^2) [28]. All central thrombi but none of the segmental thrombi were depicted. Sensitivity was 70%, and specificity was 100% (Table 1). Meaney and coworkers then compared a superior MR angiography technique (Table 2) with conventional angiography in 30 patients with suspected pulmonary embolism [29]. Sensitivity and specificity of 100 and 95% were obtained for segmental arteries. This limitation of evaluation to the segmental level and their conclusion that failures were mainly due to inability to breath hold both serve to highlight the need for shorter scan times and higher resolution imaging.

In a more recent study 36 patients with intermediate- or low-probability V/Q scans and a high clinical suspicion for pulmonary embolism were included. This led to a relatively high proportion of segmental and subsegmental emboli. Nevertheless the results of two observers were encouraging on a per-patient basis: sensitivity 85%, specificity 96%, positive predictive value 92%, and negative predictive value 92% [30]. On a per-embolus basis, however, the sensitivity was only 68%. In this study, Gupta et al. used a technique which

Table 2 Dynamic Gadolinium Sequence Parameters

Meaney et al. [29]	Carr et al. [31]
TR 6.5 msec	1.64 msec
TE 1.8 msec	0.6 msec
FA 40°	15°
Matrix 256 × 128	(140–180) × 256
FOV 320 mm	270–360 mm (phase) × 360 mm (frequency)
Thickness 3–4 mm	Slab thickness is 100–120 mm with 12 to 24 partitions, interpolated to 24–48 respectively,
Acquisition 27 sec	2–3 sec

acquires a 3D data set in 23 sec. However, even breath-hold periods of this length are undesirable in the typically dyspneic patients with suspected PE disease, and wide acquisition windows preclude time-resolved sequential imaging of the pulmonary arteries, parenchyma, and veins. The most current gradient technology and system bandwidth allow much shorter TRs than previously achievable, and this can be harnessed to expedite data acquisition proportionately.

Time-Resolved Dynamic Gadolinium Magnetic Resonance Imaging

Preliminary reports from investigators at Northwestern Memorial Hospital, Illinois, implementing ultrafast, multiphase 3D gadolinium vascular imaging have illustrated exciting applications of these new capabilities in the evaluation of PE [31]. This technique succeeds in imaging the pulmonary vasculature impressively quickly while maintaining sufficient resolution to visualize to the critical subsegmental level (Fig. 5).

Their technique (J. Carr, personal communication, 2000) again takes advantage of the recent developments in gradient amplifier and gradient coil technology which allow significant shortening of the pulse repetition time (TR) (Table 2). They have implemented an ultrashort TR/TE (1.6/0.65 msec) spoiled 3D gradient-echo pulse sequence on a 1.5T scanner with a high-performance gradient system (40 mT/m amplitude, 200 T/m/sec slew rate) (Siemens Sonata, Iselin, NJ).

Up to 16 sequential measurements are made in each study, each lasting 2–3 sec. Patients hold their breath during the image acquisition to reduce motion artifact and facilitate satisfactory subtraction. The entire study lasts around 24 sec. However, for evaluation of the pulmonary arterial and perfusion phases, only a short breath hold on the order of 7 sec is needed. The first 3D volume serves as the precontrast mask and is then subtracted from subsequent volumes so that the output includes the partitions from all measurements, a full set of subtractions, and a coronal maximum intensity projection (MIP) image for each of the subtracted sets.

Their technique offers increased temporal and spatial resolution while using a shorter breath hold compared to previous reports. Moreover it also provides the ability to define multiple pulmonary and systemic phases of enhancement. This phased visualization of the pulmonary vasculature should simplify interpretation of arterial disease by eliminating overlapping venous structures. Some earlier studies have used similar spatial resolution but acquisition times per single 3D volume have typically been 20 sec or longer. High-

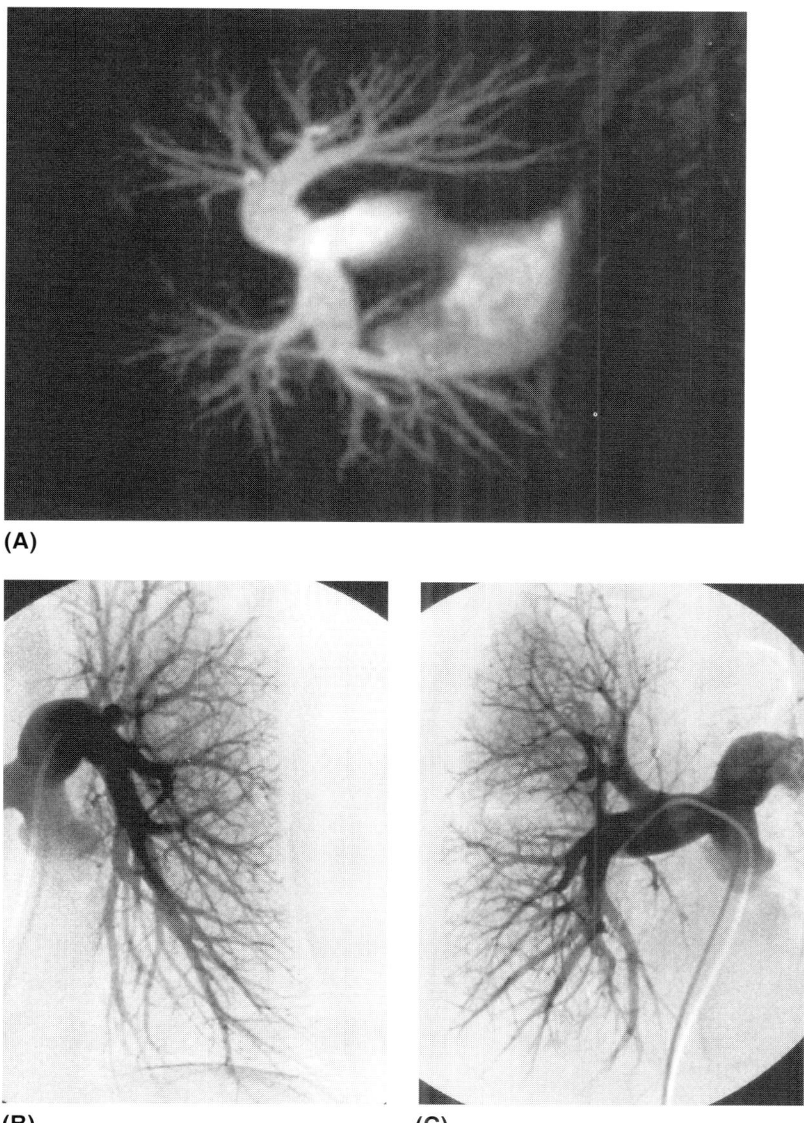

(A)

(B) (C)

Figure 5 Example of normal gadolinium 3D MRA (A) with corresponding normal conventional digital subtraction angiograms of right and left lungs (B and C). (Courtesy of J. Carr and P. Finn, Northwestern Memorial Hospital, Illinois).

temporal-resolution techniques in humans have also typically employed 2D acquisitions [32,33] but these Northwestern studies are achieving 3-sec temporal resolution using a 3D technique while maintaining spatial resolution. Ultrashort TR times, asymmetric K-space ordering, and data interpolation have been effectively combined to greatly decrease the minimum acquisition window achievable per 3D volume.

Initial reports from Finn and Carr at Northwestern University indicate that, using ultrashort TR pulse sequences, time-resolved 3D vascular imaging of the lungs is feasible. Although their technique requires high-performance gradients and high-bandwidth electronics, all the components used in their method are now commercially available. The ability to perform high-quality imaging with high temporal resolution in short-breath-hold periods is an exciting development for imaging of pulmonary embolism and the results of controlled trials of the technique's accuracy are eagerly awaited.

V. FUNCTIONAL IMAGING OF THE LUNG

A. Perfusion Imaging

New MR technologies incorporating contrast and noncontrast methods have resulted in major advances in pulmonary perfusion imaging.

Contrast Enhanced Pulmonary Perfusion Magnetic Resonance Imaging

Pulmonary perfusion can be imaged by using an inversion recovery turbo FLASH sequence with an ultrashort TE and 1 msec temporal resolution following gadolinium administration [34]. Serial enhancement of the systemic veins, right atrium, right ventricle, and pulmonary arteries to beyond the segmental level can be tracked followed by a gradual diffuse increase in signal intensity of the lung parenchyma over 4–7 sec (Fig. 6). Preliminary reports show the feasibility of this MR perfusion technique in the evaluation of patients with PE. Both 2D and 3D techniques have now been demonstrated. The Beth Israel Deaconess group has performed quantitative analysis on the indicator dilution principle using a pig model of pulmonary embolism [32]. The results were compared with the absolute pulmonary perfusion obtained with colored microspheres. The inverse of apparent mean transit time [1/tau(app)], distribution volume (*V*), and *V*/tau(app) correlated well with the absolute lung perfusion. Dynamic contrast-enhanced MRI also appears capable of demonstrating gravitationally dependent differences in lung perfusion [35].

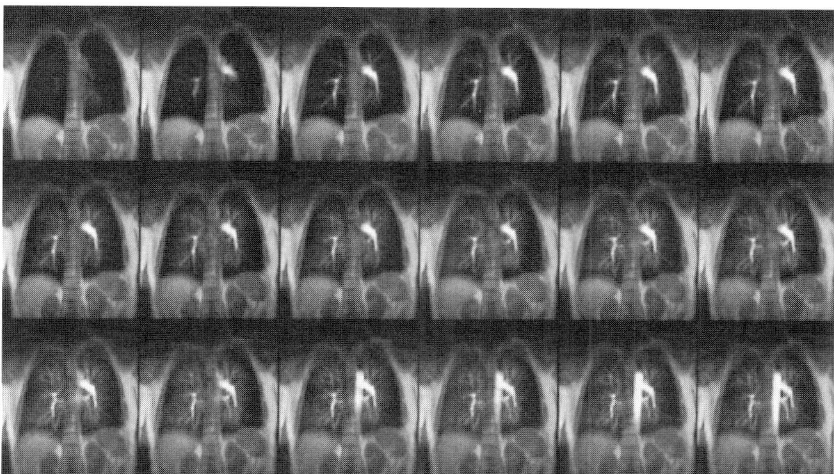

Figure 6 Magnetic resonance perfusion imaging with gadolinium DTPA demonstrating serial enhancement of pulmonary arteries, segmental arteries, lung parenchyma, and aorta.

Berthezene and colleagues assessed the accuracy and potential of lung MR perfusion imaging compared with perfusion scintigraphy in the evaluation of patients with suspected lung perfusion defects [36]. Their technique also used an inversion recovery turbo-FLASH sequence with ultrashort TE (1.4 msec). The dynamic study was acquired in the coronal plane and consisted of 10 images of 6 slices (a total of 60 images/series). The average sensitivity and specificity of MR were 69 and 91%, respectively. The overall agreement between MR and scintigraphy was good, with a good correlation between the two modalities ($\kappa = 0.63$). Their study confirmed the promise of lung MR perfusion techniques in detecting perfusion defects.

Perfusion defects post artificial embolization (Fig. 7) have been described in animal models using a multiphasic 2D technique [33] and a single-phase 3D technique [37]. Multiphasic pulmonary parenchyma perfusion in Carr and Finn's time-resolved 3D study was demonstrated as a dynamic change in signal-to-noise over time with well-defined wash-in and wash-out phases and several temporal frames of parenchyma enhancement. By acquiring 3D volumes in these multiple phases, it is possible to identify and assess each bronchopulmonary segment directly using multiplanar reconstructions. The ability to assess the pulmonary arteries, together with pulmonary parenchyma

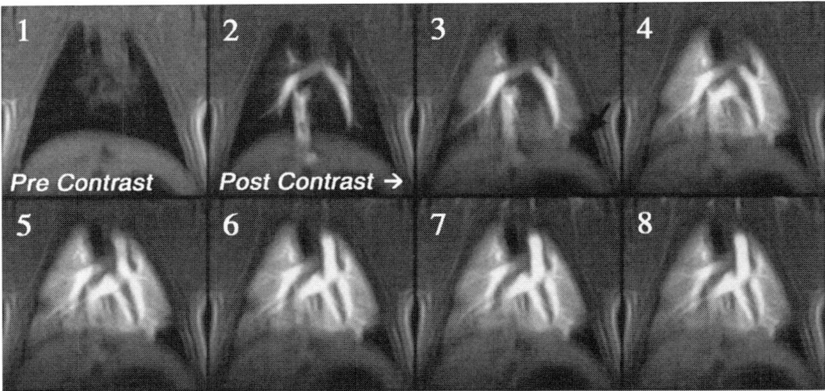

Figure 7 Pulmonary embolism model: multiple slices from dynamic gadolinium perfusion imaging showing reduced perfusion in several areas bilaterally due to PE.

perfusion, has the potential to increase detection of thromboembolic disease by drawing attention to the specific arteries supplying the regions of reduced perfusion. However, this attractive hypothesis remains to be evaluated in clinical studies.

Pulmonary Perfusion Magnetic Resonance Imaging with Star Techniques

Non-contrast-dependent techniques demonstrating parenchymal perfusion have been developed by Edelman and coworkers using modifications of the signal targeting and alternating radiofrequency (STAR) sequence [38]. For each breath hold, two sets of images are acquired. In one set of images, an inversion recovery pulse is applied to the right ventricle and main pulmonary artery to invert the magnetization of blood within these structures. After an inflow period (TI), data are acquired using a HASTE pulse sequence. The subtraction of the two images is the perfusion image. A further development based on this principle is the flow-sensitive alternating inversion recovery with an extra radiofrequency pulse (FAIRER) sequence (Fig. 8).

Mai et al. have reported on the FAIRER sequence, which also involves acquiring two images: a control and a tagged image [39,40]. A spatially selective inversion pulse, followed by a selective 90° pulse, precedes the control image. A nonselective inversion pulse, followed by a selective 90° pulse prepares the tagged image. Image acquisition is then performed after a time delay.

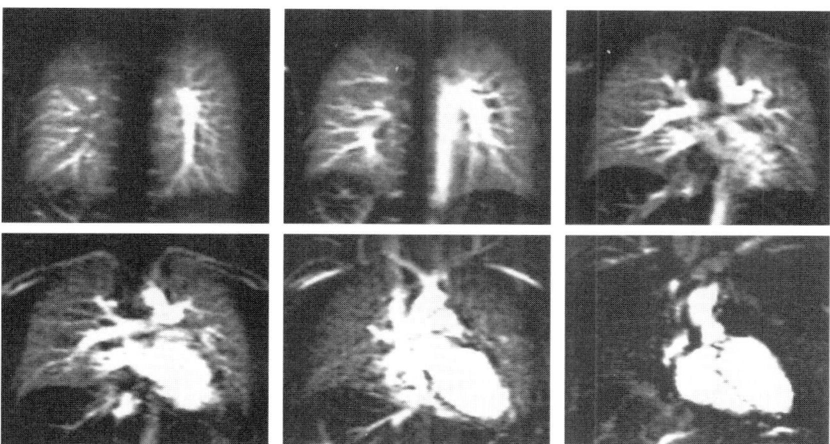

Figure 8 Six coronal images using flow-sensitive alternating inversion recovery with an extra radiofrequency pulse (FAIRER) technique with normal perfusion to both lungs.

Perfusion-weighted images are obtained by subtracting the tagged image from the control. Image acquisition of both images is interleaved and performed within a breath-holding period. Cardiac triggering is used to ensure that all images are acquired at the same phase of the heart cycle, thereby reducing motion artifacts. The time delay between triggering and commencing image acquisition is 1600–2000 msec depending on the heart rate of the patient.

A HASTE sequence, which has an intrinsically reduced susceptibility to heterogeneous magnetic environment, is used with an effective TE of 36 msec. The short echo spacing is 4.5 msec, which minimizes the effect of field inhomogeneities. A total of 72 differently phase-encoded spin echoes is acquired for a HASTE read-out, with the eight extra lines being used for phase correction in the half-Fourier image reconstruction. This example of a pulsed arterial spin labeling technique is a promising novel method to assess pulmonary parenchymal perfusion.

B. Ventilation Magnetic Resonance Imaging for Pulmonary Embolism

This chapter focuses on MR ventilation techniques as they apply to the assessment of PE, as the general subject of MR ventilation is covered in a separate chapter. Recent work has highlighted the potential of ventilation imaging with MRI using molecular oxygen and hyperpolarized ^{129}Xe and ^{3}He. Edelman and coworkers have demonstrated the use of 100% oxygen as a T1 contrast agent for ventilation imaging in humans [41–43]. Oxygen modulates MR signal in blood and fluid by the paramagnetic properties of both deoxyhemoglobin and of molecular oxygen. Deoxyhemoglobin has the property of shortening T2* with little T1 effect. This effect is exploited in the blood oxygenation level dependent technique, which has been widely used throughout the body to evaluate local blood flow and tissue oxygenation [44]. In ventilation imaging, however, the effect taken advantage of is the T1 shortening effect of dissolved oxygen in blood, and the spin echo sequences employed minimize any T2* effect.

The technique of Edelman and colleagues employs a T1-weighted inversion recovery single-shot turbo spin-echo sequence while the patient is ventilated with 100% oxygen. In their comparative study, room air was also inhaled and the delay time TI (600–1100 ms) was adjusted to obtain the maximum signal difference between the two gas inhalations. For each slice, 40–80 coronal images were acquired with images obtained every 5 sec (Fig. 9). Oxygen is inexpensive and readily available in most MR units as a standard and its administration is generally safe under supervised conditions. Edelman's group have also shown that MR oxygen-enhanced ventilation imaging of the lung is possible with an open-configured 0.2 T MR system [43]. This oxygen venti-

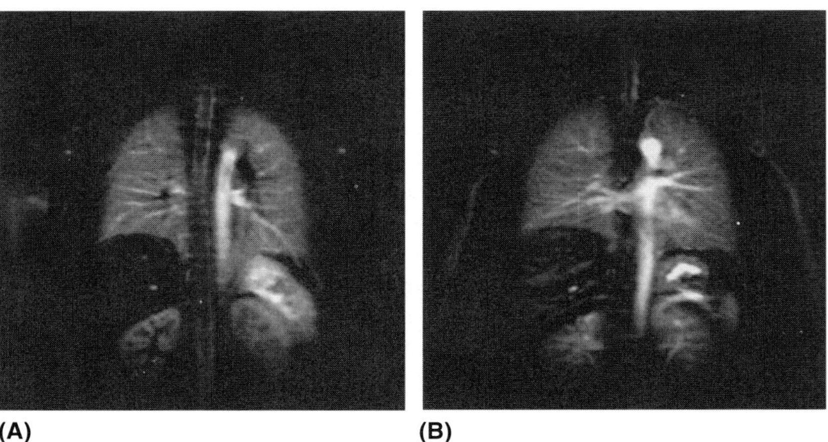

(A) (B)

Figure 9 Oxygen-enhanced ventilation MRI calculated ventilation maps (A and B) following 100% O_2 inhalation.

lation approach clearly shows considerable potential as a complement to the perfusion and angiographic techniques already described for evaluation of patients with suspected PE.

Inhaled ^{129}Xe and ^{3}He gases have also been employed for ventilation MRI [44–49]. These inert noble gases are hyperpolarized using optical pumping techniques, which increase their MR signal by 100,000 times compared with that in a thermal equilibrium state. Such strong signal allows for direct data acquisition using inhaled gases themselves, thus making lung imaging of the airways possible. Excellent results have been achieved in both animal and human studies. Hyperpolarized gas MR scans can be acquired rapidly because there is no need for recovery to thermal equilibrium, and ultrafast functional MR imaging is now possible. While highly promising, these methods have some drawbacks. The administration of these gases in severely ill patients has not been evaluated for safety and the gas polarization apparatus and special MR imaging hardware are costly. The gases all differ in weight to oxygen and thus their behavior in the lungs may also differ due to gravitational effects.

C. Combined Ventilation/Perfusion Magnetic Resonance Imaging

The fundamental difficulties of lung imaging with MR can thus be overcome by these new imaging techniques that are fast, have high signal-to-noise ratio, and are insensitive to local magnetic field inhomogeneities. For example, we have seen how the use of a single-shot TSE sequence for ventilation MRI dramatically reduces the impact of local magnetic field inhomogeneity and motion artifacts. Similarly, we have described how the use of FLASH sequences with ultrashort TE (0.9 msec) for perfusion MRI overcomes the short T2* found in lung tissue. Combining these MR techniques, Chen and colleagues have been able to accomplish integrated pulmonary ventilation and perfusion MRI using oxygen and gadopentetate dimeglumine as contrast agents, respectively [33,50].

The perfusion sequence used by Chen et al. balanced temporal resolution with the amount of lung imaged. A temporal resolution of under 300 msec could be obtained for a single slice acquisition or of 2–3 sec for any given slice in a multislice acquisition. The overall coverage comprised 60 mm in the coronal plane and could be increased by reducing temporal resolution or administering further contrast. The duration of the sequence was sufficient to evaluate both the first pass of contrast medium as well as recirculation.

The use of centrically reordered phase encoding scheme in ventilation MRI has significantly improved signal-to-noise ratio. A 2.5-fold increase in

SNR has been observed when compared to regular HASTE sequences. The short effective time (TE_{eff} = 4.2 msec) resulting from the centric reordering method maximized the signal contribution from short T2 lung tissue, but this increase in signal occurred at the expense of some loss of spatial resolution. The discontinuity of MR signals at the center of K space causes image blurring and the later echoes obtained are mainly noise due to the long acquisition time (538 msec) and short T2 values in the lung. When these noisy echoes are in the periphery of k space, spatial resolution information is poor. The perennial MR trade-off between signal-to-noise and between coverage and resolution again needs to be balanced. Advances in parallel imaging, including simultaneous acquisition of spatial harmonics (SMASH) and sensitivity encoding (SENSE) methods, may help in this regard. These new techniques, which exploit the properties of arrays of multiple receiver coils, may thus play a role in the future of pulmonary MR imaging. The SMASH technique exploits spatial information inherent in a phased array coil. Several lines of K space are acquired simultaneously, and this technique can be used to reduce imaging time or increase resolution without any requirement for improved gradient performance [51]. SENSE is also based on the fact that receiver sensitivity generally has an encoding effect complementary to Fourier preparation by linear field gradients. Thus, by using multiple receiver coils in parallel, scan time in Fourier imaging can be considerably reduced and MRI performance potentially greatly enhanced [52].

The study by Chen and colleagues clearly demonstrates the ability of MRI to assess both regional pulmonary ventilation and perfusion. In their model of airway occlusion, a mean 11-fold increase in ventilation signal enhancement was seen in the normal lung compared with the obstructed lung. This indicates that oxygen is a feasible MR contrast agent for the evaluation of regional ventilation impairment. In the same experiment, MR perfusion imaging showed an associated decrease in perfusion signal enhancement in the obstructed lung, likely reflecting hypoxic vasoconstriction. The ability to image the basic functions of the lung with this precision is highly promising.

In their model of pulmonary embolism, mismatched ventilation and perfusion patterns were observed in all animals. Perfusion defects were seen in regions distal to the thrombi, whereas no ventilation abnormalities were detected in any animals (Figs. 10 and 11). Mismatched ventilation/perfusion abnormalities (reduced perfusion with normal ventilation) suggest a high likelihood of PE, whereas perfusion defects accompanied by abnormal ventilation are unlikely to represent pulmonary emboli.

This same concept has also been applied to a rat model of pulmonary embolism by Berthezene et al. using MRI [53]. In their study, pulmonary

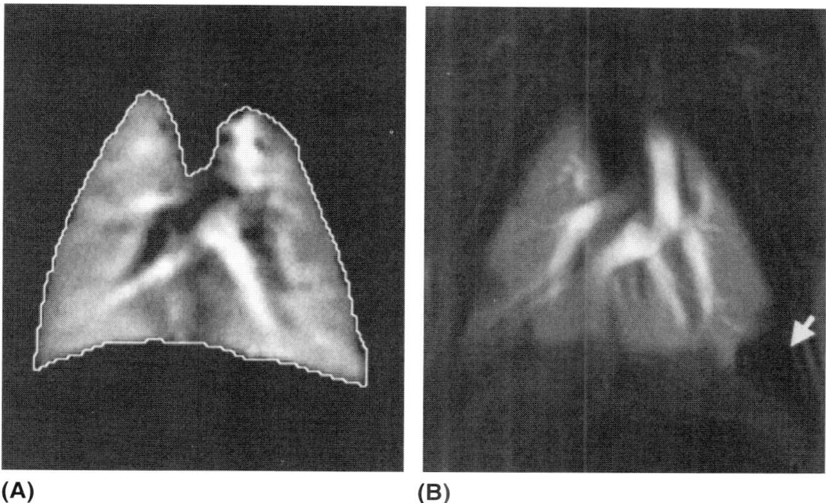

Figure 10 Pulmonary embolism model: mismatch of normal O_2 MR ventilation (A) and gadolinium DTPA MR perfusion (B) with perfusion defect in left base (arrow).

ventilation was assessed using aerosolized gadopentetate dimeglumine as a T1 contrast agent and pulmonary perfusion was assessed with intravenous administration of polylysine gadopentetate dimeglumine. Their results confirmed that simultaneous assessment of ventilation and perfusion improved the specificity of contrast-enhanced perfusion MR imaging. The same group has also used hyperpolarized ^{3}He as the inhalation agent to assess lung ventilation function, along with lung perfusion proton imaging using contrast agent injection. Both imaging techniques have been implemented using projection-reconstruction sequences with free induction decay signal acquisitions. Their projection-reconstruction sequences allowed 3D data set acquisition in several minutes without high-performance gradients. They have also demonstrated normal lung ventilation associated with defective lung perfusion on an experimental rat model of pulmonary embolism [54].

The use of combined MR ventilation and perfusion imaging has the potential to have a major impact on the evaluation of pulmonary embolism and a host of other pulmonary disorders. To date, evaluation of pulmonary embolism using MR perfusion and ventilation techniques has generally been employed on a very limited basis. Combined with pulmonary MR angiography, this technique can demonstrate both ventilation/perfusion mismatches

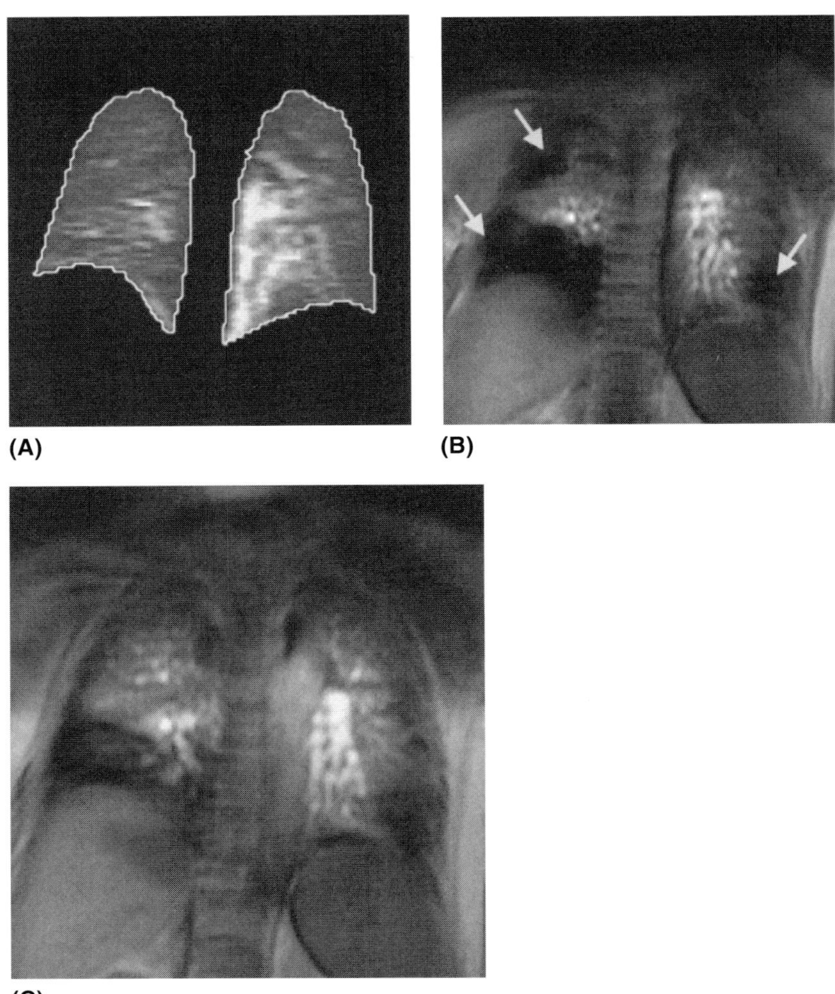

Figure 11 Pulmonary embolism in a patient with iodinated contrast allergy. Mismatch of normal O_2 MR ventilation (A) and gadolinium MR perfusion (B and C) showing reduced perfusion in several areas (arrows).

and the accompanying emboli. However, difficulties may be encountered from the presence of concomitant lung disease. For example, the presence of atelectatic lung leads to an alteration in signal intensity of the lung parenchyma. The effect of this factor upon the detection of small emboli will need to be evaluated in future studies.

VI. FUTURE DEVELOPMENTS

Improvements in the MR evaluation of PE has been driven by the increasing capacities of modern MR systems and underpinned by researchers' innovative approaches on multiple fronts. The possibilities of combining high-resolution imaging of perfusion, ventilation, and angiographic anatomy with MRI are intriguing and could confer a unique advantage in aiding the diagnosis of pulmonary embolic disease. In particular, advances in blood-pool contrast agents, functional imaging, and parallel imaging will likely propel MRI into a larger role in the diagnosis of PE (Fig. 12).

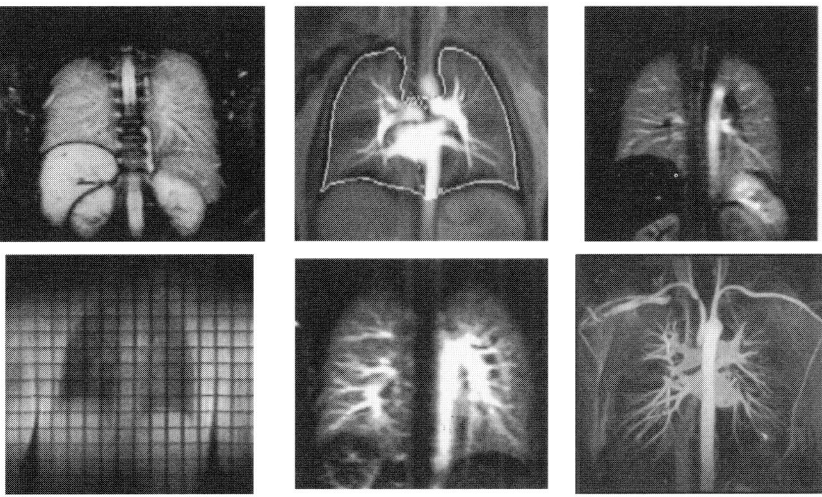

Figure 12 Six-image montage demonstrating potential complete evaluation of pulmonary embolism with examples of anatomic imaging (MIR HASTE), first pass perfusion, ventilation, mechanical deformation (SPAMM), arterial spin labeling (FAIRER), and MR angiography.

VII. CONCLUSION

Magnetic resonance has the ability to simultaneously image pulmonary arteries and the deep venous system for evidence of thromboembolism without iodinated contrast use or radiation exposure. Clinical studies have demonstrated sensitivity in the range of 75 to 100% and specificities between 42 and 90%, depending on the technique employed. MRI technology is still rapidly advancing and clinical accuracy will likely improve as experience with new techniques develops. In present clinical practice, MRI mainly plays a complementary role to conventional methods of diagnosing PE disease. Its lack of ionizing radiation is appealing to subgroups of patients such as pregnant women and young children and absence of iodinated contrast is helpful for assessing patients with renal failure or iodinated contrast allergy.

While CTA is an excellent technique for evaluation of PE, the CT diagnosis is purely morphological and based on relatively limited density information. In contrast, MR can avail of multiple parameters to characterize pathology based on relaxation times, proton density, ventilation, perfusion, diffusion, and susceptibility-induced T2* changes. The improved ability to perform high-quality imaging with high temporal resolution in short-breath-hold periods is clearly an exciting advance. Although the precise role of MRI in the diagnosis of PE remains to be clarified, we believe advances in fast and functional imaging will ensure a place for MRI in the standard diagnostic evaluation of PE in the near future.

Acknowledgment

The authors thank James Carr and Paul Finn of Northwestern Memorial Hospital, Illinois, for their generous help in the preparation of this manuscript.

REFERENCES

1. Bell WR, Simon TI. Current status of pulmonary embolic disease: pathophysiology, diagnosis, prevention and treatment. Am Heart J 1982; 103:239–262.
2. Remy-Jardin M, Remy J, Watinne L, et al. Central pulmonary thromboembolism: diagnosis with spiral volumetric CT with the single breath-hold technique—comparison with pulmonary angiography. Radiology 1992; 185:381–387.
3. Van Rossum AB, Pattynama PM, Tjin ER, et al. Pulmonary embolism: validation of spiral CT angiography in 149 patients. Radiology 1996; 201:467–470.
4. Mayo JR, Remy-Jardin M, Müller N, et al. Pulmonary embolism: prospective

comparison of spiral CT with ventilation-perfusion scintigraphy. Radiology 1997; 205:447–452.

5. Kim K, Müller N, Mayo JR. Clinically suspected pulmonary embolism: utility of spiral CT. Radiology 1999; 210:693–697.
6. Drucker EA, Rivitz SM, Shepard JO, et al. Acute pulmonary embolism: assessment of helical CT for diagnosis. Radiology 1998; 209:235–241.
7. Goodman LR, Curtin JJ, Mewissen MW, et al. Detection of pulmonary embolism in patients with unresolved clinical and scintigraphic diagnosis: helical CT vs angiography. Am J Roentgenol 1995; 164:1369–1374.
8. Remy-Jardin M, Remy J, Deschildre F, et al. Diagnosis of pulmonary embolism with spiral CT: comparison with pulmonary angiography and scintigraphy. Radiology 1996; 200:699–706.
9. Loud PA, Katz DS, Klippenstein DL, et al. ZD Combined CT venography and pulmonary angiography in suspected thromboembolic disease: diagnostic accuracy for deep venous evaluation. Am J Roentgenol 2000; 174(1):61–65.
10. Hidajat N, Maurer J, Schroder R, et al. Radiation exposure in spiral computed tomography—dose distribution and dose reduction. Invest Radiol 1999; 34:51–57.
11. PIOPED Investigators. Value of the ventilation/perfusion scan in acute pulmonary embolism: results of the prospective investigation of pulmonary embolism diagnosis (PIOPED). J Am Med Assoc 1990; 263:2753–2759.
12. Perrier A, Demaris S, Goehring C. D-Dimer testing for suspected pulmonary embolism in outpatients. Am J Respir Crit Care Med 1997; 156:492–496.
13. Zuckerman DA, Sterling KM, Oser RF. Safety of pulmonary angiography in the 1990s. J Vas Interven Radiol 1996; 7:199–205.
14. Remy-Jardin M, Remy J, Artaud D, et al. Peripheral pulmonary arteries: Optimization of spiral CT acquisition protocol. Radiology 1997; 204:157–163.
15. Oser RF, Zuckerman DA, Gutierrez FR, et al. Anatomic distribution of pulmonary emboli at pulmonary angiography; Implications for cross-sectional imaging. Radiology 1996: 199:31–35.
16. Bergin CJ, Glover GH, Pauly JM, Lung parenchyma: magnetic susceptibility in MR imaging. Radiology 1991; 180:845–848.
17. Erdman WA, Peshocj RM, Redman HC, et al. Comparison of MR images with radionuclide and angiographic studies. Radiology 1994; 190:499–508.
18. Fischer MR, Higgins CB. Central thrombi in pulmonary arterial hypertension detected by MR imaging. Radiology 1986; 158:223–226.
19. Posteraro RH, Sostman HD, Spritzer CE, et al. Cine gradient refocused MR imaging of central pulmonary emboli. Am J Roentgenol 1989; 152:465–468.
20. Hatabu H, Gefter WB, Axel L, et al. MR imaging with spatial modulation of magnetization in the evaluation of chronic central pulmonary thrombo-emboli. Radiology 1994; 190:791–796.
21. Foo T, MacFall J, Hayes C, et al. Pulmonary vasculature: single breath-hold MR imaging with phased-array coils. Radiology 1992; 183:473–477.
22. Schiebler M, Holland G, Hatabu H, et al. Suspected pulmonary embolism: pro-

spective evaluation with pulmonary MR angiography. Radiology 1993; 189:125–131.
23. Grist T, Sostman H, MacFall J, et al. Pulmonary angiography with MR imaging: preliminary clinical experience. Radiology 1993; 189:523–530.
24. Wielopolski P, Haacke E, Adler L, et al. Three-dimensional MR imaging of the pulmonary vasculature: preliminary experience. Radiology 1992; 183:465–472.
25. McFall JR, Sostman HD, Foo TK, et al. Thick section, single breath-hold magnetic resonance pulmonary angiography. Invest Radiol 1992; 27:318–322.
26. Creasy J, Price R, Presbrey T, et al. Gadolinium-enhanced MR angiography. Radiology 1990; 175:280–283.
27. Prince M. Gadolinium-enhanced MR aortography. Radiology 1994; 191:155–164.
28. Loubeyre P, Revel D, Douek P, et al. Dynamic contrast-enhanced MR angiography of pulmonary embolism: comparison with pulmonary angiography. Am J Roentgenol 1994; 162:1035–1039.
29. Meaney J, Weg J, Chenevert T, et al. Diagnosis of pulmonary embolism with magnetic resonance angiography. N Engl J Med 1997; 336:1422–1427.
30. Gupta A, Frazer C, Ferguson J, et al. Acute pulmonary embolism: diagnosis with MR angiography. Radiology 1999; 210:353–359.
31. Carr JC, Laub G, Simonetti O, et al. Time resolved pulmonary angiography and perfusion imaging with MR. Am J Roentgenol (Abstract Supplement) 2000; 174(3):83.
32. Hatabu H, Gaa J, Kim D, et al. Pulmonary perfusion: qualitative assessment with dynamic contrast-enhanced MRI using ultra-short TE and inversion recovery turbo FLASH. Magn Reson Med 1996; 36(4):503–508.
33. Chen Q, Levin D, Kim D, et al. Pulmonary disorders: ventilation-perfusion MR imaging with animal models. Radiology 1999; 213:871–879.
34. Chen Q, David V, Levin DL, et al. Ventilation-Perfusion MRI of Pulmonary Embolism. Proceedings of the Sixth Annual Meeting of the International Society for Magnetic Resonance in Medicine 1998; 1:453.
35. Stock KW, Chen Q, Levin, D, et al. Demonstration of gravity-dependent lung perfusion with contrast-enhanced magnetic resonance imaging. Journal of Magnetic Resonance Imaging. 1999; 9(4):557–61.
36. Berthezene Y, Croisille P, Wiart M, et al. Prospective comparison of MR lung perfusion and lung scintigraphy. J Magn Reson Imag. 1999; 9(1):61–68.
37. Hatabu H, Gaa J, Kim D, et al. Pulmonary perfusion and angiography: evaluation with breath-hold enhanced three-dimensional fast imaging steady-state precession MR imaging with short TR and TE. Am J Roentgenol 1996; 167:653–655.
38. Hatabu H, Wielopolski PA, Tadamura E. An attempt of pulmonary perfusion imaging utilizing ultrashort echo time turbo FLASH sequence with signal targeting and alternating radio-frequency (STAR). Eur J of Radiol 1999; 29(2):160–163.
39. Mai VM, Berr SS. MR perfusion imaging of pulmonary parenchyma using pulsed

arterial spin labeling techniques: FAIRER and FAIR. J Magn Reson Imag 1999; 9:483–487.
40. Mai VM, Hagspiel KD, Christopher, JM, et al. Noninvasive MR perfusion imaging of pulmonary parenchyma using flow-sensitive alternating inversion recovery with an extra radiofrequency pulse (FAIRER). Magn Reson Imag 1999; 17: 355–361.
41. Edelman RR, Hatabu H, Tadamura E, et al. Noninvasive assessment of regional ventilation in the human lung using oxygen-enhanced magnetic resonance imaging. Nature Med 1996; 2(11):1236–1239.
42. Chen Q, Jakob P, Griswold M, et al. Oxygen enhanced MR ventilation imaging of the lung. MAGMA 1998; 7:153–161.
43. Stock K, Chen Q, Morrin M, et al. Oxygen-enhanced magnetic resonance ventilation imaging of the human lung at 0.2 and 1.5T. J Magn Reson Imag 1999; 9: 838–841.
44. Turner R, Lebihan D, Moonen CT, et al. Echo-planar time course MRI of cat brain oxygenation changes. Magn Reson Med 1991; 22:159–166.
45. Schreiber WG, Weiler N, Kauczor HU, et al. Ultrafast MRI of lung ventilation using hyperpolarized Helium-3. Rofo Fortschr Geb Rontgenstr Neuen Bildgeb 2000; 172:129–133.
46. Kauczor HU, Hofmann D, Kreitner KF, et al. Normal and abnormal pulmonary ventilation: visualization at hyperpolarized He-3 MR imaging. Radiology 1996; 201(2):564–568.
47. Bachert P, Schad LR, Bock M, et al. Nuclear magnetic resonance imaging of airways in humans with use of hyperpolarized 3He. Magn Reson Med 1996; 36(2):192–196.
48. Mugler JP III, Driehuys B, Brookeman JR, et al. MR imaging and spectroscopy using hyperpolarized 129Xe gas: preliminary human results. Magn Reson Med 1997; 37(6):809–815.
49. Johnson GA, Cates G, Chen XJ, et al. Dynamics of magnetization in hyperpolarized gas MRI of the lung. Magn Reson Med 1997; 38(1):66–71.
50. Chen Q, Jakob PM, David V, et al. Oxygen enhanced ventilation MRI of the human lungs. Proceedings of Fifth Annual Meeting of the International Society for Magnetic Resonance in Medicine. Vancouver, Canada, 1997.
51. Sodickson DK, Manning WJ. Simultaneous acquisition of spatial harmonics (SMASH) fast imaging with radiofrequency array coil arrays. Magn Reson Med 1997; 38:591–603.
52. Pruessmann KP, Weiger M, Scheidegger MB, et al. SENSE: sensitivity encoding for fast MRI. Magn Reson Med. 1999; 42(5):952–962.
53. Berthezene Y, Vexler V, Clement O, et al. Contrast-enhanced MR imaging of the lung: assessments of ventilation and perfusion. Radiology 1992; 183:667–672.
54. Cremillieux Y, Berthezene Y, Humblot H, et al. A combined 1H perfusion/3He ventilation NMR study in rat lungs. Magn Reson Med. 1999; 41(4):645–648.

13
Digital Chest Radiography

Matthew Freedman
Georgetown University
Washington, DC

I. THE IDEAL CHEST IMAGE

The chest radiograph is a complex image containing information on many structures in the thorax. In this image, one can see the lungs and their diseases; the pulmonary vessels and their diseases; the heart; the mediastinum; the bony thorax; the chest wall; and portions of the neck, abdomen, and arms. Because of the great differences in the absorption and inherent tissue contrast in these regions, the ideal chest radiograph has conflicting requirements. All current chest radiographs, both analog and digital, represent compromises to accommodate these conflicting optimal requirements. Digital radiography currently comes closer to meeting these requirements than analog radiography, but current systems are still not able to produce the ideal image and further developments are needed.

In the ideal chest image, one would want to be able to assess each structure in the chest with sufficient contrast to detect disease and sufficient resolution to define the structural features of what is seen. The fundamental problem in chest radiography is that the absorption of different parts of the chest varies widely and the inherent contrast of different structures—the inherent differences in absorption of different tissues—varies widely. To ''create'' an ideal chest radiograph, one must consider both general regional differences in absorption and the local differences in the absorption of the tissues within the region. One needs an image that accommodates the large differences in regional absorption within the mediastinum and the local differences in absorption, such as visualization of the structures within the lung. For the bedside chest examination, we need one that either has some method for automatic exposure control (AEC) or that uses some method of postprocessing of the image to correct for exposure differences among images that are very difficult to control in standard chest radiography where both under- and overexposure are common.

Digital radiography helps to overcome this problem of varying exposures in bedside radiography [1,2]. In one study, beside screen–film radiographs had a mean lung optical density of 2.43 with a standard deviation of 0.31. High lung optical density was used to provide adequate mediastinal density to visualize the tubes within the mediastinum, an important part of the evaluation of post-cardiac-surgery patients. Digital radiographs had an average lung density of 1.44, standard deviation 0.13 [2]. Digital chest radiographs were closer to the optimum optical density recommended by the International Labor Organization (hilar regions at a minimum of 0.2 optical density units above fog; parenchymal regions at a maximum of 1.8 units of optical density above fog) [3] and showed less variation film to film and patient to patient, allowing easier comparison.

Image processing of digital chest radiographs allows one to adjust partially for the regional differences in absorption and to enhance the contrast of specific structures within the lung. While such corrections can improve the image, they are only a partial solution to the problems in projection chest radiography. There are three main substances that absorb and scatter X-ray photons: air, water, and calcium. The variable absorption and scattering encode the original X-ray beam with information. Only those X-ray photons that reach the detector are used to form the image, so if the photons are absorbed or scattered sufficiently, they do not reach the detector. Air absorbs and scatters the least, calcium the most. The thickness of each of these substances also affects absorption; the more there is of any of these substances in the path of the X-ray beam, the more it absorbs and scatters. For each portion of the chest, the proportion of the X-rays reaching the image recording system will depend on the types of substances in the X-ray beam and their combined thickness for each location in the projected image. The chest has a wide range of absorption differences. If one attempts to display the entire range of absorption differences, two things can happen: either the image is of low contrast, or some areas are of high contrast and others of low contrast. The standard screen–film chest radiograph is generally presented as an image where the contrast in the lungs is moderately high and that in the mediastinum and projected over the upper abdomen is relatively low. The areas of lower contrast, however, may contain important details in the image. Digital chest radiography can be adjusted so that these areas of lower contrast are altered to become regions of higher contrast, while leaving the contrast of the lungs nearly unchanged.

A. Requirements for the Lungs

In the region of the image where the lungs are projected, there is far less water density material to absorb and scatter the X-rays than there is in the mediastinum and lateral chest wall. For this reason, the lung regions need less X-ray exposure than the mediastinum to produce an image of appropriate optical density (for an analog system) or appropriate signal-to-noise (for a digital system). Ideally, the maximum contrast between the vessels, interstitium, and the air in the lungs is desired. Current analog and digital images must compromise on this because of the differences in the thickness and absorbing characteristics of different parts of the chest. In general, because there is less air and more water and calcium absorption in the lateral and apical portions of the lung, the region projected behind the heart and in the lung area projected behind the diaphragm, these areas require more exposure. Unfortunately, the exposure level necessary for these regions to have an ideal exposure is excessive for the lungs and would make them very dark, sufficient to obscure disease. With digital chest images, different settings can be used to adjust the density range of the image, allowing one to gain optimum settings for each of these regions, but at a cost of the time required to make these separate adjustments.

Special Requirements for the Lung Apices

The clavicles and the upper ribs (which are more closely spaced than the lower ribs) overlie the lung apices. The presence of these bony structures can obscure underlying lung disease. In addition, the apical lung is relatively small, so that processes are more likely to reach a pleural surface. When a process reaches a pleural surface, it tends to extend along the surface, thus losing its sharp edge, making it harder to identify. In the ideal image, one would want to decrease the degree to which the bony structures obscure the apical lung. There are two current and one future method that can help accomplish this. The first is to obtain the chest radiograph at the highest kilovolt peak possible since the absorption differences between calcium and water decrease with increasing kilovolts. With a higher kilovolt peak, any lung process becomes more equal in density to the bone projected over it. The second method is to use energy subtraction. With this method (described below), special image acquisition and image processing can form an image in which the bone is largely subtracted away. Special equipment and image processing are necessary for this technique. Third, experimentally, several groups are developing temporal subtraction chest radiography. If one has two chest radiographs that are similar in their positioning, it is possible to process them so that they are nearly superimposed. Once superimposed, the computer can subtract one image from the other. The bony structures are unlikely to change, while the lung can develop pneumonias, cancers, and so on. Thus, the subtraction image provides a potentially better view for the detection of change in the apical lung. This technique is demonstrated below.

Special Requirements for Lateral Margin of the Chest

Because of the generally ovoid shape of the lungs, there is less lung and there are more chest wall structures near the edges of the chest. This increase in soft tissue and bony structures results in the lungs appearing more opaque (whiter) peripherally than centrally. This factor, combined with the shadows from female or male breast tissue, makes it harder to show lung detail with maximum contrast. If one chooses maximum contrast centrally, the lung periphery may be underexposed. Equalizing these lung densities across the chest should enhance the ability to use higher contrast imaging of the lungs.

Special Requirements for the Region Projected behind the Heart and Diaphragm

Portions of the lungs project behind the heart and behind the diaphragm. These areas are difficult to visualize on screen–film chest radiographs because of the larger amount of water density absorbers there than over the central portions of the lungs and because there is less lung tissue. A lateral view of the chest partially compensates for this, but not completely. Moreover, with bedside chest radiographs, a lateral view is often not feasible. Image processing can partially correct this density difference. One method is to increase the optical density of the entire image when one looks at these regions and then use a different processing setting to look at the central portions of the lungs (Figs. 1a and 1b). A second technique is to use regional density equalization methods to enhance these regions (Figs. 2a and 2b). Because the blackness of a film can be adjusted by image processing, it can be more difficult to assess whether there is disease behind the heart or whether this region is simply underexposed (since image processing can make it as black as one could desire). A useful guide is that the region is adequately exposed for lung disease if one can see

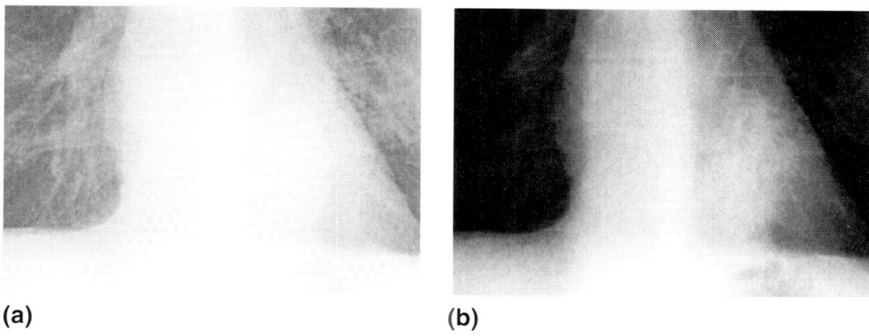

Figure 1 (a and b) Improved detection of retrocardiac pneumonia using image processing. A small area of pneumonia behind the heart can be seen on both images, but is more conspicuous on the image that has been processed to be darker (b).

the ribs projected through the heart. If the ribs cannot be seen, the image is underexposed and the failure to see normal lung vessels is not a sign of disease (Fig. 3). The same rule applies for the assessment of mediastinal tubes. If the spine can be seen, the exposure should be adequate for the detection of tubes and lines. Be aware, however, that some noise-suppression algorithms can obscure tubes while maintaining some degree of visibility of larger structures, such as the spine.

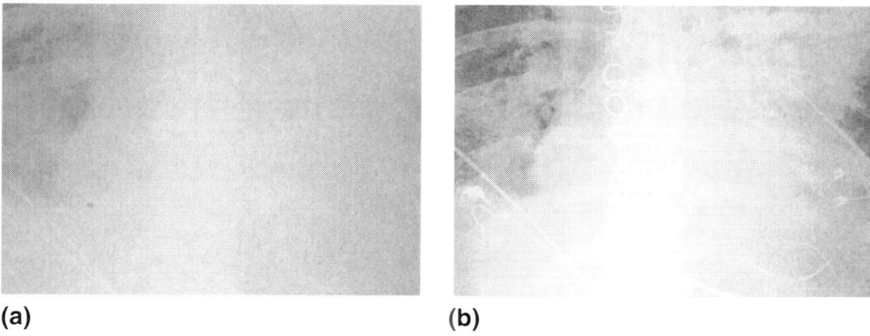

Figure 2 (a and b) Improved visualization of retrocardiac tubes and lines by using optical density equalization algorithm. The tubes and lines are better visualized on image b, in which optical density equalization has been applied.

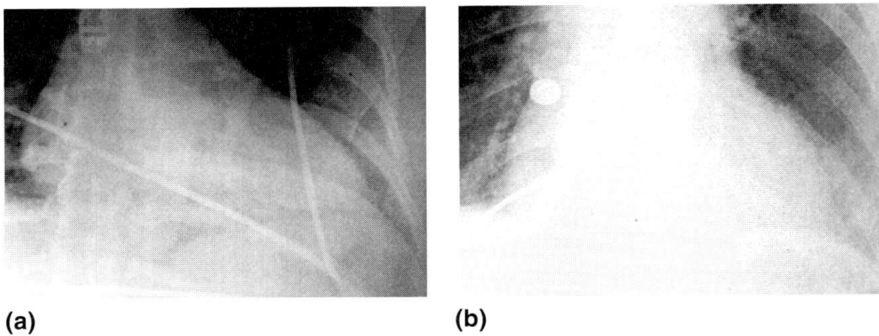

(a) **(b)**

Figure 3 Effect of exposure factors on assessment of the retrocardiac region. (a) Retrocardiac atelectasis is visible; the ribs can be seen. (b) Retrocardiac area cannot be evaluated; the ribs cannot be seen. Underexposed film with Fuji ''S'' of 8955 (the ''S'' number of a properly exposed chest radiograph is approximately 200–400). Due to underexposure, one cannot tell whether there is retrocardiac airspace disease or effusion. The system has, however, permitted overcorrection of the density of the lungs to be blacker than those of a properly exposed bedside chest radiograph.

B. Special Requirements for Specific Disease Processes

Pneumothorax

On both screen–film and digital chest radiographs, pneumothoraces may be difficult to detect. Detection of a pneumothorax depends on the detection of two findings: the first is the radiolucency of the lung outside of the edge of the lung; the second is the detection of the lung edge. Because digital image processing can change the density of regions of the image, density equalization programs may make the radiolucency harder to detect. The pleural edge can be very thin and can be superimposed on the ribs. Detection of the edge of the lung depends somewhat on the thickness of that edge, which varies among individuals. Using a slight degree of image processing to enhance edges increases the conspicuity of the lung edge and makes it easier to see the pneumothorax (Fig. 4). When the edge of the lung is superimposed on a rib, a low-kilovolt-peak chest X-ray technique may make it harder to see the lung edge because the relative radiodensity of the lung is increased, therefore a high-kilovolt-peak technique is preferred. The outer 2 cm of the lungs are more radiolucent than the more central portion since there is less lung, fewer blood vessels, and therefore less tissue density. If the image is too dark, it may become quite difficult to see detail in this region. If you are using a workstation to look at the image, making the image lighter can enhance the conspicuity of a pneumothorax. In carefully controlled settings, the detection of pneumothoraces on screen–film and digital images has been shown to be equivalent [4,5,6].

Emphysema

The edges of emphysematous bullae and blebs are often very fine curved lines. Such lines can be blurred by the penumbra resulting from the X-ray tube focal spot. Small degrees of edge enhancement can enhance the conspicuity of these structures. For this reason, it can be easier to detect small amounts of emphysema on digital images (Fig. 4).

Interstitial Disease

Edge enhancement will increase the conspicuity of normal lung structures and interstitial lung disease. With edge enhancement, several reports document no difference in detection of interstitial lung disease [4,7,8]. Without edge enhancement, one study [9] showed that interstitial disease is less conspicuous (Figs. 5a–5c).

Interstitial disease is composed of fine and coarse lines and nodules. The conspicuity of these can be increased by a small amount of edge enhancement. The interstitial disease seen on digital chest radiographs, when minimal, may be quite difficult to see on conventional screen–film chest radiographs.

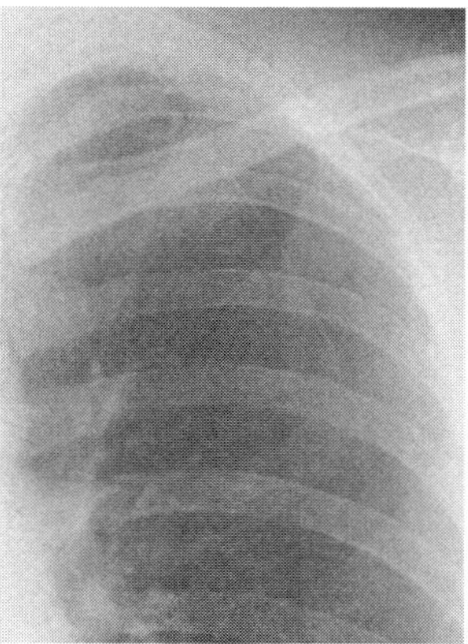

Figure 4 Pneumothorax detection in a 22-year-old male with a spontaneous pneumothorax. The pneumothorax is visible laterally. A few very small blebs are minimally visible at the apex of the lung.

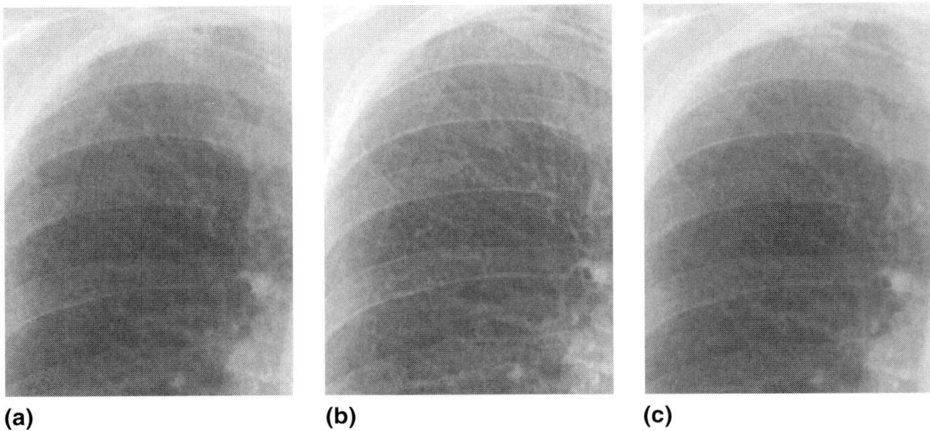

Figure 5 Effect of edge enhancement algorithm on detection of interstitial lung disease in patient with methotrexate induced interstitial lung disease. Interstitial disease shown with no edge enhancement (a), standard edge enhancement (b), and exaggerated edge enhancement (c). Increasing enhancement accentuates the fine curved fibrotic lines. However, the small nodules are better seen in the less enhanced images. A small degree of edge enhancement (b) shows the pattern of interstitial disease best.

Thus, one is likely to detect minimal interstitial disease more often on the digital images. At the same time, the vessels may be more conspicuous on digital chest radiographs, so it is important to carefully assess visible lines. In general, if the lines branch, they are vessels; if they fail to branch, they are likely interstitial lines. On underexposed images, the noise can become visible and may simulate very small, miliarylike nodules. Figure 3b shows the nodular appearance of noise on a severely underexposed film. Conversely, the use of a blurring algorithm to decrease the visibility of noise may also blur fine interstitial lines and nodules decreasing their conspicuity, particularly if they are in lighter areas of the image.

Masses and Nodules

Digital chest radiography has not resulted in problems in the detection of small lung nodules [4,7,8,10,11]. Nodules superimposed on the mediastinum have been shown to be easier to detect on digital compared to screen–film chest radiographs [10,12]. Because the contrast scale on digital chest radiographs can be changed, it may be more difficult to tell if a nodule is calcified. However, when techniques of image processing are standardized, this problem does not occur. The detection equivalence of lung nodules is seen when appropriate image processing is used [12]. Inappropriate image processing of digital chest radiographs, however, can decrease the visibility of lung nodules. The conspicuity of lung nodules is equivalent with high-kilovolt-peak, high-contrast images. On the other hand, if the image processing produces a low-contrast image or if a low-kilovolt-peak image results in increased conspicuity of the ribs, nodules may be less visible (Fig. 6).

The detection of large lung masses and large areas of pneumonia may appear different on digital images when regional density equalization algorithms are used. These density equalization algorithms may partially equalize their density so they may not appear as dense for their size as they would on screen–film images.

Detection of Calcium in Lung Nodules. Digital image processing allows one to change the contrast of the chest image. Calcium in lung nodules is detected by two findings: first, the identification of the irregular shape of the calcifications and second by the greater density of nodule for its size than would be expected for a noncalcified nodule. While the first sign remains unchanged with digital images, image processing can change the contrast of a nodule compared to its background, making it appear more radiodense or less radiodense. If techniques for image processing are standardized, there is usually no problem, but if one varies the image processing technique for different patients, it may be confusing to the radiologist.

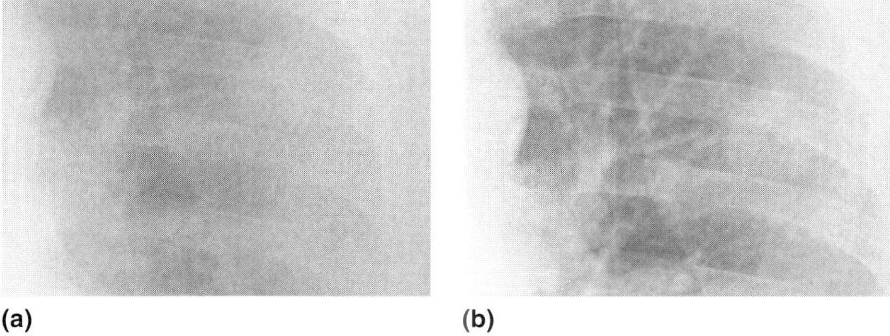

(a) (b)

Figure 6 Effect of edge and contrast enhancement on lung nodule detection. Non-small-cell primary lung cancer in the periphery of the left upper lobe shown (a) without and (b) with minimal edge and contrast enhancement. The mass is more easily seen with the edge and contrast enhancement.

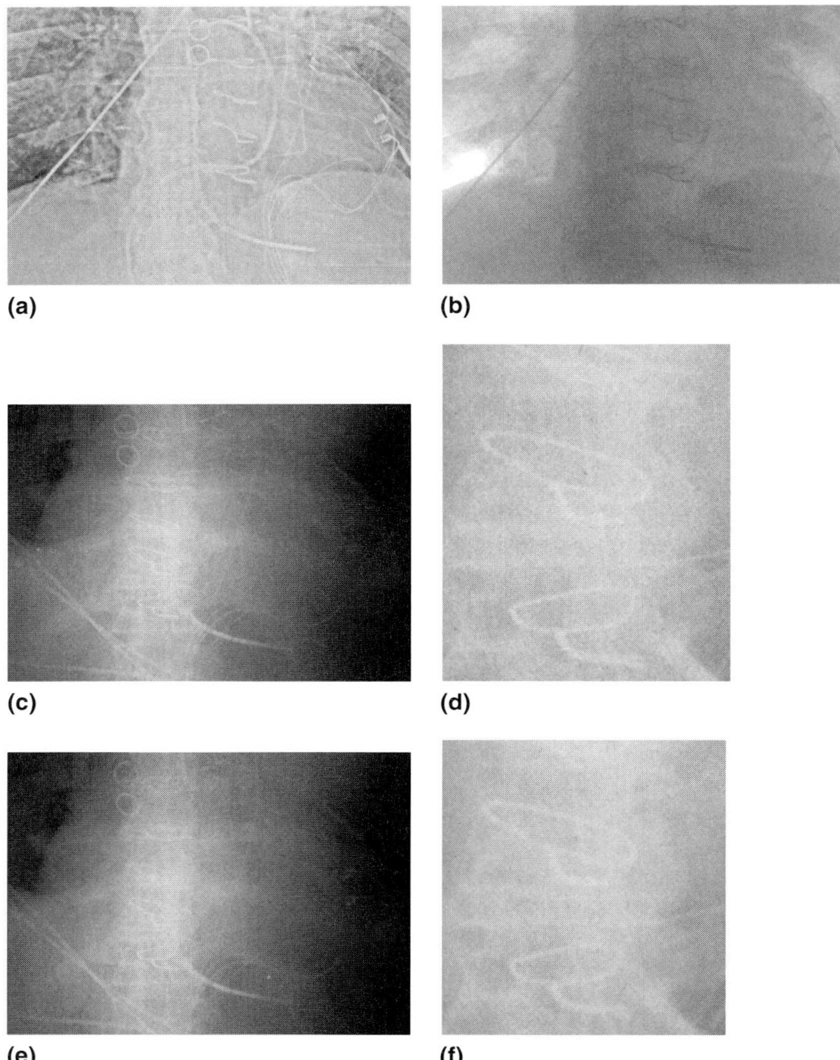

Figure 7 Assessment of lines and tubes using digital radiography. Retrocardiac tubes shown with DRC plus edge enhancement (a) and black/white inversion (b). (c) Same patient, different day. Film is underexposed. Noise is more visible on local view shown in d. (d) Same image as c, but a local view. The noise is visible, but the edges of the lines can be seen. (e) Image blurring has been used to decrease visible noise. (f) Same image as (e), but a local view. Lines blurred by image smoothing, and less noise is visible. The edges of the lines are harder to see as compared to those in d.

Requirements for the Mediastinum

In the mediastinum and chest wall, there is much more water density material to absorb and scatter the X-rays. The absorption difference between normal structures and the findings of mediastinal disease (such as lymph nodes) is relatively low. For this reason, one would ideally want to have high contrast to see the anatomic changes in the mediastinum and a higher exposure than we need to see the lungs. Digital chest radiographs have been shown to enhance the visibility of mediastinal structures [10,13].

Special Requirements for Seeing Tubes and Devices in the Mediastinum. Especially in bedside examinations, identifying the location of tubes and lines within the mediastinum is of great importance since a misdirected line may have serious consequences for the patient. Digital chest radiography allows one to enhance the identification of the locations of these tubes and lines using three different methods (Fig. 7a–c). The first is to increase the optical density of the image so that the mediastinum is projected in the maximum contrast density of the film or monitor one is using. The second is to black/white invert the image. The third is to use density equalization algorithms. If the film is properly exposed, any of these techniques will usually suffice. If the image is underexposed, the necessary information may not have been captured.

Digital radiography software allows one to smooth the image to make the noise that occurs in regions of low exposure less visible. This smoothing may also smooth the edges of tubes and lines making them less visible (Fig. 7c–f). For this reason, we prefer to have a somewhat noisy-appearing mediastinum on our images since that increases the chance that we will be able to identify the edges of the tubes and lines.

II. DIGITAL RADIOGRAPHY VERSUS ANALOG RADIOGRAPHY

A. Analog Chest Radiography

Analog radiography is the commonly used method of acquiring chest radiographs using an X-ray machine, a phosphorescent screen that generates light when exposed to x-rays, and film that is exposed by the light generated by the screen. The film is then processed in chemicals and is viewed on a viewbox or lightbox.

Relationship of Intensity of X-Ray Exposure to Degree of Blackness on Film

In the standard form of chest radiography, the degree of blackness in each part of the film is related to the exposure of the phosphorescent screen to X-ray photons. The response of the film is determined by its characteristic curve of response, a curve that is usually S-shaped. This characteristic curve is usually divided into three parts, the bottom (or toe), the midportion, and the top (or shoulder). Exposure of the film in the midpoint results in a near-linear relationship of exposure to film blackening. Exposures in the bottom (or toe) region and the top (or shoulder) region have nonlinear responses. Most importantly, in these regions, the degree of darkening for any set amount of increase or decrease in exposure results in less change in blackening than the same exposure change in the midportion. This means that the contrast in the bottom and top of the curve is less than that in the midportion.

Factors Affecting Contrast

The phosphorescent screens used in analog chest radiography vary in the amount of light they produce for each unit of X-ray exposure and in their resolution. Films vary in their contrast scale (how steep the mid portion of the characteristic curve is) and in the shape of that curve. They also vary in resolution, but it is the screen rather than the film that has the greatest effect on resolution.

Contrast in analog radiography depends on the contrast inherent in the film used, in the screen used, on the kilovolt peak used to form the image, and on the methods used for film processing. One can choose a specific level of contrast for the entire image by selecting an appropriate screen–film combination or a specific set of film development parameters. One can change the contrast on a specific film by adjusting the kilovolt peak. A higher kilivolt-peak range produces a lower contrast image. These traditional methods, however, do not allow one to specifically alter the contrast in a specific region of the image.

Asymmetric Screen Film Analog Methods

Special asymmetric screen–film combinations have been developed that have different characteristics on their front and back surfaces. In these special combinations, the back screen and the back side of the film emulsion have been made to provide increase blackening predominately in regions of low intrinsic exposure, such as in the mediastinum and behind the heart. These regions are enhanced by the special systems, but with lower contrast than the remainder of the image. They provide at least some of the advantages of digital optical density equalization algorithms [14].

Size of Analog Images

Depending on the analog methods used, the image can be close to life size, enlarged, or decreased in size.

B. Digital Methods

Digital chest radiography is a method by which a chest radiograph is obtained as or converted into computer readable form. There are three basic forms (1) digitization of an analog chest radiograph (sometimes called digitized radiography), (2) storage devices that capture the exposure with delayed extraction of image data [computed radiography (CR) or storage phosphor radiography are common names for one type; digital selenium radiography is a competing type], and (3) exposure capture systems that in near real-time convert the analog exposure information to digital data [these are sometimes called direct radiography (DR) systems]. Each of these three methods for obtaining digital images provides generally similar advantages, but they are not equivalent.

The advantages of digital methods is that they allow the separation of four different parts that are included in an analog system: acquisition of image data representing different amounts of X-ray exposure, image processing (or enhancement), image storage, and image display. Image processing and enhancement by computer provides the main disease detection and diagnostic advantage of digital methods. Image storage and retrieval provides the main economic argument for its benefit.

Film Digitization

Film digitization was the first method applied to obtain digital chest data and still has specific indications. It is by far the cheapest in equipment costs, but because of film handling, it has the highest labor costs.

In film digitization, the film is placed in a special machine that shines light through the film. The light may be broad spectrum, narrow spectrum, or laser light. In regions of the film radiograph where the image is more transparent, more light is transmitted, and in regions where the image is more opaque (blacker areas), less light is transmitted. Because the signal-to-noise ratio varies with the amount of light transmitted, there is more noise in dark areas of the original image. In general, in chest radiography, this is not a problem if the original image was of high quality, since there should be no very dark regions of the image. If the lungs are too dark, however, information may be lost. More important is the effect in the more transparent parts of the chest image (for example, behind the heart). In these regions, the original film image is often of low contrast and this low contrast is maintained in the digitized image. Image processing may not be sufficient to restore the contrast.

Application of Film Digitization. Film digitization provides an important economic advantage in providing teleradiology from low-volume sites. If one starts with high-quality radiographs, the transmitted images can be interpreted with an accuracy similar to that for the original film. A high-quality original image is a necessity.

Chest films, once digitized, can also be used for digital storage and for use in computer aided diagnosis systems.

Techniques to Enhance the Quality of Digitized Film Chest Radiography. Analog chest radiographs have regions of high contrast and low contrast, high optical density and low optical density. Film digitizers will produce the best digital data for teleradiology in regions of high contrast and medium optical density. The best way to achieve an optimal analog image for teleradiology is to acquire the image with a lower contrast scale than would normally be used for nonteleradiology purposes. One can do this by using a screen–film system with relatively low contrast. If one acquires relatively low-contrast data, one can use image processing to recreate a high-contrast image and can process it for both the mediastinum and lungs. If one starts with a high-contrast image, the region behind the heart and in the mediastinum may be underexposed and image processing may not provide sufficient enhancement. Film digitizers are designed to capture information from a specified range of film optical densities. If one exceeds the optimal range, the digitizer may not capture all of the information. Different digitizers have different optimal ranges. In general, less expensive digitizers have a more limited optimum range. The type of film digitizer selected should be based on the optical density of the films to be digitized.

Digital Systems That Capture the Image Data for Delayed Data Extraction: Computed Radiography and Digital Selenium Radiography

In this second type of digital chest radiography system, the X-rays produce a change in the charge in a flat plate of material that can then be moved to a reader that extracts the image. Currently, most available commercial systems use special phosphor imaging plates to store the data. The X-rays are encoded with information as they pass through the patient's body and interact with a special phosphor material that both produces some light but also stores an electron charge in its molecules. When this plate with stored data is exposed to a laser, the electron charges are released, producing a new flash of light that can be detected, amplified, and used to create an image. To produce the image, the laser is scanned over the imaging plate and the light emitted at each point is recorded along with its location. The initial flash of light is measured using analog methods but is then converted to digital format through a device called an analog-to-digital converter. From that point on, it is handled as digital data. Systems are available from several sources and some of these systems are called computed radiography.

The Imaging Plates Are Usually Placed in a Cassette. The advantages of this type of system are that it uses cassettes that are the same size as standard screen–film cassettes and these cassettes can be transported from many radiographic rooms to one plate reader. The use of cassettes also allows use of the system for bedside chest radiographs. Because one system can serve as the imaging plate reader for multiple rooms, this technique is the most cost-effective current method for digital chest radiography. Once the equipment is purchased, it may have a small cost advantage compared to screen–film systems in that the number of repeat films for incorrect exposure decreases. The system records a wider range of exposures than the analog screen film systems normally used for chest radiography. It therefore provides a better set of data than digitized screen–film radiographs for image processing.

The disadvantages of this system compared to standard screen–film radiography are its equipment costs. Its disadvantage compared to "direct" digital systems is that it has only a small effect in decreasing labor costs.

There are also digital storage systems that do not use cassettes. These cassetteless systems use an imaging plate or imaging cylinder. Once this plate or cylinder is exposed, it is moved to a different position in the same device where the stored data is extracted. The cylinder system uses a thin layer of selenium on a drum to temporarily store the encoded X-ray information [11].

Data Capture Devices with Near Real-Time Analog-to-Digital Conversion: "Direct" Digital Radiography

The third general type of digital chest radiography system is designed to provide for more immediate output of the digital data. This type is designed so that the X-ray-encoded data is detected by a system into which is embedded the method for extracting the data and converting it to digital format. In this type of system, there is no need for the technologist to move a cassette from the site of acquisition to a separate image plate reader. These devices are based either on selenium or silicon. The silicon methods resemble transistors in their structure. Some use a layer of phosphor to convert the X-ray photons into light that is then detected by the device, and others directly capture the X-ray photon and then extract the stored data. These systems are composed of a tightly packed array of smaller cells. Each of these has a charge produced in it either from direct X-ray photon interaction or from the light produced by the X-ray photon interaction with a phosphor. The charge is extracted as an analog signal and then converted within the device into a digital signal by an analog-to-digital converter.

These devices provide an important advantage in that they provide digital data in near real-time. This allows the technologist to rapidly survey the image to see if it needs to be repeated. Because of this time-saving aspect for the technologist, productivity can be increased. In theory, the efficiency of the detection of X-rays can be greater than that of the phosphor storage systems.

The main disadvantage of these systems is that each X-ray room must have its own detector system, thus increasing costs. Currently, these systems are not suitable for bedside examinations, but this is likely to change in the near future.

The main unknown is that these devices are relatively new and their durability in clinical use is not yet established. These devices are still likely to be in a phase of moderately rapid improvement.

Advantages and Disadvantages of the Various Digital Methods

Briefly, each method for digital chest radiography has advantages and disadvantages. Digitized film is the lowest costs method. It is suitable for low-volume sites. High-quality films are necessary for good-quality results. In particular, the exposure factors must be carefully controlled. This method is moderately labor intensive. The resulting imaging quality can be good to very good.

The Image Storage systems are of intermediate cost and are suitable to moderate to high volume. It can accept images obtained under less optimal conditions and is therefore very well suited for bedside chest radiography. It provides images of very high quality when used for either in-department or bedside examinations. There is a low to moderate improvement in technologist productivity compared to standard screen–film chest radiography.

Near real-time digital radiography systems (''direct'' digital radiography) require that the image recording system is duplicated for each room in which it is used. It is therefore of higher initial cost if several rooms are to be equipped. It provides a greater improvement in technologist productivity that may in some settings justify its cost. It is not currently suitable for bedside chest radiography, but likely will be in the future. Images are of very high quality.

Special Methods of Image Acquisition Using Digital Systems: Dual Energy Methods

Digital techniques make it possible to obtain two separate images with different energy spectra. Calcium shows more of a decrease in X-ray photon absorption than water as the energy of the X-ray photons increases. Because of this difference, if one obtains radiographs with two different X-ray photon energy spectra, it is possible to produce a bone-emphasis or a soft-tissue-emphasis image. Digital acquisition, because of the linear response of the data to X-ray exposure, makes it easier to create these emphasis images. Devices have been built for the storage phosphor systems and could be built for the near real-time systems to produce these images. These images have their main advantage in the apices where the lungs are extensively covered by bone, but may have advantages elsewhere by removing the clutter of the ribs and thereby improving the conspicuity of lung lesions. Dual energy methods are further discussed and examples are shown below.

X-Ray System Effects on Acquired Data

The X-ray system used to produce the X-ray photons for chest radiographs has a major effect on the quality of the resulting analog or digital chest radiograph. Three effects are of greatest importance: kilovolt peak (kVp), penumbra based on focal spot size, and patient motion (related to exposure time). Because image processing can make images look better, one could be misled to think that these postprocessing methods of contrast and edge enhancement available on digital images can correct for technical flaws in image acquisition. Image processing only partially corrects for image acquisition errors; thus, high-quality X-ray technique remains very important.

Kilovoltage Peak. In analog systems, high-kilovolt-peak technique is often used to decrease the conspicuity of the ribs based on the relatively lower absorption of X-ray photons by calcium at high compared to low photon energies. For digital chest radiography with storage phosphor methods, lower kilovolt peaks are often recommended since these enhance the absorption of X-ray photons by the imaging plate. One can then reduce the conspicuity of the ribs by image processing. Unfortunately, this method can also decrease the contrast of lung disease and normal lung structures. For this reason, I have chosen to use 125 kVp for my chest radiographs. Three phase systems produce a better energy spectrum for chest radiography. There does not appear to be a diagnostic accuracy study [such as a receiver operating characteristic (ROC) study] to determine the benefit of a higher vs a lower kilovolt peak.

X-Ray Focal Spot. The X-ray focal spot size and patient motion are the main factors in image blurring. To detect disease, the sharpest image is desired. The focal spot size affects the penumbra along the margins of lung structures. A larger focal spot size will decrease the edge sharpness of lung objects. When these objects are thin interstitial lines, these lines will become less distinct. Digital image processing using edge enhancement methods will restore some of this edge sharpness, but high-quality initial acquisition is more important. For both analog and digital images, one should use the smallest focal spot size that provides sufficient output for a properly exposed image. A maximum focal spot size of 1.2 mm is preferred [15].

Stopping Patient Motion. The second major effect resulting in edge blurring is patient motion. Not all patients can completely stop lung motion when asked to take in a deep breath and hold it. Vessel pulsation is always present and some patients have slight tremors or unsteadiness. The shorter the exposure time, the less likely these factors are to have an effect on the image. For this reason, one should use the highest kilovolt peak, highest milliamperage (mA), and shortest time (s) possible for both analog and digital chest radiography systems. In an individual patient, the best radiograph may result from the use of a larger focal spot with a shorter exposure rather than from the use of the smallest available focal spot.

X-Ray Exposure. One of the great advantages of digital chest radiography is the ability to correct for underexposure and overexposure through digital image processing. The digital receptors have a wider range of acceptable exposure than the screen–film systems used for chest radiography. Importantly, this factor allows them to accommodate variations in exposure to a greater degree than conventional systems. This accommodation, image processing to correct the optical density of the final image, is acceptable for a single image, but careful control of exposure is still important since image processing may not restore the full information content of an underexposed image or, conversely, systematically overexposed images will result in patients receiving higher than necessary X-ray exposures.

The Risk from Overexposure: Overexposure on a digital chest radiograph contains three potential problems. First, the patient is not receiving a dose meeting the "as low as reasonably achievable (ALARA)" recommendation. Second, at sufficiently high exposures, the digital detectors become nonlinear and image quality deteriorates. Third, digital imaging systems are very sensitive to low exposures of radiation. Scatter and backscatter increase as exposure increases. This scattering may produce detectable artifactual images from the back of the cassette or from the back of the digital detector with high exposures. Scatter and backscatter on a collimated image may be sufficiently intense to confuse the part of the computer algorithm that determines the edge of the collimated field. This can result in the computer algorithm overestimating image size, underestimating exposure, and thereby adjusting the image to one in which the lungs are too dark. When using screen–film systems, technologists adjust their exposure settings according to the blackening seen on the resulting films. In digital radiography, the digital system adjusts the resulting image to correct for under- and overexposure. This could result in a risk of systematic overexposure. We have not found this to happen in our facility, but intermittent monitoring of this parameter is recommended [16].

The Decrease in Image Quality from Underexposure: Underexposure increases the noise in the image by decreasing the signal. The digital system provides image processing with smoothing parameters to make the noise less visible. It does this by decreasing the high-spatial-frequency component of the image in regions with low exposure. The problem with this method is that the edges of catheters are of high spatial frequency and this image smoothing may cause them to have low conspicuity or even disappear. When there are very high levels of noise, the noise may start to resemble high-spatial-frequency information in the lungs, either concealing fine interstitial disease or causing the radiologist to report interstitial disease when it is not present.

The Proper Exposure for Digital Systems: The proper level for digital chest radiographic exposures has been established by testing for the Fuji CR® FCR 9000 system to be in the range of a 200- to 400-speed screen–film radiographic system. At lower exposure levels, noise in the mediastinum can obscure the edges of catheters. Systems with improved X-ray photon capture including newer Fuji systems may be usable at lower exposures, but the appropriate exposure range would have to be established for each of these systems through observational or experimental clinical trials.

Automatic Exposure Control and Digital Chest Radiography Systems: The storage phosphor digital systems rely on the AEC device built into the chest cassette holder. Some cassettes used for digital radiography are lead backed.

This can result in an increase in patient exposure compared to a standard screen–film system because the lead will absorb some of the radiation so that the AEC senses less of the exposure that the patient received and does not stop the exposure at the same low level used for conventional screen film–radiographs. When changing to a storage phosphor digital system, the exposure levels used should be checked. On the Fuji system, the average ''s'' number for each technologist should be in the 200–400 range. If it is outside of this range and an AEC device is used, then the AEC device needs to be reset. Intermittent monitoring of technologists as they use the system is recommended to avoid exposure drift. A method for this has been proposed [16].

For the near real-time systems, it is possible for the system to monitor on-line the exposure reaching each cell and to stop exposure once a certain minimum exposure has reached each cell or once an average preset exposure has been reached. Thus, a near real-time digital detector can serve as its own AEC device. In theory, the near real-time devices could be designed to select exposure measurements from any group of cells, potentially enhancing the image quality by better compensating for unusual patient anatomy or extensive disease affecting only one lung (like a severe unilateral pneumonia).

III. IMAGE PROCESSING

Image processing is the computer manipulation of digital image data done with the goal of enhancing image quality. Sometimes the image processing is done to enhance the attractiveness of the image, sometimes it is done to enhance disease conspicuity, and sometimes both attractiveness and conspicuity result at the same time. Image processing is discussed in three different parts: standard commercial methods, special commercial methods, and experimental methods that may potentially provide additional benefits.

A. Currently Available Commercial Image Processing Methods

Currently available image-processing methods produce six different effects on image appearance. They define the ''window of clinically useful exposure data,'' they affect the degree of image blackness and image contrast, they equalize image blackness in different parts of the image, and they provide edge enhancement or provide blurring of noise in parts of the image. The steps described below have been written in a logical progression, but may or may not be actually carried out in this way or in this sequence. More detail on these methods is available [17,18,19].

Defining the "Window of Clinically Useful Exposure Data"

Digital acquisition systems are designed to record data from a wide range of X-ray exposures in a relatively linear relationship of exposure to pixel value. This wide range of recorded exposure is desirable because it can correct for X-ray exposure errors and for patients with different body builds. If one used this "raw" data to create the images, they would be of very low contrast. By design, the width of the window of pixel values set for accepting this information is set very wide.

The raw data that has been received by the imaging device contains both useful and nonuseful exposure data. Nonuseful data, for example, include the exposure that occurs from X-ray photons that passed through the area outside of the patient and areas outside of the collimated field. Because the imaging device received unimportant exposure data, the digital data will contain unimportant exposure data. To cope with this, the first step in image processing is to define what data is likely to represent the data encoded as the X-ray photons pass through the body.

At least two different methods are involved in this analysis. One defines the edge of the collimated field and excludes the data outside of the collimated field from further analysis. Different companies use different proprietary methods for this purpose and these methods are moderately effective.

The second method uses information from the exposure histogram. The exposure histogram is a map of the different intensity values of the picture elements (pixels) that form the image. The algorithm selects those pixel values from the exposure histogram that are likely to contain clinically relevant information. For this step, the computer uses a search algorithm that is seeking the region of the remaining data that looks like chest radiograph data; one can think of this as a search for the shape within the exposure histogram that matches the shape of a chest radiograph histogram. The data for different parts of the body are different. The algorithm has been set to look for the data patterns seen in different body parts and the different common variations that are seen for each body part. Once the algorithm identifies the appropriate shape, it then uses this to defines the upper and lower boundaries of exposure data to be included in the formation of the image. This subset of the original data is then used to direct the next steps in image processing.

Poorly processed digital chest images usually result from problems occurring at these stages of the process. The most common causes are a failure to instruct the digital system as to the type of image to be processed or excessive scatter outside the edge of the collimated field. The digital system has to be told that the data set it is looking for is a chest radiograph. If it is told that a different part of the body is being imaged, it will look for data that looks like that body part and process the image data incorrectly. If there is a lot of scatter in the area outside the collimated field, it may not correctly define the edge of that field and may incorporate the scattered exposure into its defined exposure boundary. This is one of the reasons why it is important to avoid overexposure. On an overexposed image, the algorithm is more likely to include data that is due to scatter and is therefore not in the clinically relevant region of exposure.

Adjusting the Data for Differences in Exposure: The Fuji "S" Number, the Initial Adjustment for Display Optical Density

The method used by the system to define the ''clinically relevant data'' does not depend on the exposure used to obtain the original data set. In order to display the ''clinically relevant data'' as an image with proper display optical density or luminance, the system must correct for exposure differences. It does this by comparing the pixel values for the ''clinically relevant data'' to a stored expected range of pixel values. It then adjusts the ''clinically relevant data'' to lie within the range for proper display. The degree of adjustment is related to a number called ''S.'' If the extracted ''clinically relevant data'' is underexposed compared to the range of pixel values for display, the ''clinically relevant data'' will be adjusted so that it falls within the display range by amplifying each pixel value. If it is overexposed, then the computer program will decrease each pixel value. The Fuji system was designed so that an ''S'' value of 200 corresponds to the correct level for display of the image. The ''S'' value is not the speed of the system. The ''speed'' of an analog system is defined as the exposure level required for a specific degree of film optical density. In the digital systems, the optical density of the display is not determined by the exposure of the digital receptor. There is no way to equate the speed of a screen–film system to the proper exposure for a digital system. An ''S'' of 200 may have originally been based on the exposure required for a 200-speed screen–film system, but as the Fuji systems evolved, the imaging plates have become more sensitive to X-ray photons while the ''S'' number system has remained the same.

Final Adjustment for Image Mean Optical Density

The "S" number adjustment will usually place the image data set close to the range for proper display. There is, however, some variability in laser printers and in soft-copy display devices, so the system makes it possible to adjust the final optical density or luminance and then store this change so it can be used for subsequent radiographs. In the Fuji system, this factor is called the GS factor.

Adjustment for Display Contrast

In the process of selecting the "clinically relevant data," the computer program selected the highest and lowest pixel values of this data. This constitutes an initial estimate of the contrast range for the final image. It does not define the shape of the contrast curve or the steepness of its midportion. The final adjustment is made by use of a conversion method called a look-up table. In this method, there is either a stored table or a stored formula that says for a data pixel value of "*x*," use a value of "*y*" for the display. The companies recommend specific look-up tables for specific parts of the body. The radiologist can accept the companies' recommendations or choose different look-up tables. Once chosen, this selection can be stored in the computer memory so that the same look up table can be consistently chosen. In the Fuji system, this factor is called the GT factor.

Once this overall look-up table has been selected, one can accept the company's default setting or one can adjust the slope of the midportion of the characteristic curve. This factor is called the GA factor in the Fuji system. The higher the GA, the steeper the slope of the midportion of the characteristic curve, and the less steep the bottom and top of the characteristic curve.

High-Spatial-Frequency Enhancement: Edge Enhancement

Mathematically, all images can be transformed (using the Fourier transform) into groups of sine and cosine waves. The waves are of different frequencies and it is therefore possible to describe images as having different spatial frequencies. All images are composed of parts with different spatial frequencies. High spatial frequencies are seen in where there are sharp edges; lower spatial frequencies are seen where there are blurred or unsharp edges. Filtering methods exist to enhance or diminish the intensity of specific groups of spatial frequencies in an image. By enhancing high spatial frequencies in an image, sharp edges are enhanced and appear sharper, but since image noise is also of high spatial frequency, it is also enhanced. If high spatial frequencies are filtered from the image, then the edges of sharply defined objects and visible noise are decreased.

Edge enhancement is an important part of the image processing of digital chest radiographs. The edges of all objects in standard chest radiographs are somewhat blurred because of the penumbra caused by the X-ray tube focal spot size and often by slight patient motion and cardiac pulsation. Slight edge enhancement restores these edges toward the appearance they would have in a specimen radiograph with a very small focal spot X-ray tube. It enhances the conspicuity of blood vessels, interstitial markings, surgical staples, and pneumothoraces (Fig. 8). This method also enhances the edges of catheters, making them easier to see. It is normally included as part of the recommendation for image-processing settings for film display. Some soft-copy display systems, however, do not provide the capabilities for edge enhancement and diagnostic accuracy in these systems may be less (20).

High-Spatial-Frequency Blurring: Noise Blurring

High-spatial-frequency blurring can be used to decrease the visibility of noise in digital images. Because noise from quantum mottle makes some digital images appear grainy, image processing methods were provided so that the images would look smoother, more like screen–film images. If such processing were applied to the entire image, then fine interstitial lines would also

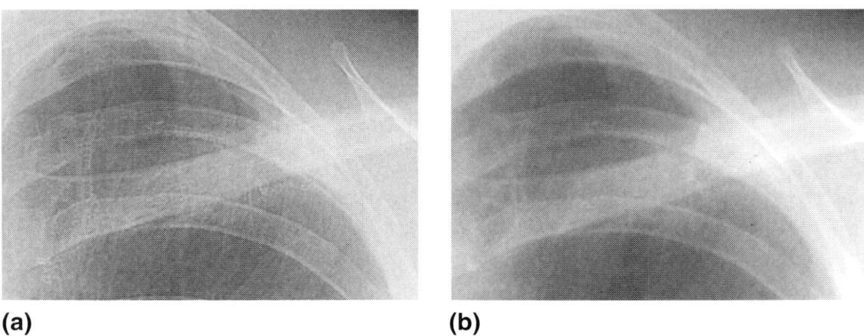

(a) **(b)**

Figure 8 Improved visibility of pneumothorax using edge enhancement in a patient status post surgery for recurrent spontaneous pneumothoraces. The surgical clips and the small residual pneumothorax are more conspicuous in (a) with mild edge enhancement than in (b) with no edge enhancement.

blur and be more difficult to detect. For this reason, some programs apply the image blurring only to areas of relatively low pixel values (more transparent regions of the original image. The use of these noise concealing programs unfortunately also blurs the edges of high-frequency structures, such as catheters in the mediastinum (see Figs. 7d and 7f).

Optical Density Equalization: Methods to Bring the Entire Image to an Optical Density Where High-Contrast Display Is Possible

The range of optical densities on a chest radiograph is quite wide. This is the result of the differing proportions of water, calcium, and air in the path of the X-ray photons in different parts of the image. Because of this wide range of densities, all chest images represent a compromise: To have the lungs at a proper display density, the mediastinum is too light. If one wants to see tubes in the esophagus behind the heart, then one can increase the exposure, but the lungs become too dark. Optical density equalization image processing is used to partially correct for these density differences. Current methods are moderately good, but in the future, newer methods will probably be better.

The fundamental concept underlying methods for optical density equalization is that one can separate an image into components of different spatial frequencies. High spatial frequencies show the edges of objects, medium spatial frequencies demonstrate the shape of moderate sized structures, and low spatial frequencies tend to show broad effects across an image. It is the low-spatial-frequency information that is modified in optical density equalization. While different methods are used by different companies, in concept, if one takes the low-spatial-frequency image and changes areas that are black to white (and vice versa) and then partially adds it back into the original image, then larger areas of density differences will be decreased in their intensity and the whole image will show a lower range of optical densities. The resulting image will show a lower range of optical densities across the image allowing one to then enhance the contrast across the entire image. Enhancing the contrast results in smaller details being more conspicuous. This method is very helpful for enhancing interpretation of bedside chest radiographs. It has the disadvantage that large areas of lung consolidation or large pleural effusions will also be affected by the processing, making them less intensely white. Sometimes faint but larger areas of air space disease will be less conspicuous on these images. Also, the area over the liver sometimes looks more radiolucent and could appear similar to the radiolucency that can occur on supine films with free abdominal air.

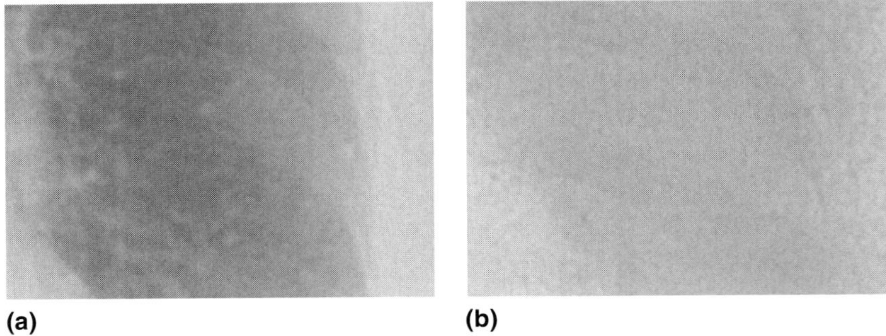

(a) (b)

Figure 9 Energy subtraction used to confirm calcification in nodules. (a) A digital chest image with standard processing shows several small lung nodules. (b) The calcium emphasis image is shown and the small nodules can be seen to contain calcium.

Energy-Subtraction Imaging

Energy-subtraction imaging is based on the kilovolt dependence of absorption of calcium and water. At lower kilovolt levels, calcium absorbs or scatters moderately more X-ray photons than water. At higher kilovolt levels, the absorption levels are more similar. By obtaining a chest radiograph at two different energy spectra, one can process the images to create a bone-emphasis and a soft-tissue-emphasis image. This acquisition can be done either using one exposure where two imaging plates are exposed, but with a layer of copper

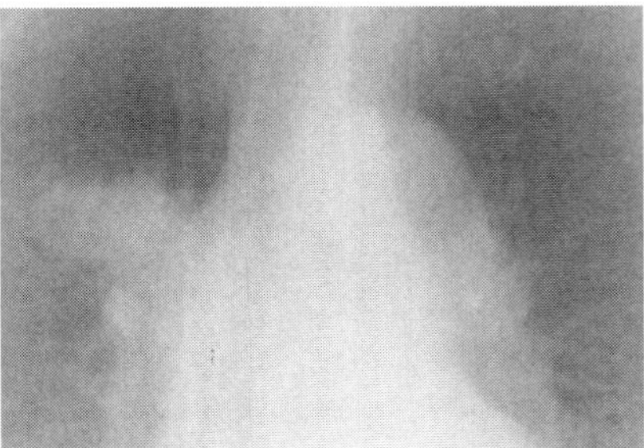

Figure 10 Energy subtraction used to enhance visibility of a central mass. A squamous-cell lung cancer involving the right upper hilum is seen. The energy subtraction processing has greatly decreased the visibility of the ribs and enhance the conspicuity of the mass.

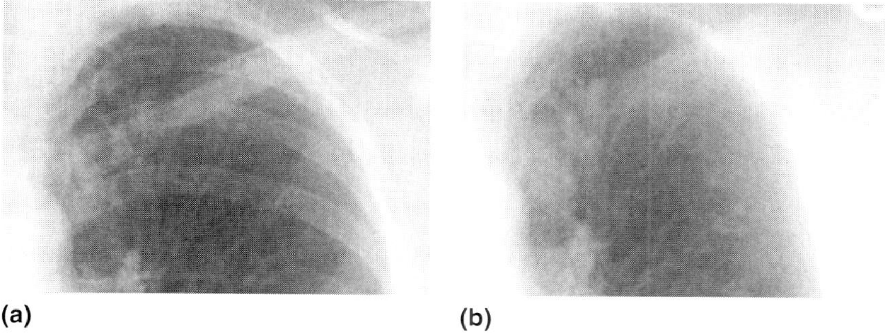

Figure 11 Energy subtraction used to enhance visibility of airways disease. Digital chest radiographs with (a) standard and (b) soft-tissue-emphasis energy-subtraction processing in a patient with mucus plugs and bronchiectasis from cystic fibrosis. The soft-tissue-emphasis image largely eliminates the conspicuity of the ribs. The lung disease is more conspicuous.

or other absorber between them so that the energy spectra are different, or by taking two exposures one right after the other at different kilovolt peak settings. The images must then be closely matched so that the chest is exactly the same size and position. This is done by a process called warping, where one image is distorted (warped) to be the same size and shape as the other. Subsequently, the images are registered (matched in position) as closely as possible. They can then be processed through a complex series of steps that eventually yield the bone-emphasis and soft-tissue-emphasis images (Figs. 9–11). With the current commercial system, slight image blurring occurs in this process, so that the finest intersitial lines may be less conspicuous, but at the same time, areas of infiltrate and small masses become more conspicuous. It is likely that future developments both in acquisition devices and software will improve the quality of energy subtraction and increase its value.

AMBER system

The AMBER system is a special type of digital chest radiographic system that scans the chest adjusting the intensity of the X-ray beam according to how much radiation has penetrated the chest. It continually adjusts the amount of exposure so that more radiation is applied where there is more absorption (as in the mediastinum) and less over the lungs. It produces very high quality images.

IV. IMAGE PROCESSING: FUTURE METHODS

Future developments in the image processing of digital chest radiographs are likely. While the following section cannot be complete, it describes several approaches that appear promising.

A. Image Segmentation for Anatomic Definition of Processing Parameters

Segmentation of an image is the process whereby an image is divided into separate regions, either by hand or computer, based on some identified differ-

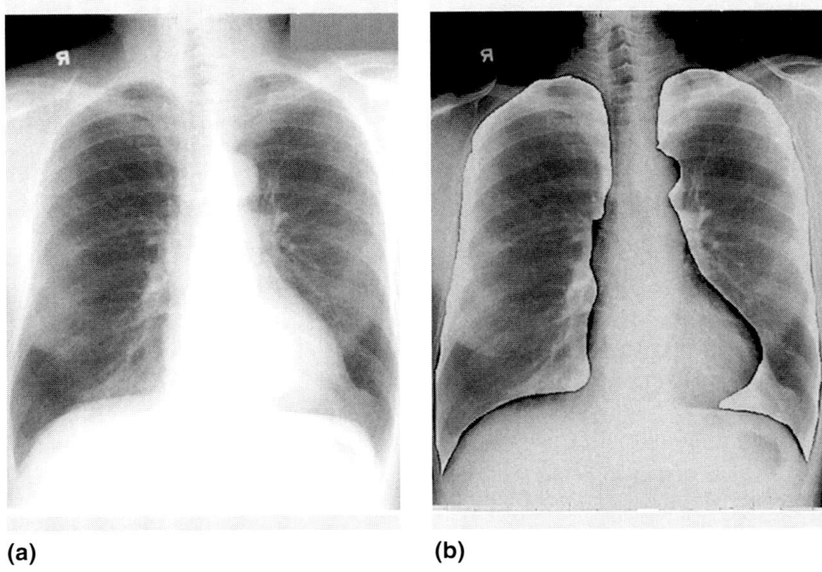

Figure 12 Segmentation for anatomy-based image processing. In this study, a normal screen–film chest radiograph has been digitized (a). It has then been processed so that the lungs are segmented from the image for organ-specific image processing (b). By doing this, the processing for the mediastinum and the lungs can be different. In this case, the mediastinum and upper abdomen were processed to have a greater optical density and more edge enhancement than the lungs. The retrocardiac region (particularly the vessels), chest wall, and abdomen have been enhanced. (Experimental work of the author, S. C. B. Lo, and H. Zhao.)

ence between them. In the chest, work is underway to segment the mediastinum, rib boundary of the lungs, and the lungs themselves [21,22,23]. Once these areas are segmented, different image-processing techniques could be applied to these different regions (Fig. 12). The segmented areas could be adjusted to have different black/white scales, different degrees of edge enhancement, and/or different contrast scales.

B. Computer-Aided Detection and Diagnosis

Once the chest radiograph has been converted into a computer-readable form, the computer can be used to search for signs of specific diseases. Experimentally, computer-aided detection methods have been used to identify lung nodules, interstitial disease, and cardiomegaly [24,25,26,27,28,29]. The first commercial system for assisting radiologists in the detection of small pulmonary nodules has received FDA Pre-Market Approval [30]. The clinical trial showed that radiologists using the system, using retrospective data, detected an average of 5% more lung cancers when they used the system than they did without the system. The greatest benefit was seen for the smallest nodules (those 9–14 mm in size), with slightly less benefit for those 15–19 mm, and with almost no benefit for those larger than 20 mm. The average size of lung cancers found retrospectively is 14 mm, but missed prospectively in one of the large lung cancer-screening programs that used chest radiographs (the author of this chapter worked on the development of this system and is both a patent holder and stockholder in the company). It is expected that future work in computer-aided detection will demonstrate that radiologists will have improved detection of other disease with the use of future computer programs.

C. Sequential Subtraction: Change Detection

Computer programs are under development to enhance the detection of changes from one film to the next as a method to aid radiologists in their detection of disease [31,32]. The processes involved include warping, registration, and subtraction. Because most nonobvious disease occupies only a small portion of the chest, the algorithms which function on the whole chest can warp one image to match the other in spatial dimensions, register them, and subtract them, enhancing only the area that showed local change (Fig. 13). These techniques are still relatively immature and experimental, but it is likely that they will become commonly used in the future.

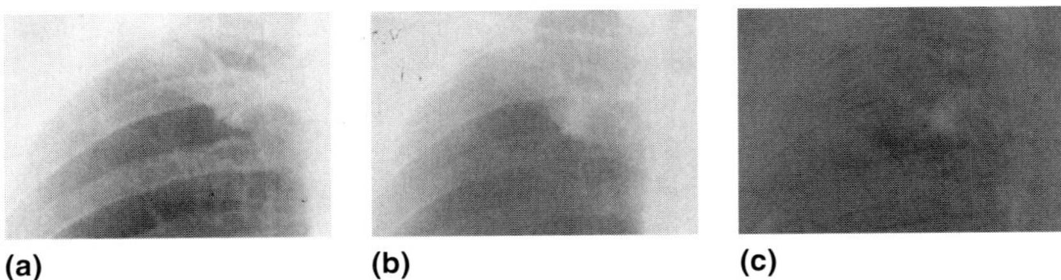

Figure 13 Sequential subtraction used to aid detection of lung nodule. (a) The lung apex 1 year before b was taken. (c) The subtraction image obtained after the images have been warped and registered. This subtraction image shows (as a white region) a change between the two films, which represented a small non-small-cell lung cancer projected over the first-rib calcified cartilage. (Experimental work of the author, S. C. B. Lo, and H. Zhao.)

D. Disease-Specific Algorithms

A disease-specific algorithm is a preselected method for image processing that is optimized to identify a specific disease. An example would be that if one knows that a patient is at risk for a pneumothorax, one could have the computer enhance the image so that any pneumothorax would become more conspicuous. While disease-specific image-processing settings do not yet exist, situation-specific image-processing algorithms are commonly used. The clearest example is the use of histogram equalization to enhance the visibility of tubes and lines within the mediastinum and upper abdomen. The settings used enhance this visibility, but with some probable loss of information for subtle disease in the lungs. In the past, optimization methods have emphasized the desire to find image-processing settings that maximize the value of the chest radiograph for all diseases based on both how common the diseases are and their importance to the patient. In the future, it will be possible to have a system in which each chest radiograph goes through several different image-processing methods, each optimized for detection of a specific group of diseases. It has been proposed that one would use the input of clinical information to decide which image-processing method should be applied to each film. There is an inherent risk in this method in that if one only looks for what is expected, then one may fail to detect an unsuspected disease until it is more severe. Thus, I think that more than one image-processing method should be used on all films rather than a single method tailored to look for a specific diagnosis. In the future, computer-detected disease patterns are likely to be used to adjust the image processing or display parameters so that the detected disease is emphasized. The research goal is to have the computer adjust the image so that the radiologist is unlikely to miss the disease rather than have the computer place an arrow on the image directing the radiologists attention to a specific location.

V. DISPLAY METHODS

A. Printed on Film versus Soft-Copy Display

Digital chest radiographs can be viewed either by printing them on film or by viewing them on a computer screen. With current technology, there is no firm evidence that one method of viewing provides greater accuracy than the other. Display on film is a more mature technology and only limited technical improvements that would affect diagnostic quality are foreseen. Computer screen (or monitor) display is a moderately mature technology, but one where technical innovation is more likely. If the changes in computer screen display are favorable to the display of chest radiographs, then this method of display may eventually surpass that of the display on film. Some of the future advances that could make soft-copy display the diagnostically superior method are the ability to rapidly switch between image-processing settings, the incorporation of computer-aided detection and diagnosis, and the ability to label an image that will be incorporated into the report to the patient's treating physician. The optimum report in the future is likely to consist of annotations on an image with a final impression rather than the word-based descriptions currently used.

B. Image Size and Viewing Distance

Digital chest radiographs can be printed life-size or at a decreased size. Studies have shown that diagnostic accuracy on two-thirds-size images is equivalent to screen–film chest images [4,8,33]. One study showed no problems at 56% of life-size with a selenium detector system [34]. On the other hand, half-size images have been reported to limit disease detection [35,36]. When smaller images are used, the radiologist viewing them should be closer to see the fine detail. If one normally views a standard chest radiograph at 3 feet, the two-thirds-sized image should be viewed at 1½ to 2 feet, for example.

VI. SUMMARY

Digital chest radiography is a rapidly evolving method for imaging the chest. In its current form, it has been shown to be diagnostically equivalent to conventional chest radiography. Since analog screen–film chest radiography is technologically mature and digital chest radiography is still in a process of moderate innovation, it is likely that the diagnostic quality of digital chest radiography will, in the future, be superior to that of conventional chest radiography, replacing it for many uses. Digital chest radiographs can be produced by three competing methods: film digitization, systems that store the energy of the encoded X-ray photons for later extraction, and near-real-time systems for extracting the encoded X-ray information. For each of these methods, there are trade-offs in labor versus machine costs. To date, there is no evidence that any one method is diagnostically superior to the other, although digitized film requires that the original film be of high quality to achieve a high-quality digitized image. The two other types of digital acquisition are more robust to exposure differences. Once in digital form, image processing provides important advantages in correcting and improving disease conspicuity. Digital images are the input data for computer-aided detection systems. They allow digital storage, transmission, retrieval, and soft-copy display. There are likely to be continued improvements in image quality based on improved image-processing methods, energy subtraction, and temporal subtraction.

REFERENCES

1. Schaefer CM, Greene RE, Oestmann JW, et al. Improved control of image optical density with low-dose digital and conventional radiography in bedside imaging. Radiology 1989; 173:713–716.
2. Freedman M, Lo SCB, Nelson MC, Pe E, Mun SK: Comparative test of two storage phosphor plate imaging systems: The Agfa ADC and the Fuji AC- 1+. In: Brody W, Johnston G, eds. Computer Applications to Assist Radiology. Carlsbad, CA: SCAR 92, Symposia Foundation, 1992.
3. International Labor Organization. Guidelines for the Use of the International Classification of Radiographs of Pneumoconiosis. Geneva: International Labor Organization, 1992.
4. MacMahon H, Sanada S, Doi K, et al. Direct comparison of conventional and computed radiography with a dual-image recording technique. RadioGraphics 1991; 11:259–268.
5. Marglin SI, Rowberg AH, Godwin JD. Preliminary experience with portable digital imaging for intensive care radiography. J Thorac Imag 1990; 5:49–54.
6. Kehler M, Albrechtsson U, Andresdottier A, Larusdotti H, Lundin A. Accuracy of digital radiography using stimulable phosphor for diagnosis of pneumothorax. Acta Radiol 1990; 31:47–52.
7. Schaefer CM, Green RE, Oestmann JW, et al. Digital storage phosphor imaging

versus conventional film radiography in CT-documented chest disease. Radiology 1990; 174:207–210.
8. Kehler M, Albrechtsson U, Andersson B, Larusdotti H, Lundin A, Pettersson H. Assessment of digital chest radiography using stimulable phosphor. Acta Radiol 1989; 30:581–586.
9. Schaefer CM, Greene RE, Llewellyn HJ, et al. Interstitial lung disease: impact of postprocessing in digital storage phosphor imaging. Radiology 1991; 178:733–738.
10. Schaefer CM, Greene RE, Hall DA, et al. Mediastinal abnormalities: Detection with storage phosphor digital radiography. Radiology 1991; 178:169–173.
11. Woodard PK, Slone RM, Sagel SS, et al. Detection of CT-proved pulmonary nodules: comparison of selenium-based digital and conventional screen-film chest radiographs. Radiology 1998; 209:705–709.
12. Kim JH, Im JG, Han MC, Min BG, Lee CW. Improved visualization of simulated nodules by adaptive enhancement of digital chest radiography. Acad Radiol 1994; 1:93–99.
13. Garmer M, Hennigs SP, Jager HJ, et al. Digital radiography versus conventional radiography in chest imaging: diagnostic performance of a large-area silicon flat-panel detector in a clinical CT-controlled study. Am J Roentgenol 2000; 174: 75–80.
14. Muller RD, Wahling S, Hirche H, et al. ROC analysis of detection performance by analogue and digital plain film systems in chest radiography. Acta Radiol 1996; 37:847–854.
15. American College of Radiology. Standards 1999–2000. Reston VA: American College of Radiology, 2000.
16. Freedman MT, Pe EV, Mun SK, Lo SCB, Nelson MC. Potential for unnecessary patient exposure from the use of storage phosphor imaging systems. SPIE Med Imag 1993; 1897:472–479.
17. Freedman MT, Mun SK, Pe EV, Lo SCB, Nelson MC. Image optimization procedures for the Fuji AC-1. SPIE Med Imag 1993; 1897:480–502.
18. Freedman M, Artz DS. Image Processing in Digital Radiography. Semin Roentgenol 1997; 32:25–37.
19. Freedman M, Artz DS: Digital Radiography of the Chest. Semin Roentgenol 1997; 32:38–44.
20. Kosuda S, Kaji T, Kobayashi H, Watanabe M, Iwasaki Y, Kusano S. Hard-copy versus soft-copy with and without simple image manipulation for detection of pulmonary nodules and masses. Acta Radiol 2000; 41:420–424.
21. Hasegawa A, Lo SCB, Lin JS, Freedman MT, Mun SK. A shift-invarant neural network for the lung field segmentation in chest radiography. J VLSI Sign Proc Sys 1998; 18(3):241–250.
22. Tsujii O, Freedman MT, Mun SK. Anatomic region-based dynamic range compression for chest radiographs using warping transformation of correlated distribution. IEEE Trans Med Imag 1998; 17:407–418.
23. Tsujii O, Freedman MT, Mun SK. Lung contour detection in chest radiographs using 1-D convolutional neural networks. J Electron Imag 1999; 8:46–53.

24. Xu XW, Doi K, Kobayashi T, et al. Development of an improved CAD scheme for automated detection of lung nodules in digital chest images. Med Phys 1997; 24:1395–1403.
25. MacMahon H, Engelmann R, Behlen FM, et al. Computer-aided diagnosis of pulmonary nodules: results of a large-scale observer test. Radiology 1999; 213: 723–726.
26. Lo SCB, Freedman MT, Lin JS, Mun SK. Automatic lung nodule detection using profile matching and back-propagation neural network techniques. J Digit Imag 1993; 6:48–54.
27. Lo SCB, Chan HP, Lin JS, Li H, Freedman M, Mun SK. Artificial convolutional neural network for lung nodule detection. IEEE Trans Med Imag 1995; 14:711–718.
28. Lin JS, Lo SCB, Hasegawa A, Freedman M, Mun SK. Reduction of false positives in lung nodule detection using a two-level neural classification. IEEE Trans Med Imag 1996; 15:206–217.
29. Lin JS, Hasegawa A, Freedman M, Mun SK. Differentiation between nodules and end-on vessels using a convolutional neural network architecture. J Digit Imaging 1995; 8:132–141.
30. Freedman M, Lo SCB, Lure F, Xu XW, Lin J, Zhao H, Osicka T, Zhang R. Computer aided detection of lung cancer on chest radiographs: algorithm performance vs radiologists' performance by size of cancer. SPIE Med Imag 2001; in press.
31. Difazio MC, MacMahon H, Xu XW, et al. Digital chest radiography: effect of temporal subtraction images on detection accuracy. Radiology 1997; 202:447–452.
32. Katsuragawa S, Tagashira H, Li Q, MacMahon H, Doi K. Comparison of the quality of temporal subtraction images obtained with manual and automatic methods of digital chest radiography. J Digit Imag 1999; 12:166–172.
33. Kehler M, Albrechtsson U, Arnadottier E, et al. Digital luminescence radiography in interstitial lung disease. Acta Radiol 1991; 32:18–23.
34. van Heesewijk HP, vad der Graff Y, de Valois JC, Vos JA, Feldberg MA. Digital chest imaging using a selenium detector: the impact of hard copy size on obsever performance: a computed tomography-controlled study. Invest Radiol 1997; 32: 363–367.
35. Schaefer CM, Prokop M, Oestmann JW, et al. Impact of hard-copy size on observer performance in digital chest radiography. Radiology 1992; 184:77–81.
36. Fisher PD, Brauer GW. Impact of image size on effectiveness of digital imaging systems. J Digit Imag 1989; 2:39–41.

Index